Cleft Palate and Its Associated Speech Disorders

McGRAW-HILL

Series in Speech

Glen E. Mills, *Consulting Editor in General Speech*
John J. O'Neill, *Consulting Editor in Speech Pathology*

Armstrong and Brandes: *The Oral Interpretation of Literature*
Baird: *American Public Addresses*
Baird: *Argumentation, Discussion, and Debate*
Baird and Knower: *Essentials of General Speech*
Baird, Becker, and Knower: *General Speech Communication*
Carrell and Tiffany: *Phonetics*
Gibson: *A Reader in Speech Communication*
Hahn, Lomas, Hargis, and Vandraegen: *Basic Voice Training for Speech*
Hasling: *The Message, the Speaker, the Audience*
Henning: *Improving Oral Communication*
Kaplan: *Anatomy and Physiology of Speech*
Kruger: *Modern Debate*
Ogilvie: *Speech in the Elementary School*
Ogilvie and Rees: *Communication Skills: Voice and Pronunciation*
Powers: *Fundamentals of Speech*
Reid: *Teaching Speech*
Robinson and Becker: *Effective Speech for the Teacher*
Wells: *Cleft Palate and Its Associated Speech Disorders*

CLEFT PALATE AND ITS ASSOCIATED SPEECH DISORDERS

Charlotte G. Wells
University of Missouri-Columbia

McGraw-Hill Book Company

New York St. Louis San Francisco Düsseldorf Johannesburg
Kuala Lumpur London Mexico Montreal New Delhi Panama
Rio de Janeiro Singapore Sydney Toronto

CLEFT PALATE AND ITS ASSOCIATED SPEECH DISORDERS

Library of Congress Catalog Card Number 77-139567

07-069243-2

3456789 KPKP 79876

Contents

PREFACE vii
ACKNOWLEDGMENTS xi

1 THE HISTORY AND INCIDENCE OF PREPALATAL AND PALATAL CLEFTS 1

Introduction 1
Clefts of the prepalate and palate 2
Multidisciplinary care 2
Terminology 3
Treatment of acquired and congenital clefts 7
Incidence of clefts of the prepalate and palate 26

2 DEVELOPMENT AND FUNCTION OF THE PREPALATAL AND PALATAL AREAS 39

Normal growth and development of structures 39
Use of normal structures in speech 60
The mechanism of normal velopharyngeal closure 60
Major functions of the velopharyngeal valve 63

3 CAUSES OF CLEFTS OF THE PREPALATE AND PALATE 70

Parental inquiries 70
Early superstitions and theories 71
Two major questions: "Why?" and "How?" 74
Etiology: "Why?" 77

	Agreement on causal factors	92
	Pathogenesis: "How?"	98
	Differences between prepalatal and palatal clefts	102
4	**TYPES AND EFFECTS OF CLEFTS**	**103**
	Classifications of clefts	103
	Effects of clefts	115
	Specific effects on children	124
	The "typical" cleft palate child	140
5	**THE CLEFT PALATE TEAM**	**143**
	Efforts in the management of clefts	143
	The surgeon as a member of the team	147
	The orthodontist as a member of the team	163
	The prosthodontist as a member of the team	167
	The speech pathologist as a member of the team	171
	Additional team functions	174
6	**ASSESSMENT OF SPEECH**	**176**
	The responsibility of the specialist	176
	Factors to be considered by the speech pathologist	177
	Accumulating and coordinating information	183
7	**REMEDIAL PROCEDURES**	**222**
	Evaluation and therapy	222
	Goals of speech training for children born with clefts	225
	Plans for the remedial process	227
	Conclusion	274
	BIBLIOGRAPHY	**275**
	INDEX	**305**

Preface

The disorders of oral communication associated with congenital clefts of the orofacial area present a special challenge to the speech pathologist and audiologist. The interdisciplinary approach that now characterizes the management of those with congenital clefts of the prepalate or palate includes speech pathologists and audiologists as valuable members of the team.

My interest in the speech problems of cleft palate children began in 1941, when I directed one of the first intensive training programs for children with congenital clefts at the request of Robert West of the University of Wisconsin and Frank V. Powell of the Wisconsin Bureau for Handicapped Children. Faced with a group of twenty-five children, all with surgically repaired clefts of the palate, none with pharyngeal flaps or obturators, I found that some procedures used to modify the speech behavior of the normal child were not appropriate for a group with structural anomalies. I developed a special concern for these children, who resemble their peers yet present individual and group variations, who are intelligent or slow to learn, who may be well-behaved or undisciplined, whose common characteristic is the congenital lack of complete structures of the lip, alveolus, hard palate, or soft palate. To contribute to the habilitation of these children has been rewarding, and this opportunity to share with others some of the information gathered through study and experience has been gratifying.

In this book, the sequence is from general to specific, from background information to application of principles and theories. Chapter One presents the history of the cleft palate problem and some of the ways in which certain disciplines have dealt with it. The chapter also presents figures on the incidence of clefts, as reported from many sources, and on the variations in incidence that result from differing categorizations.

Chapter Two traces the normal development and growth of structures in the prepalatal and palatal areas. The mechanism of normal velopharyngeal closure and the major functions of the velopharyngeal valve are also discussed in this chapter. The illustrations were designed and adapted to help the reader comprehend the relative size of the various structures as they develop prenatally.

Chapter Three considers the causes of clefts, with two basic emphases: the reasons for the failures of prenatal development that result in clefts and the ways in which these failures occur. Here, as in other chapters, "prepalate" refers to the area anterior to the incisive foramen and "palate" to the area posterior to that point. The etiology and pathogenesis of clefts are more readily understood, I believe, if the prepalate and palate are differentiated.

Chapter Four discusses the types and effects of congenital orofacial clefts. The illustrations were derived from drawings that accompanied the classifications presented by the Nomenclature Committee of the American Cleft Palate Association in 1960, but they have been given additional dimensions that should make them more meaningful. The final section of this chapter describes the "typical" cleft palate child, who probably does not exist but whose characteristics are cited to summarize the effects of congenital clefts.

The interdisciplinary efforts being made to habilitate the cleft palate child are described in Chapter Five. No attempt has been made to provide the details of the work of the surgeon, orthodontist, prosthodontist, or speech pathologist; but the major contributions of each are pointed out, and some of the terminology used in team conferences or correspondence has been cited. The work of other specialists is also acknowledged, but I have emphasized those who work most closely and directly with children and adults whose oral communication may be affected by congenital clefts.

Plans for assessing the communicative skills and disabilities of individuals with congenital clefts, as presented in Chapter Six, are specific and detailed. The importance of good communication among those who are involved in the habilitation of such children, stressed in Chapter Five, was given careful consideration in preparing the forms for obtaining and recording information from team members. These forms, in booklets on pages of appropriate size for filing, may be purchased from the author.

The procedures for remediation in Chapter Seven should be adapted to the situation and the individuals concerned. However, the variety of approaches to the modification of speech behavior will permit the clinician to select the most suitable techniques or to use the ideas as guides to others more suited to the patient, the clinician, and the setting.

Throughout the text, I have defined terms that might be unfamiliar to some readers. In addition, I have tried to refer to individual authorities, past and present, in such a way that the reader will feel that these persons existed outside the books, articles, or techniques with which their names are associated. Hence, when an individual is cited for the first time in a chapter, except in a parenthetical reference to source material, his first name as well as his last is given, in the hope of making him seem more real. Their lives have been chronicled in biographies of various kinds, and their contributions have been described in detail in many books and journals.

Charlotte G. Wells

Acknowledgments

Management of the child born with a cleft of the prepalate or palate requires the concerted efforts of many individuals. So, too, this discussion of congenital clefts and their effects on oral communication is the result of multiple efforts. I am particularly grateful to all those who assisted in the preparation of this book. My colleagues at the University of Missouri-Columbia in administrative offices, the Department of Speech and Dramatic Art, the Area of Speech Pathology-Audiology, the Medical Center and Medical Library, and the Illustration Section of Medical Educational Services assisted me in many ways. W. Francis English, Loren Reid, and Clifton Cornwell were instrumental in obtaining a sabbatical leave for me, during which Thelma Trombly and Donald Williamson carried unusually heavy administrative and teaching loads in the Area of Speech Pathology-Audiology. The staff at the Medical Library furnished work space, obtained reference materials, and provided help in research tasks. Edward Lowrance, of the Department of Anatomy, reviewed the section on embryology and made valuable suggestions for improving the presentation of information in the first part of Chapter Two. Ruth Wakerlin, who prepared the illustrations, brought imagination as well as artistic skill to her work. Students in my classes asked pertinent questions, read portions of the manuscript, and helped me to find a better focus for some of the discussion.

To Donna Crockett, who typed the manuscript, to staff members in the libraries of the dental schools at the University of Texas and the University of Missouri-Kansas City, and to many others, I am grateful for encouragement, advice, and assistance.

Most of all, I acknowledge my indebtedness to the many children with congenital clefts who have taught me while I tried to teach them, children for whose benefit this book was intended. If my efforts in preparing this material enable any of them to acquire better oral communication and thus have more opportunity for optimum personal achievement, my time will have been well spent and my purpose fulfilled.

Charlotte G. Wells

CHAPTER ONE

The History and Incidence of Prepalatal and Palatal Clefts

THE SECOND HALF OF THE TWENTIETH CENTURY HAS BROUGHT, TO THOSE WITH HANDICAPS THAT MAKE THEM DIFFERENT FROM THEIR PEERS, OPPORTUNITIES FOR HELP THROUGH MANY AGENCIES.

Now, as never before, the deaf, blind, hard of hearing, crippled, mentally retarded, emotionally disturbed, and culturally deprived are receiving, through local, state, and federal programs, the kinds of services that enable them to reach their maximal levels of achievement and become self-sustaining members of society. Physical and mental differences, present at birth or acquired, can often be minimized or overcome through concerted efforts by the handicapped themselves, their families, their communities, and the groups of professional workers who combine their skills to provide diagnostic and therapeutic management of these differences.

AMONG THE PHYSICAL ANOMALIES PRESENT AT BIRTH AND HENCE AMENABLE TO EARLY CORRECTIVE MEASURES ARE CLEFTS OF THE PREPALATE AND PALATE.

These congenital malformations are not, in every sense, "crippling" conditions. The child with a cleft in the lip, the alveolus, the hard palate, or the soft palate can, in the absence of other physical and intellectual deficits, attend to his personal needs, run and walk, and develop physically and mentally as he might if he had no deviations in mouth structure. Nevertheless, he is different from his siblings and playmates. He may have a scarred lip or deformed nose; he may undergo surgery at an early age; he must keep regular appointments for continuing evaluation and remediation. He may have experienced separation from his family and may have heard comments about his appearance from friends and strangers. He faces a number of years of remedial procedures that will take his time and require his cooperation. Although his needs and interests may be similar to those of other children, his ability to speak normally may be impaired; and he may encounter the frustrations of being unable to communicate easily with those in his environment. In spite of the multiple problems enumerated above, the child with a congenital cleft of the palate has the opportunity to reach his individual potential and to lead a rich, full life if he receives adequate care.

THIS CARE, SO ESSENTIAL TO THE HABILITATION OF THE CHILD WITH A CONGENITAL DEFORMITY OF THE PREPALATE OR PALATE. IS MULTIDISCIPLINARY IN NATURE.

Any discussion of the child, the cleft, or the management of both involves several professional fields; the group of specialists concerned with assessment and management of the child with a congenital cleft is usually called a team. The personnel of the team and their specific functions will be considered in Chapter Five. Those with primary responsibilities include the surgeon, the dentist, the speech pathologist, and the audiologist. With other specialists, they provide the treatment needed by the child with a congenital malformation of the prepalate or palate. They also conduct research programs designed to improve their procedures, and they seek preventive measures that have the aim of reducing the incidence of anomalies of the facial area.

WHEN ANY OF THESE SPECIALISTS READS THE LITERATURE OUTSIDE HIS OWN FIELD, HE MAY ENCOUNTER TERMS HE DOES NOT KNOW; OR HE MAY FIND THAT WORDS HAVING ONE MEANING FOR HIM ARE USED IN A DIFFERENT WAY BY OTHERS WRITING ABOUT THE SAME ANOMALY.

Problems of terminology are the result of specialization, of the explosive growth of research, and of the ever-increasing number of translations of articles and texts into languages other than the original. In some instances, technical language can interfere with the free flow of ideas and the retrieval of information. To avoid such barriers, the members of the several disciplines concerned with services to individuals with oral clefts need to discuss these patients without misunderstanding and to use terminology that facilitates communication. Throughout this discussion of clefts of the prepalate and palate, many of the terms will be defined as they are used.

Two basic terms recur in all the literature and all the discussion of congenital malformations of the lip, the alveolus, and the palate. The history and the variant forms of "cleft lip" and "cleft palate" suggest that even these words, used so commonly by several groups of specialists, may need definition and explanation.

A congenital fissure in the upper lip is often called "harelip" in historical and current literature, although the analogy with the rabbit is inexact. Clefts in human lips are, except in rare instances, on one or both sides of the upper lip, not in the center. However, in most of the writing prior to 1925, the term "harelip" was used far more commonly than "cleft lip." Pierre Franco, a French surgeon of the sixteenth century, is credited with coining the term "cleft lip," although he also described a kind of cleft that he called "hare's tooth." In this type of cleft, both the lip and the palate were affected (Barsky, 1964). The use of "harelip" by Franco's more famous contemporary, Ambroise Paré, may account for the popularity of that term (Dorrance, 1933); and French writers have been consistent in their use of the term "harelip" even to the time of Victor Veau. German writers have used "harelip" or "hare's fissure," but they have also written about "split lip" (*Lippenspalte*).

Truman W. Brophy, an American surgeon, used the term "cleft lip" in 1923; but his bibliography and entries in government documents from the Surgeon-General's Office in the nineteenth century show clearly that "harelip" and its equivalents—French *bec de lièvre,* German *Hasenlippe* or *Hasenscharte,* Italian *labbro leporino,* and Danish *hareskaar*—were terms used most frequently by writers from the Middle Ages to the early part of the twentieth century.

Francis Mason in 1877, James Berry and T. Percy Legg in 1912, and James V. Neel in 1958 referred to labial clefts as "harelips"; and that term appeared after 1965 in reports from the World Health Organization (Stevenson and others, 1966) and the International Symposium and Workshop on Craniofacial Anomalies (Longacre, 1968). Medical terminology is not entirely consistent, but the term "cleft lip" now appears frequently in medical dictionaries and is used as a separate entry rather than as a synonym for "harelip." Such words as "cheiloschisis" and "split lip" also appear in the literature, although infrequently.

The transition to more general use of "cleft lip" probably took place between 1940 and 1960. The term "harelip" was used by Poul Fogh-Andersen in 1942 and Richard Stark in 1954, for example; and the more current term appeared in articles by these same authors in 1961 and 1962. Publications such as *Plastic and Reconstructive Surgery,* the *Cleft Palate Journal,* and current editions of American medical dictionaries use the term "cleft lip," which is preferred by modern writers who deal with congenital anomalies of the face.

Recent modifications in classifications of congenital facial clefts, discussed in Chapter Four in some detail, have led to the introduction of such terms as "cleft of the primary palate" (Kernahan and Stark, 1958; Stark and Kernahan, 1959) and "prepalatal cleft" (Harkins and others, 1960) to indicate a defect in the area including the upper lip and the alveolar ridge. Because "prepalatal" encompasses both lip and alveolus, the term "prepalatal cleft" will be used in this text to indicate a cleft in the upper lip, the alveolar ridge, or both, with the incisive foramen serving as the posterior boundary of the prepalatal area. Figure 1-1 shows the prepalatal area and the location of the incisive foramen.

Use of the term "prepalatal" has several advantages. It permits reference to "labial clefts"—clefts of the lip with no involvement of the alveolus—and thus avoids the necessity for speaking of "isolated cleft lip." It also allows consideration of clefts of the alveolus—"alveolar clefts"—if these occur independently of labial clefts. It conforms to terminology now being used by many of those who report their investigations of congenital anomalies of the facial area. Furthermore, as later chapters will show, it is a useful term in discussions of current theories on the etiology and morphology of orofacial anomalies. Finally, it provides for reference to clefts of the area posterior to the incisive foramen as "palatal clefts" rather than as "isolated

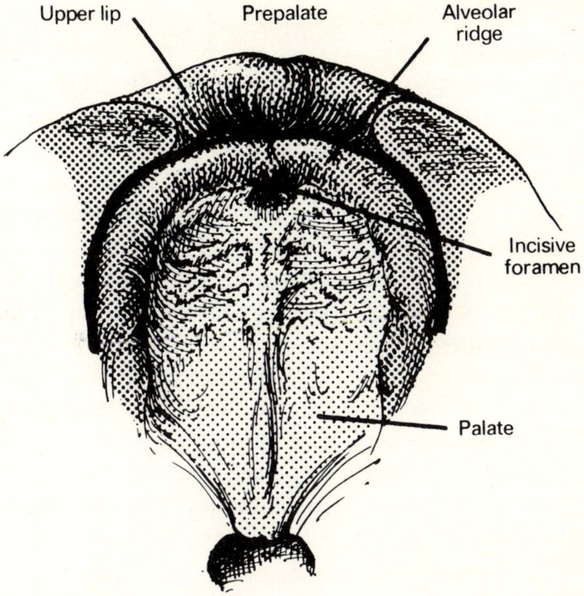

FIGURE 1-1 Location of incisive foramen

palatal clefts," with indications, if necessary, of the specific location of clefts in the hard or soft palate.

The term "cleft palate" has been used consistently throughout the past several centuries to designate clefts in the hard or soft palate, although it has sometimes included clefts in the alveolar ridge, particularly in the absence of a labial cleft. The French *division palatine* and the German *Gaumenspalte* also have been commonly used. Words that suggest analogy with animals have not been popular in connection with palatal clefts, except for one descriptive term, possibly coined to describe the combination of protruding premaxilla and cleft of the prepalate and palate. This term—*gueule de loup* in French, *Wolfsrachen* in German, *gola lupino* in Italian, and *boca de lobo* in Spanish—indicates that, at least to some observers, the appearance of the individual with this kind of cleft was like that of a wolf. Veau (1938) reserved the term *gueule de loup* for complete bilateral cleft of the lip, alveolus, and palate, which he called the most severe form. "Uranoschisis," "palatoschisis," "staphyloschisis," and "split palate" also are used in the literature to refer to palatal clefts; but the terms "cleft palate" or "palatal cleft" will be used here to indicate defects in the hard and soft palate posterior to the incisive foramen.

The specialists in surgery, dentistry, speech pathology, and audiology make use of certain procedures in the management of clefts that may also need definition. The surgeon, for example, uses cheiloplasty, palatoplasty, and pharyngoplasty to repair or revise the lip, alveolus, palate, or pharynx. Other names for these procedures include cheilorrhaphy and cheilostomatorrhaphy for surgery to the lip; uranoplasty, uranorrhaphy, and palatorrhaphy for the operations on the palate; and pharyngorrhaphy for modifications of the pharyngeal area. Members of the medical profession who are specially trained in these surgical techniques are usually called plastic surgeons. Their field of specialization, which extends beyond revisions of the labial, alveolar, and palatal areas, is plastic, reconstructive, or reparative surgery. This field was defined by Earl C. Padgett as "that branch of general surgery which deals with the repair of defects and malformations of both a congenital and acquired nature." The object in undertaking such reparative procedures, Padgett added, is "the restoration of function, or the improvement of appearance, or both" (in Bankoff, 1952, p. 16).

The member of the dental profession who provides special services for those with clefts of the prepalate and palate may be called a prosthodontist or an orthodontist, depending on his particular training and contribution to the habilitative process. The prosthodontist may use a prosthesis, an obturator, or both to assist the child with a palatal cleft to obtain improvement in speech, appearance, and management of food. In some instances, the prosthesis (a replacement for some missing part) or the obturator (a device used to close an opening) includes an extension or bulb to facilitate closure of the velopharyngeal passageway. In some instances, only the bulb serves as an obturator; this is sometimes referred to as a speech aid or a speech bulb. The orthodontist modifies the form of the dental arch and the relationships of the teeth. He uses appliances, which are neither prostheses nor obturators, to change the positions of the teeth, the shape of the dental arch, or the relationships between the upper and lower arches and the teeth they contain. The terms "orthodontics" and "prosthodontics" are used to describe these areas of specialization within the field of dentistry. The oral surgeon, whose title suggests his function, is usually a member of the dental profession who is qualified, through special training, to perform surgery in the mouth area. Although some oral surgeons repair palatal defects, many restrict their activities to secondary procedures following management of the clefts by plastic surgeons.

Speech pathologists and audiologists are concerned with bringing to adequacy the speech and language of the child with a congenital cleft of the prepalate or palate. The title of speech pathologist indicates specialization in evaluating and minimizing disorders of speech and language. The audiologist is specially qualified to evaluate auditory capacities and to provide assistance for those whose primary communicative disability is in audition. In some settings, those who conduct speech training sessions are known as speech clinicians; and the person who provides remedial assistance in a clinical setting for the deaf and hard of hearing may be called a hearing clinician.

Those who study abnormal development and congenital malformations work in an area called teratology, which had the original connotation of the study of monsters but is now applied to consideration of any anomaly that results from abnormal prenatal development. The teratologist investigates the production, development, anatomy, and classification of congenital deformities. The plastic surgeon, orthodontist, prosthodontist, speech pathologist, and audiologist, in their study of children or adults with congenital prepalatal or palatal clefts, share in the interests of the teratologist.

ANOMALIES OF THE HUMAN PREPALATE AND PALATE, REGARDLESS OF THE TERMS USED TO NAME THEM, HAVE APPEARED THROUGHOUT MAN'S HISTORY; AND SPECIALISTS, WHATEVER THEIR TITLES, HAVE TREATED THESE ACQUIRED AND CONGENITAL CLEFTS.

Some writers have mentioned the discovery of an Egyptian mummy with a perforated maxilla, probably the result of an injury (Baden, 1955); but no evidence of the use of prostheses or of dental surgery has been found in Egyptian skulls (Lufkin, 1938). Aulus Cornelius Celsus, writing in the first century of the Christian era, indicated that plastic surgery, undoubtedly for acquired defects, was practiced at that time (Mettler, 1947); he also described ulcers that spread over the entire mouth and involved the palate and uvula (Lufkin, 1938). Skulls of ancient Peruvians have provided evidence of the appearance of palatal clefts in that early civilization (Weinberger, 1948). A Chinese text from the fourth century reported surgical repair of a labial cleft (Boo-Chai, 1966). Other writers have provided additional information on the existence of facial clefts, congenital or acquired, in ancient times and have described the ways in which specialists in various fields attempted to modify these deformities (Dorrance, 1933; Vaughan, 1940; Gordon, 1959; Warkany, 1959; Rogers, 1967; others).

The surgical correction of acquired facial deformities was not unknown in ancient and medieval civilizations. The Hindus, for example, found a need for plastic surgery to improve the appearance of those who had their noses cut off as a punishment for adultery (Maltz, 1946). Rhinoplasty was a specialty in some European countries in the Middle Ages, when the nose was particularly vulnerable to sword wounds (Garrison, 1917). Gaspare Tagliacozzi, an Italian, has been considered the perfecter of rhinoplasty; and some have designated him as the creator of the specialty of plastic surgery (Zimmerman and Veith, 1967). Tagliacozzi used a skin flap from the patient's arm to reconstruct his nose, but the operation met with serious objections from other surgeons and from the Church. In fact, Tagliacozzi's body was removed from consecrated ground as a condemnation of his surgical procedures; but the surgeon's home city of Bologna, defying the Church, erected a statue in his honor, showing him holding a nose in his hand (Maltz, 1946).

Little evidence of surgical procedures for facial clefts appeared until the sixteenth century, when printing made texts on various medical subjects available. Rhinoplasty continued to be popular; but a fourteenth-century physician, Jan (or Jehan) Yperman, was said to have closed clefts of the lip by suturing. Hieronymus Brunschwig described lip repair in the fifteenth or early sixteenth century (Rogers, 1967); and Jacques Houllier described the closure of a perforation of the palate that resulted from "a violent discharge," advising the use of a wax or sponge plug if the surgery was not entirely successful (Maltz, 1946).

During the Dark Ages, the surgeons were looked down on by the physicians; and the barbers, whose functions were quite different in those times, were not recognized by either the surgeons or the physicians (Lufkin, 1938). Surgery was separated from medicine in the fourteenth century, and French medical students at that time had to promise not to perform "manual surgery" (Barsky, 1964). Before the sixteenth century, when the physicians and barber-surgeons began to provide remedial attention for those with clefts, surgery was undertaken chiefly by barbers, bathers, and bonesetters; but several sixteenth-century surgeons gave assistance to individuals with clefts of the facial area. Their attention was chiefly to acquired clefts; but, like Yperman, they also closed congenital clefts of the lip.

Surgical repair of congenital prepalatal clefts, chiefly those of the lip, probably took place before surgical modification of congenital clefts of the palate. Two Frenchmen of the sixteenth century, Franco and Paré, contemporaries who drew on each other's works, gave special attention to clefts of the lip. Paré is more famous than Franco, perhaps because he served the nobility while Franco worked in the provinces and because the Huguenot wars gave him the opportunity to present some revolutionary ideas on the treatment of wounds. Both men left lasting impressions on their own generation and on succeeding generations of surgeons.

Franco used the term "cleft lip" (*lèvre fendue*) and recognized that labial clefts could be congenital (Barsky, 1964). He also described congenital clefts of the palate, stating that they were difficult to treat and that some people were convinced that this birth defect should remain unchanged because it had been given by God. Franco described the presence of the anteriorly positioned premaxilla in bilateral clefts of the prepalate and palate, but he gained unfavorable attention by recommending removal of the premaxilla if it protruded. Excision of the premaxilla resulted in severe problems in dentition and appearance, and Franco's suggestion was not well accepted by his contemporaries or his successors.

The father of modern surgery, Paré, cited in histories of dentistry as well as of medicine, introduced procedures that foreshadowed those used several centuries later. His modification of the surgical methods of his day, when wounds were customarily treated with boiling oil or hot irons, began what has been termed the actual renaissance of surgery. Paré began as a barber-surgeon, served an internship in Paris, joined the army of the Duke of Montejan in 1537, and returned to practice in Paris in 1538. He was licensed as a master barber-surgeon in 1541 and as a Sworn-surgeon thirteen years later (Hamby, 1967). Although Paré may have given most of his attention to matters other than congenital defects of the lip, his works indicated that the father of modern surgery was at least aware of such anomalies. He referred, for example, to "lips which are cleft from the first conformation in the womb by the errors of the forming faculty" (in Holdsworth, 1963, p. 38).

Attention to labial clefts has thus been part of medical history from early times. The labial cleft was obvious, it could be managed more easily by surgery than by prosthesis, the site for operation was accessible, and the surgical procedures did not seem so drastic as those for repair of a palatal cleft. Hence, although in some Oriental cultures a cleft lip was considered a mark of distinction, surgical repair of the prepalatal area undoubtedly preceded surgical modifications of congenital palatal clefts.

Congenital clefts of the palate must have existed in earlier civilizations, but practically no surgical treatment for them was provided prior to the eighteenth century. Several factors were probably responsible for the lack of attention to congenital palatal clefts. The chief of these were the limitation of the number of individuals who presented such an anomaly, the prevalence of palatal clefts that were acquired rather than congenital, the opinion that congenital clefts of the palate were unoperable, the presence of syphilis as a cause for many acquired clefts, the lack of ability to control infection and pain, and ecclesiastical rulings that prohibited the invasion of the cavities of the body by the physician.

Throughout the ages, children born with the physical anomaly of cleft palate were permitted to die or were unable to survive because of lack of nutrition. Thus, although little information is available on the early incidence of such deformities, many children born with cleft palates must have died in early infancy and did not come to the attention of the surgeons.

Arrow and gunshot wounds and disease caused destruction of the palate that required immediate attention from the surgeons who served in the armies of the nobles or the courts of the kings in the Middle Ages; only these acquired defects were cited in the few texts that referred to clefts before the seventeenth century. Heinrich von Pfolspeundt, a Bavarian surgeon, wrote in 1460 about plastic surgery for the face to repair injuries incurred in battle; but he did not repair congenital clefts of the palate. Paré and others, of course, were well aware of the damage to the roof of the mouth that could be caused by "the shot of an arquebus." However, one review of the evolution of plastic surgery stressed the point that Paré did not mention or treat cleft palate and added, "As a matter of fact, he merely used obturators for closing acquired defects resulting from disease" (Maltz, 1946, p. 185).

Apparently, the great surgeon-physicians of the Middle Ages considered congenital palatal clefts to be unoperable. Some writers as late as the eighteenth century held this opinion; and so the earlier barber-surgeons may well have thought that a palatal cleft in a child who survived was something to be accepted, not remedied.

Although syphilis was not clearly identified and named until the fifteenth century, it affected many people during the Middle Ages and the Renaissance. As early as the fourth century, a treatise on "venereal poison" included a dramatic description of the effects of the disease on the teeth, mouth, and voice (Riesman, 1935). Syphilis of the head often attacked the palate; and, according to one opinion, surgical correction of congenital clefts of the palate was delayed many centuries because physicians and surgeons thought that most palatal defects were syphilitic lesions (Rogers, 1967).

As late as the nineteenth century, those who had congenital clefts of the palate without accompanying labial clefts were suspected of having acquired the lesions as the result of syphilis. The eminent French surgeon Philibert Roux hesitated to inquire about the cause of the deviant speech of a medical student because he believed that the young man's speech defect was the result of syphilis that had destroyed the palate. John Stephenson, the medical student, described his congenital cleft in the thesis for his degree; he reported his conversation with Roux as follows:

> When in Paris pursuing my professional studies I was talking one day to Dr. Roux, most famous of the French surgeons, about something quite unrelated to my affection. He suddenly took notice of the harshness of my voice and rightly dropping his politeness, enquired if I had ever had a syphilitic ulceration of the palate, for there was no external sign of the disease; whereupon I showed him the lesion and explained it all. He immediately thought it operable and spoke to me of the possibility. [Stephenson, 1820, in Francis, 1963, p. 213]

Stephenson, explaining why the British surgeons with whom he studied had never asked him about the cause of his deviant speech, said that all his medical friends suspected that his trouble was syphilitic but had never examined his throat and so were unaware of the cleft in his palate (Francis, 1963; A. B. Wallace, 1966).

Later, when Roux wrote about his examination of Stephenson, he said:

> I had never seen a cleft of the soft palate alone and now (since that first case) I have seen several hundreds of this type. I recognized it from the few descriptions in the scientific literature under the name of bifid uvula. Till I observed the young Mr Stephenson I had seen only cleft palate associated with a unilateral cleft lip; the horrible deformity known under the name of "Gueule-de-loup." [Roux, 1854, in A. B. Wallace, 1966, p. 13]

The reluctance of the early surgeons to undertake operations on the palate can be understood when one recalls that infection was difficult to control prior to the Listerian age, which began shortly after the American Civil War, and that anesthesia was not available until 1846. Surgery prior to the nineteenth century was mostly an emergency procedure necessitated by trauma or disease. The surgeon, unable to control infection or pain, did not repair congenitally cleft palates even if he was aware of them.

One of the factors that encouraged the development of medieval medicine may also have served to delay the emergence of surgery to palatal clefts.

The Church encouraged the study of medicine and science but ruled that physicians could not invade the cavities of the body or draw blood. Hence, operative techniques were not evolved; and, until the nineteenth century, the child born with a cleft palate, if he lived, was destined to exist without surgical intervention to close the cleft.

Even if they did not provide surgical closure for congenital clefts of the palate, the physicians of the sixteenth century led the way in designing obturators for acquired clefts. Some proposed the use of wax, sponge, cotton wool, or oakum to plug the opening in the palate; others suggested that plates to fit over such an opening could be made from leather, silver, gold, or ivory (Platt, 1947). Credit for introducing the palatal obturator has been assigned to two sixteenth-century physicians—one Italian, one French. Amatus Lusitanus may have been the inventor of the artificial palate (Leibowitz, 1958); Paré was acclaimed the inventor by some (Lufkin, 1938; Vaughan, 1940).

Whether or not he was the first to construct a palatal obturator, Paré made use of this device for those to whom "it happeneth that a portion or a part of the bone of the Palat, being broken with the shot of a Gun or corroded by the virulency of the *Lues Venerea* falls away" (Paré, probably 1575, in Gibson, 1955, p. 5). The descriptions of his obturators were accompanied by drawings that showed the ingenuity of the devices, one of which was made with a sponge, "which when moistened with the moisture distilling from the brain will become more swollen and puffed up, so that it will fill the concavity of the Palat that the artificial Palat cannot fall down" (Paré, probably 1564, in Gibson, 1955, p. 5). Paré's lack of understanding of some physiological matters did not detract from the skill he showed in devising this obturator and another that was held in place by a turnbuckle rotated by a forceps after the apparatus was in place.

These devices, introduced by surgeons of the sixteenth century and constructed or recommended by such men as Geronimo Fabrizio, Etienne and Bernard Bourdet, Pierre Fauchard, and Richard Wiseman in the two centuries that followed, were for palatal clefts acquired by disease or injury (Kingsley, 1880; Denton, 1935; Lufkin, 1938; Rogers, 1967). In fact, according to one opinion, from Paré in the sixteenth century to James Snell in the nineteenth, "all prosthetic attempts were restricted to acquired palatal deformities" (Harkins, 1960, p. 5). However, reports that Hendrick von Roonhyse and John Ward wrote about cleft lip as well as cleft palate in the seventeenth century suggest that these men, and perhaps others of their time, recognized the existence of congenital clefts (Vaughan, 1940; McNeil, 1954).

Although, during the Middle Ages and even later, the surgeons had designed the obturators, one of the first reported surgical repairs of a palatal cleft was performed by a dentist. One description of the event, which took place about 1764, read: "A child had the palate cleft from the velum to the incisor teeth. M. le Monnier, a skillful dentist, endeavored and succeeded in reuniting the two borders of the cleft. . . . The child was perfectly cured" (Robert, 1766, in Dorrance, 1933, p. 3).

Such cures were rare, however; and *Cooper's Surgical Dictionary* in 1818 did not mention surgery for cleft palates (Mason, 1877). As late as 1856, the fourth edition of James Syme's *Principles of Surgery* stated: "Split palate does not admit any remedy for the division of the hard palate, except the closure of the communication between the nose and mouth by a piece of silver, enamel, or other substance, so fitted as to retain it without shifting" (in Mason, 1877, p. 63). Robert Liston's textbook of surgery, published in 1846, expressed the same idea more dramatically, saying: "When the hard palate is deficient, the patient is subjected to great inconvenience from food escaping into the cavities of the nose, and, in later life, horrible wretchedness of articulation occurs. It can readily be understood that surgery is of very little avail here. Recourse must be had to a mechanical contrivance" (p. 329).

The rapid development of medicine during the nineteenth century brought surgery to the fore, however, in the treatment of congenital clefts. Within a three-year period in the first quarter of that century, Karl Ferdinand von Graefe in 1816 and Roux in 1819 "simply undid the harmful and indifferent effects of 4300 previous years of unintentional ignorance, superstition, surgical timidity, and 'the venereal taint' by introducing, each in his own manner, a simple closure of the congenitally cleft soft palate" (Rogers, 1967, p. 15).

The Frenchman Roux and the German von Graefe were the first in a group of surgeons who gave special attention to palatal repair during the nineteenth century. Others whose names would appear on any roster of well-known surgeons of the time included Johann Dieffenbach, Bernhard von Langenbeck, Theodor Billroth, and Philippus Gustavus Passavant in Germany; Guillaume Dupuytren, Jean-Nicholas Demarquay, Alfred Velpeau, and Philippe Blandin in France; Thomas Alcock, Sir William Fergusson, Joseph Lister, and Robert Liston in England; and Alexander Stevens, John Collins Warren, and Jonathan Mason Warren in the United States.

These men were more than contemporaries in time. Many of them were colleagues in universities and hospitals in Europe and America. At one of the famous Berlin hospitals, for example, von Graefe was succeeded as chairman of the department of surgery by Dieffenbach, who improved on the work of his distinguished predecessor by extending surgery to the hard palate (Dorrance, 1933; Goldwyn, 1968b). Dieffenbach's successor was von Langenbeck, teacher of Billroth, author of an article on the surgical treatment of "stammering," and editor of a journal in which several of these men published (Goldwyn, 1969).

The leading surgeons in France in 1835 took part in an exchange of appointments, a sort of "medical musical chairs," described in *Lancet* in April of 1835:

> The vacancy at the Hotel Dieu, caused by the decease of Dupuytren, has, as we have already announced, caused the removal of M. Roux to the Hotel Dieu and of M. Velpeau to La Charité. The vacant place at La Pitié, quitted by Velpeau, has since been conferred on M. Blandin.

All these men, with Demarquay, who supplemented Roux's description of patients with submucous clefts, were prominent in France in the nineteenth century.

The English surgeon Liston taught Fergusson, who was the teacher of Mason, author of one of the earliest texts devoted entirely to surgery for clefts. Alcock was reported to have performed the first operation on the palate in England in 1821, just a few years after Roux and von Graefe had introduced staphylorrhaphy in France and Germany (Vaughan, 1940). Lister performed a series of operations on the clefts of a five-year-old child in 1881 (Pickerill, 1950–1951).

In the United States, the first chairman of the Department of Surgery at Harvard was John Collins Warren, also cited as the founder of Massachusetts General Hospital in Boston (Goldwyn, 1968b). His son, Jonathan Mason Warren, often identified as "the younger Warren," studied with Sir Astley Cooper and Dupuytren (Garrison, 1917). Stevens, the younger Warren, and T. D. Mütter performed the first operations for closure of the soft palate in the United States.

Scientific advances during the nineteenth century facilitated the work of the surgeons. The establishment of medical schools and societies, the increase in number and scope of publications, the use of anesthetics, and the introduction of antiseptic surgery encouraged the development of new and improved surgical techniques (Bankoff, 1952).

During the first half of the nineteenth century, medical schools opened in England, Canada, Germany, France, and the United States; dental schools were founded in Maryland and Ohio; and the medical associations of America and Britain were begun. One of the founders of the American Medical Association, N. S. Davis, published two articles on surgical repair of cleft lip, one in 1841 and the other in 1847, the year in which he and John Collins Warren participated in the establishment of the AMA.

Journals in the fields of science and medicine supplemented texts and pamphlets issued during the nineteenth century, and many of these publications were directly concerned with clefts of the prepalate and palate. More than 150 books and monographs on these anomalies and treatment for them were published between 1803 and 1900, at least ten of them in America. Covering a range of topics that included abnormalities of the palate, surgical procedures, unusual forms of labial clefts, and artificial palates, these books, together with more than 1,200 articles in professional journals, provided information in several languages for the surgeons of the nineteenth century.

In spite of some differences in reported dates, a method to relieve the pain of surgery was achieved before the American Civil War. Chloroform, known since 1831, was used as an anesthetic in 1847. A year before that, John Collins Warren introduced ether anesthesia into surgery. A group made up of two physicians and two dentists also claimed the credit for discovering the use of ether as an anesthetic in the same year; and the term "anesthesia" was coined at that time by the physician-author Oliver Wendell Holmes (Maltz, 1946). The initiator of the use of ether may not have been identified without question; but the use of anesthetics permitted better surgery, encouraged operative procedures in place of prostheses for palatal clefts, and led such surgeons as Fergusson in England and the Warrens in the United States to recommend surgery to the cleft palates of children three or four years of age.

Another barrier to successful surgical practice was eliminated when Lister succeeded in convincing his colleagues that application of his antiseptic principles in the practice of surgery would solve the problem of wound infection. Lister changed operative surgery from a hazardous lottery to a safe and soundly based science (Truax, 1944), and his principles undoubtedly affected the surgical attention given to congenital clefts.

Once they had begun to treat palatal clefts, the surgeons of the nineteenth century apparently developed considerable skill. Fergusson reported 400 operations for cleft lip with only three failures and 134 operations for cleft palate with only five failures in the period from 1828 to 1864 (Garrison, 1917), although "failure" was not specifically defined. In America, Mütter said that he was successful in repairing lips and palates in eighteen out of twenty cases; and Jonathan Mason Warren, reporting success in thirteen out of fourteen cases before 1834, introduced procedures to close clefts of the anterior palate instead of limiting surgery to clefts in the posterior part of the mouth (Vaughan, 1940). Just before the end of the century, Robert Abbe of New York City described the procedure that he used for surgical correction of lips "which had extreme flatness and scantiness of the upper lip with an enormous pouting and redundance of the lower one" (Abbe, 1898, p. 477).

As travel and communication improved, the plastic surgeons in many parts of the world exchanged ideas through visits and correspondence as well as in publications. The procedures of the great surgeons were studied and observed; and between 1875 and 1925, such men as Germanicus Mirault, George van Ingen Brown, William Rose, Thomas Annandale, George Dorrance, Vilray P. Blair, T. Pomfret Kilner, Harold Vaughan, Warren B. Davis, Sir Harold Gillies, Sir William Arbuthnot Lane, W. E. M. Wardill, Brophy, and several others modified and improved techniques to such an extent that surgery for congenital clefts of the prepalate and palate has become a major means of solving the problems of those to whom cheiloplasty, palatoplasty, and pharyngoplasty can bring improved appearance, better management of food, and more intelligible speech.

During ancient and medieval times and until the eighteenth century, care of the teeth was in the province of medicine; but, when he wrote a two-volume work on the treatment of teeth in 1723, Fauchard became the father of modern dentistry. Dental literature was almost unknown until Fauchard's time; and his book *Le Chirurgien Dentiste,* although its title stressed the blend of professions that had been in existence for many years, was the first publication on dentistry by a man with special skill in that field (Taylor, 1922; Denton, 1935). Perhaps Fauchard did not originate all the ideas attributed to him, and perhaps he was not the sole author of *Le Chirurgien Dentiste;* but he put down, for many to read, matters that had not been written about before.

Within 150 years after Fauchard's book, the profession of dentistry had become recognized, the first dental school in America had opened in Baltimore, and dentists were publishing articles about artificial palates. Following the example of a French dentist who attached ligatures to the teeth to hold a plate over a palatal opening and of Christophe-Francois Delabarre, who introduced "mechanical dentistry" and an artificial velum of soft gum rubber, American dentists became deeply interested in the construction of obturators.

Warren Rowell of New York built a prosthesis with a bulb above a plate that supported artificial teeth. S. P. Hullihen described a four-part obturator that permitted the patient to control the amount of air he desired to send through the nares. J. D. White wrote, in 1858, about an obturator with a nearly entire set of artificial teeth, in which gutta-percha, a rubberlike substance, was used over a plate of silver to make knobs to plug the openings into the nasal cavity and antrum (Kingsley, 1880).

As newer materials became available, the gutta-percha was replaced by a substance introduced by Charles Goodyear, who called it "vulcanite" (Lufkin, 1938). An American physician, C. H. Stearns, who had a congenital cleft of the soft palate that had not been successfully closed by surgery, decided to make an appliance for himself. Using some of Goodyear's soft, elastic material, he evolved what his colleagues called "a marvel of ingenuity." Edwin Sercombe and Snell of England worked out similar devices at about the same time. Norman W. Kingsley (1880) used the term "artificial palates" for all these devices but divided them into two categories: obturators that fitted into an opening with a well-defined border and artificial vela that moved under the control of surrounding muscles. Calvin S. Case, in his description of "a new artificial palate" in 1903, used the same classifications. Other well-known dental specialists, T. Koelliker, Heinrich Brugger, and L. Brandt, were among those who made mechanical obturators and movable vela. Wilhelm Suersen, H. J. Billeter, G. A. Stoppany, Kurt Warnekros, John J. Fitzgibbon, and N. A. Olinger designed "physiological speech-aids" that contributed to prosthetic therapy during the years following the Civil War and into the twentieth century (Baden, 1955).

Eventually, the profession of dentistry acquired even more adaptable materials for the construction of artificial palates; the modern rigid obturator, rather than the complicated artificial velum, was chosen to facilitate speech and deglutition in those with palatal clefts. As the field of dentistry developed, the orthodontist and the oral surgeon joined with the general practitioner and the prosthodontist in providing the dental care so essential to the complete management of patients with acquired or congenital clefts of the palate.

Among the several specialties concerned with habilitation of those with oral clefts, surgery and prosthetic dentistry have the longest histories. However, attention to defects of speech resulting from anomalies of the mouth began long before the twentieth century. As early as A.D. 350, Marcellus Empiricus, describing the effects of "venereal poison," stated that, in addition to damaging the teeth and mouth, this infection damaged or paralyzed the voice "by reason of the extensive destruction of the palate" (in Gordon, 1959, p. 529).

The physicians of the sixteenth century were aware of the effects of palatal clefts on speech. Paré, describing an obturator he constructed, said that he wished to help the patient who, because of injury or infection, was "disabled from properly pronouncing words and from making himself understood" (in Weinberger, 1948, p. 251). One of the books in his extensive works dealt with "means and artifices to replace that which is missing by nature or through accident"; and he described a wooden clapper, which was tied to the lower front teeth and extended over the stump of the tongue, devised "to help such as cannot speak by reason of the loss of some part of the tongue" (in Gibson, 1955, p. 6). Franco commented: "When the palate is also cleft, the patient must talk through his nose, so that he can be understood only with difficulty, all the more because the mouth, which shapes the words, is defective" (in Barsky, 1964, p. 346).

Physicians, dentists, and surgeon-dentists did little to alleviate disorders of communication during the eighteenth century; but they began to describe these deviations in specific terms. In Delaware, Matthew Wilson spoke of "aphonia" and "hypostaphyle," saying that the former came from ill configuration of the parts and the latter from a palate that was "relaxed, inflamed, ulcerated, incrossated, attenuated, or forked" (Rogers, 1967). In Germany, a writer named Siebold described the specific articulatory defects he noted in a child of three years of age who had a cleft of the soft palate (Rogers, 1967). Although the errors he listed might not be considered atypical for a three-year-old today, the observation showed an emerging interest in more than the cleft itself. This author deplored the fact that no surgical procedures could correct defects of the soft palate, but he was writing more than fifty years before the initiation of antiseptic surgery and the use of anesthesia and only a few years after people had stopped believing that cavities in the teeth were caused by worms.

Just before the American Revolution, when dentistry came to the Colonies, advertisements in the newspapers of the day showed the interest of the "surgeon-dentists" in speech. Some of these practitioners provided advice and assistance for those with clefts and suggested that the appliances they made would improve speech (Weinberger, 1948). A Doctor Fendall, announcing his availability in the *Maryland Gazette* for August 15, 1776, said, for example:

> Disorders of the teeth, as well as other more general ones of the whole system, sometimes bring on a caries of the palatal bone; in consequence

of which, the food in chewing is apt to pass into the nose, and the speech becomes disagreeable. When these thin bones are once lost they never are regenerated, and an artificial [palate] is the only remedy.

Later advertisements showed that other early dental specialists expressed an interest in oral communication, perhaps only as a means of getting patients to their offices. The Colonial citizen who read the *Pennsylvania Gazette,* the *Philadelphia Federal,* the *New York Weekly Journal,* or the handbills distributed in the cities visited by these traveling dentists learned that Mr. Clabeau, surgeon-dentist, could fix "obturators artificial palate"; that George Similier and Philip Lazarus could provide relief for persons afflicted with fistulas; that Robert Woffendale, surgeon-dentist, lately arrived from London, would perform operations on the teeth, gums, sockets, and palate; and that Josiah Flagg "sews up hare lips and fixes gold roofs and palates, greatly assisting the pronunciation and the swallow." An announcement in the *Missouri Gazette* of April 26, 1820, stated that a newly arrived dentist made "artificial palates, greatly assisting those who have lost their hard palate, in articulation and mastication." One dental historian expressed the belief that these handbills and newspapers indicated that regulating of children's teeth, repair of labial clefts, and use of gold for obturators characterized the practice of dentistry in the United States almost from its beginning (Weinberger, 1948).

Within the first decade of the nineteenth century, the newly devised procedures for closing congenital clefts by surgery provided the potential for better speech. Operations in the days of von Graefe and Roux may not have been highly successful. Closure of a cleft in the soft palate would not necessarily have solved the speech problems of those with clefts that extended through the hard palate. The beginning had been made, however; and surgery to the palate could now facilitate the improvement of speech. Roux's patient Stephenson was quite aware of the effect of the cleft in his soft palate on his speech, even though he did not recognize all the possible reasons for his difficulties in communication. Stephenson, in spite of his name, spoke French better than he spoke English; and his report that he always pronounced "th" like "s" may reveal the phonetic influence of his linguistic background rather than velopharyngeal incompetence. Even after the operation by Roux, Stephenson's speech, according to his own report, had an undue amount of nasality; and his graduation thesis, submitted the year after his surgery, contained a resolution to practice "persistently and patiently" for improvement (Francis, 1963; A. B. Wallace, 1966).

Although von Graefe's pioneering operation to close a cleft in the soft palate preceded similar surgery by Roux, his attention to speech has not been well documented. One can only judge that von Graefe hoped, by surgical intervention, to improve speech; but he did not have a Stephenson to provide a record of any attention he may have given to oral communication. Dieffenbach, however, writing in 1845, said that the principal objectives of palatoplasty were to improve speech and eliminate the difficulty in swallowing food (Goldwyn, 1968a).

Some surgeons of the nineteenth century apparently directed their patients to speech specialists for training. In one instance, the diary kept by the mother of a child with cleft palate provided information about procedures in surgery and speech training in 1881 (Pickerill, 1950–1951). The surgeon who operated on five-year-old Harold was Lister, whose worldwide reputation may have led Harold's mother to bring her child to England for the four operations performed by the famous surgeon during a fourteen-month period. Shortly before the mother and boy were to return to New Zealand, they saw a "Dr. van Praach," who thought he could improve Harold's speech. Lister recommended six lessons, each of which apparently cost as much as a visit to the surgeon's office; and, in June of 1881, Harold evidently had the speech training recommended by the surgeon and provided by the speech specialist. This 1881 speech pathologist was undoubtedly William van Praagh, who was neither a physician nor a dentist and whose name and title were inaccurately recorded by Harold's mother. In an address to a meeting of the Odontological Society of Great Britain in 1888, van Praagh summarized his method of speech training, saying:

> We advise gymnastics of the jaw, tongue, lips—in fact, of all the movable parts of the head; practice before a glass to improve the facial expression; exercises for teaching the patient to breathe properly; exercises for pronouncing vowel sounds, consonants, compound consonants, and all sound combinations distinctly, and when more perfect, connectedly in sentences; and lastly, we make the patient speak and read according to the recognized laws of elocution, and by so doing, he obtains proper modulation of the voice, and fluency of speech. [P. 333]

The discussion that followed van Praagh's presentation to the Odontological Society suggested that the surgeons and dentists of the late nineteenth century had not reached a point of complete agreement with one another and were not ready to give unqualified support to the elocutionists who served as speech clinicians.

Special attention to normal voice and articulation was not new in the nineteenth century, having been part of the training of public speakers since the time of the Greek orators; and treatises devoted entirely to the improvement of normal voice production had appeared during the eighteenth century. The physiology of the mechanism for speech was described by an American physician, James Rush, in 1827; and Alexander Melville Bell, whose interest in training the deaf gained him a wide reputation, published *The Science of Speech* in 1897. In Germany, Passavant presented, in 1863, the theory on the function of the area of the posterior pharyngeal wall that now bears his name. The description of Passavant's pad, bar, or cushion drew special attention to one aspect of the speech of those with congenital clefts of the palate.

Passavant's two articles, one in 1863 and another in 1869, on the role of the superior phyarngeal constrictor, had the same title, "On the Closure of the Pharynx in Speech." The second article, accompanied by three pages of diagrams, reiterated his belief that the forward movement of the superior constrictor muscle of the pharynx, in conjunction with the elevation and retraction (*Rückwartsstellung*) of the velum, closed the pharyngeal passageway. Regardless of present opinions about Passavant's theory, his ideas contributed to the stimulation of interest in the speech of patients with cleft palates in the nineteenth century.

The dentists, who had become independent of the surgeons and physicians by the second half of the nineteenth century, showed that they recognized the value of prosthetic devices in the improvement of speech. Speaking to the Massachusetts Dental Society in 1880, Henry A. Baker pointed out the differences in treating congenital and acquired palatal clefts. In the accidental clefts, he stated, the patient had learned to articulate distinctly and use the organs of speech efficiently and correctly; but "persons who are . . . deformed from birth are obliged to learn the art and methods of articulation by a slow and painful process" (p. 179). The kind of training needed for those with congenital clefts of the palate, Baker said, was similar to that needed for someone who acquires a new language; and the appliance provided by the dentist must work on the physiological principles in harmony with the natural movements and under the perfect control of the surrounding muscles.

Other dentists, too, constructed obturators with the speech of the patient in mind. J. W. Rhone (1894), suggesting that surgery was not the answer to the problem of cleft palate, said that his devices could remedy the leading difficulties—defective articulation and enunciation, the escape of solids and fluids through the nasal passages, and the difficulty of swallowing. He was less optimistic about the value of his appliances than were some of his colleagues, stating that "to promise . . . that a person under such conditions could be enabled by means of *any* appliance to speak or read without betraying the defect to an experienced ear, would simply be an *exaggeration* and a *deception*" (p. 549).

In 1880, Kingsley published his well-known treatise on oral deformities "as a branch of mechanical surgery." He was cognizant of the effects of palatal clefts on speech, saying, for example, "The only evil arising from congenital cleft palate which demands the interference of science and art is its impairment of speech" (p. 209). He also recommended procedures for speech training, advising that an artificial velum be used first to help the patient to acquire good articulation and that an obturator then be provided.

Kingsley noted, in cleft palate patients, that "in the effort to produce certain sounds, the superior constrictor would develop a ridge or roll of considerable magnitude across the pharynx." He added:

> This pharyngeal movement, important in normal articulation, becomes an essential requisite to success when articulation with an artificial palate is attempted. In a normal condition, the posterior nasal passages are closed by the combined action of the palate and the constricted pharyngeal wall. In an abnormal condition of absence of the palate, the pharyngeal action may be made to perform the office of both. [Pp. 419–420]

However, he did not refer to Passavant in his discussion of the function of the posterior pharyngeal wall in speech; and Passavant's name did not appear in the index of the book.

Kingsley's final chapter dealt with the formation of vowel and consonant sounds. Palatograms were used to illustrate the tongue positions for five vowel sounds, and diagrams showed articulatory positions for consonant sounds. Typical of all his illustrations of articulatory positioning was the presence of a protrusion on the posterior pharyngeal wall. Kingsley added a discussion of compensations and errors in the speech of those with congenital and acquired clefts of the palate, making his book one of the first to give detailed attention to speech as part of the total process of habilitation for individuals with palatal clefts.

By the beginning of the twentieth century, dental specialists and surgeons were giving a considerable amount of attention to speech in relationship to palatal clefts. Whether or not Suersen had read Passavant's 1863 article before he spoke to the Central Association of German Dentists in Hamburg in 1867, he described "a muscle which, to my knowledge, has, in connection with these operations, not yet received a sufficient amount of attention—I mean the *constrictor pharyngeus superior.*" Suersen recognized the need for separation of the nasal cavity from the oral cavity "to be able to pronounce all letters distinctly" (in Baker, 1881, p. 180).

Mason, whose 1877 publication was dedicated to his famous teacher Fergusson, reported on the improvement in voice noted in several patients after surgical repair to the palate. After describing several surgical procedures, Mason said:

> The chief object of the operation, whatever plan be adopted, is obviously to improve the voice of the patient, and I have no hesitation in saying that in many instances the voice is very materially altered for the better. It is too much to expect that the sufferer should speak as fluently as his neighbors whose palates are normally developed. Langenbeck thought that the nasal twang in cleft palate was due to want of nerve supply, but there is reason to suppose, as Passavant and Gustave Simon do, that it is attributable to the shortening of the palate. [P. 113]

Stoppany, who was from Zurich, speaking to the American Dental Society of Europe in 1909, praised Kingsley and Suerson for their work in devising obturators but stated that the results those men obtained would have been still better if their treatments "could have been followed by a course of articulation, as is given in these days, after the method of Lang and Gutzmann in Berlin" (p. 1035). This course of instruction, as Stoppany described it, began with teaching the patient how to form vowels, with the aid of a spatula that helped the tongue and lips to assume the proper positions. Additional steps in this sequence of speech training included singing of the vowel sounds, learning how to form consonants, joining the consonants to the vowels, then using the sounds in words and sentences. All the exercises were done before a mirror; and the course of instruction lasted from five weeks to three months, with fifteen to a hundred lessons. The results of the speech training, Stoppany pointed out, depended on the intelligence, the energy, and the hearing faculties of the patient. The originator of this plan of therapy, Hermann Gutzmann, served as director of a hospital for speech defects in Berlin and was the author of a series of lectures on speech disorders published in 1893. He also wrote articles and pamphlets on the teaching of the deaf and on the physiology of speech as a basis for scientific speech therapy.

Commenting on a debate held by the Surgical Section of the British

Royal Academy of Medicine, an editorial in *Lancet* for June 3, 1911, pointed out that the person with a palatal cleft might encounter problems in vocational planning because "the mere alteration of the speech is in itself sufficient to interfere seriously with his success in many occupations" (p. 1519). This evidence of recognition of the need for good speech became more and more frequent in writings in the twentieth century, by which time most of the texts on clefts of the palate included consideration of speech.

Berry and Legg, British surgeons writing in 1912, described the effects of cleft palate on speech in some detail. They explained that the main cause of the defective articulation of a cleft palate patient was that some of the air that should be expelled through the mouth escaped into the nose, and they also considered the effects of dental irregularities on speech. The aim of the surgeon, they said, should always be "to restore as completely as possible not only the shape, but also the functions of the soft palate. In proportion as he is successful in this aim, so will his patient benefit as regards speech" (p. 158).

The Chicago surgeon Brophy, finding that a section on cleft lip and palate in his 1915 text on oral surgery was very popular, published a text entitled *Cleft Lip and Palate* in 1923. He invited G. Hudson Makuen, a laryngologist who had a special interest in speech disorders, to write a chapter on the training in speech needed after surgery to the palate. Makuen had told members of the American Laryngological Society in 1901 that habits of speech formation could not be changed without special aid and instruction and that the ear "must make the discrimination and appreciate good speech before the organs can be trained to produce it" (p. 121). The sequence of training that he recommended in Brophy's book included exercises such as systematic and vigorous gargling, development of voluntary control of the muscles of the palate and pharynx, mechanical stretching of the palate with an instrument or the finger, training in phonation and in the articulation of the sounds of the "physiological alphabet," and attention to correct breathing (in Brophy, 1923, pp. 289–300). Some of these suggestions did not prove useful; others, in modified form, are part of remedial procedures used by some speech clinicians today.

Fitzgibbon, of Holyoke, Massachusetts, an outstanding dentist in the first half of the twentieth century, stressed the importance of speech training after an obturator had been provided. He constructed obturators with tailpieces that were molded by the action of the patient's muscles at the time of fitting and that were made of gold instead of the soft rubber commonly used in the preceding period. With strong personal feelings about surgery because of unsuccessful operations for his own palatal cleft, Fitzgibbon wore one of his own devices and provided a good example for his patients. He trained his own patients in speech, teaching them to imitate his muscle action in gripping and releasing the tailpiece of the obturator, to use certain sounds to improve this gripping action, to learn labial and lingual tones, and to master the dilatation of the nostrils. Fitzgibbon (1923) recommended that his patients use the newly invented disc recorders to hear their own voices and recognize their poor tones. He also advised them to modify vocabulary "so that substitute words may be used for those words difficult to produce" (p. 718). The speech training, according to Fitzgibbon, was fully as important as the proper construction of the appliance.

Continuing the practice of some of his medical colleagues, Vaughan, of New York City, wrote extensively about speech in his 1940 text on congenital clefts of the lip and palate. He acknowledged the assistance he obtained from such specialists in speech as Max Müller, John Wyllie, Richard Borden and Alvin Busse, and Sarah Stinchfield. He described and pictured "an appliance to determine velopharyngeal pressure by the blowing test." He emphasized the importance of velopharyngeal closure for good production of "oral consonants"; and he pointed out the greater difficulty in articulation when "a series of consonants must be produced, one after the other, without the interposition of a vowel" (p. 56).

Among the many dentists and surgeons who displayed considerable interest in speech training for those with palatal clefts during the first third of the twentieth century, Veau is cited as the originator of the cleft palate rehabilitation team (Converse, 1962). Veau's interest in surgery for cleft lips and palates developed during the latter part of his life, but he performed more than 3,300 operations on lips and palates. He enlisted the aid of a speech pathologist, Madame Suzanne Borel-Maisonny, who wrote the third section of the text that Veau published in 1931. The discussion included a report on the speech of 103 children on whom Veau had operated, a description of the defects of communication typical of children with cleft palates, and a listing of the procedures to be followed in speech rehabilitation for patients with surgically repaired palatal clefts.

Since 1940, many texts and articles have emphasized the relationships among dentistry, surgery, and speech pathology-audiology in the management of adults and children with clefts of the prepalate and palate. Entries in the bibliography at the end of this volume show some of the professional journals carrying articles of interdisciplinary interest. Organizations dedicated to the service of those with clefts encourage membership from several professions and give evidence of interdisciplinary discussions in the programs of their meetings. Groups of specialists in universities, hospitals, and rehabilitation centers provide service, as teams, for individuals with malformations of the lip and palate. Research projects designed to seek the causes of these malformations are staffed by representatives of many disciplines. These relationships, discussed in later chapters, started centuries ago, when a small number of dedicated men saw the multiplicity of the problem of orofacial clefts, and have grown throughout the years as members of many professions have joined together to focus their abilities on the needs of those with congenital anomalies.

TEXTS AND JOURNALS FROM THE PAST GIVE EVIDENCE OF THE INTEREST SHOWN IN INDIVIDUALS WITH PREPALATAL AND PALATAL CLEFTS; BUT, UNTIL COMPARATIVELY RECENTLY, THE NUMBER OF THOSE WITH SUCH MALFORMATIONS HAS BEEN DIFFICULT TO DETERMINE.

Data are incomplete and contradictory, and many reports have been based on records that did not show the true incidence of clefts. The range of figures is so wide that the investigator has difficulty in reaching a definite decision about the frequency with which clefts occur.

One way to learn something about the incidence of anomalies, of course, is to write to people who have firsthand experience with the problems. This was the procedure used in 1904 by R. W. Murray, a physician in England, who wrote to medical colleagues in various parts of the world, asking them to report their observations on the incidence of clefts. In the light of more recent knowledge, some of the comments were quite appropriate. The respondent from China stated that cleft lip was common there and that the Chinese paid little attention to it. Cleft palate, he said, was of rare occurrence. The correspondent in Singapore reported that cleft lip was seen occasionally among the Malays and Chinese but that these people were rather proud of the deformity and did not seek surgical correction for it. In Java, similarly, clefts were not considered a disadvantage, although they occurred commonly there and in Bombay. The reports from Africa and Jamaica foreshadowed those of the present time, stating that clefts of the lip and palate were extremely rare in those countries. Murray commented:

> I believe it to be highly probable that harelip and cleft palate accrue with varying frequency amongst all the nations of the world and that the frequency with which it is seen amongst uncivilized natives depends very largely

> upon their religious belief, which would determine whether a child born with hare-lip should be put to death or allowed to live. [P. 1423]

Information obtained from more recent investigations, although more specific than that provided by Murray's correspondents, is still incomplete. The relatively few studies of the incidence of congenital clefts of the prepalate and palate during the first quarter of the twentieth century provided data that were based on limited populations and that showed wide ranges of incidence. In London, for example, according to a frequently cited report, the incidence of clefts in 1908, based on hospital admissions, was one in each 1,742 births. Records from the United States Army showed that one in each 1,136 white and one in each 2,805 Negro draftees in World War I had a cleft of the lip or palate (Brophy, 1923). From a study of birth records in Baltimore from 1895 to 1924, John Staige Davis (1924) found that one in each 915 white and one in each 1,788 Negro babies had a cleft of the lip and/or palate. These figures sometimes vary in publications in which they are cited, possibly because of the lack of specificity of the original reports or the need to recompute some figures to obtain a consistent form for citing incidence. These early data are from such disparate populations that their actual value is less than their historical interest.

A study published in 1947 was cited frequently in the literature between 1950 and 1960. Gretchen Mueller Phair's report that one in each 770 children born in Wisconsin had cleft lip, cleft palate, or both was used as the basis for answering questions about the incidence of prepalatal and palatal clefts for almost a decade. The data were accepted because of the ten-year span of the study and because of Wisconsin's legal requirement for the reporting of congenital anomalies. Some studies since 1947 have confirmed the figure reported by Phair; others have shown different findings.

Table 1-1 shows the incidence of clefts, without differentiation of type, reported between 1960 and 1968 from widely scattered geographic areas. The figures are the results of diverse methods of collecting data; a search for patterns of similarity in terms of racial groups, climate, economic levels, and other factors did not reveal any trends that could be defended. The incidence figure near the midpoint—one in each 826 births for sixteen countries (Stevenson and others, 1966) and for twenty-seven states and two cities in the United States (Greene and others, 1965)—seems fairly representative of the incidence of clefts of the prepalate and palate in children born throughout the world today. The figures for the United States were derived from birth certificates for 1,965,400 live births; data for the countries

TABLE 1-1 INCIDENCE OF CLEFTS OF THE PREPALATE, PALATE, OR BOTH, REPORTED BY INVESTIGATORS BETWEEN 1960 AND 1968

*Incidence ratio**	*Place*	*Investigator*
1:543	Finland	Gylling and Soivio, 1962
1:546	Montana	Tretsven, 1963
1:556	New York	Milham, 1963
1:562	British Columbia	International Medical Congress, 1964
1:568	England	Wolstenholme and O'Connor, 1960
1:588	Denmark	Fogh-Andersen, 1961
1:600	England	Oldfield and Tate, 1964
1:662	Utah	Woolf and others, 1963
1:665	Denmark	Pruzansky, 1961
1:704	England	Knox and Braithwaite, 1963
1:750	United States	Public Health Service, 1966
1:762	Pennsylvania	Sesgin and Stark, 1961
1:804	Four states	Greene and others, 1964
1:812	Wisconsin	Gilmore and Hofman, 1966
1:814	Iowa	Olin, 1960
1:826	Twenty-seven states, two cities	Greene and others, 1965
1:826	Sixteen countries	Stevenson and others, 1966
1:851	California	Loretz and others, 1961
1:890	Pennsylvania	Ivy, 1962b
1:900	Brazil	Pitanguy and Franco, 1967
1:905	Brazil	International Medical Congress, 1964
1:929	Seventeen states	Donahue, 1965
1:987	Missouri	Silberg, 1968
1:1,000	England	International Medical Congress, 1964
1:1,250	New York City	Erhardt and Nelson, 1964
1:1,260	New York City	Conway and Wagner, 1966
1:1,289	New York City	Sesgin and Stark, 1961
1:1,837	Israel	Azaz and Koyoumdjisky-Kaye, 1967
1:1,887	Jamaica	Millard and McNeill, 1965

* Incidence ratios, shown from greatest to least, indicate that one child in each 543 (or 600 or 987) was born with a cleft of the prepalate, palate, or both.

that reported to the World Health Organization came from information on 416,695 single births at twenty-four different centers throughout the world. In the United States, the errors possible on birth certificates may have affected the information obtained. In some of the countries participating in the worldwide study, not all babies are born in hospitals; and the difficulties in obtaining consistent reports for those who were hospital-born may have limited the data. Nevertheless, the identity of the incidence of clefts in these two large and diverse groups suggests that Phair's 1947 estimate of one cleft in each 770 births may have been slightly high.

On the other hand, Fogh-Andersen reported an increase in the incidence of congenital clefts of the prepalate and palate in Denmark in the first third of the present century from one in 1,000 to one in 750 or even one in 500 births (in Longacre, 1968). This significant increase was documented from the records kept in Denmark, where central surgical facilities provide care for all the children born with clefts in that country. Similar information was presented by Wilhelm Tünte (1969), who reported that the incidence of cleft lip with or without cleft palate rose about 50 percent in Germany between 1901 and 1961. If these increases in the incidence of congenital clefts become evident in other countries, then Phair's figure may have been low. The variations in reports on the incidence of clefts have led to some confusion; and the data in the tables in this chapter are evidence of another of the information gaps to which Harlan Bloomer (1968) referred when he said, "Many of the answers so badly needed to promote truly effective diagnostic and treatment management of the orofacially disfigured still escape us" (p. 371).

Several books and articles published after 1960 contained tabulations showing the range of incidence of congenital oral clefts. The highest incidences reported included one in 276 births among Montana Indians, one in 373 births among Japanese, and one in 507 births in Hawaii. The lowest incidences included one cleft in 3,333 births in Switzerland and one in 4,395 births among Negroes in Pennsylvania. Table 1-2 shows the range of incidence figures presented by seventeen reporters; but these data are complicated by the differences in race, location, and date. The figures in Tables 1-1 and 1-2, therefore, like some of the early reports, have more historic than actual significance; and their range reflects the many factors that have influenced findings on the incidence of congenital clefts of the prepalate and palate.

Comparisons of even the most complete compilations of data on the incidence of clefts are limited by such factors as the sources of information, the restrictions of the studies, the geographical areas covered, the methods of reporting, and the kinds of individuals included. Each of these factors can affect the results, although the investigators have tried to control the variables.

Some investigators must depend on birth certificates or registries of births as their sources of information; and they may meet the "incompleteness, inaccuracy, illegibility, and unintelligibility with which information often is recorded on birth certificates" (Greene and others, 1965, p. 141; Greene,

TABLE 1-2 RANGE OF INCIDENCE OF ORAL CLEFTS AS REPORTED IN PUBLICATIONS BETWEEN 1960 AND 1968

Reported incidence		*Place*		
Highest	*Lowest*	*Highest*	*Lowest*	*Reporter*
1:276	1:4,394	Montana	Pennsylvania	Fukuhara, 1965
1:507	1:1,793	Hawaii	Baltimore	Greene, 1963
1:507	1:1,837	Hawaii	Israel	Azaz and Koyoumdjisky-Kaye, 1967
1:514	1:1,290	Hawaii	New York	Milham, 1963
1:543	1:1,525	Finland	Russia	Conway and Wagner, 1966
1:543	1:1,525	Finland	Russia	Holdsworth, 1963
1:543	1:1,742	Finland	London	Gylling and Soivio, 1962
1:550	1:1,742	Hawaii	London	Sesgin and Stark, 1961
1:550	1:1,742	Hawaii	London	Stark, 1962
1:565	1:3,030	Chile	South Africa	Stevenson and others, 1966
1:588	1:1,234	South Sweden	New York City	Drillien and others, 1966
1:624	1:1,681	Montana	South Carolina	Donahue, 1965
1:638	1:1,742	Germany	London	Morley, 1967
1:638	1:1,742	Germany	England	Olin, 1960
1:650	1:4,097	Montana	Louisiana	Olin, 1960
1:724	1:2,013	Pennsylvania	Pennsylvania	Ivy, 1968
1:1,400	1:4,395	Los Angeles	Pennsylvania	Altemus, 1966

1968). The value of the birth record depends on the efficiency with which it is made out; and, although some states and countries require by law the reporting of congenital anomalies, many either make no such requirement or provide space on the birth certificate for a report of anomalies without requiring the physician or midwife to provide the information. Lack of communication between the physician and the person who fills out the certificate may make for incompleteness, and some who are responsible for making out certificates hesitate to stigmatize a child by listing a congenital anomaly in a record that might be available for inspection (Wallace and Fisher, 1966).

In some instances, birth certificates are made out by nonmedical attendants at births; some of these assistants may not check carefully to determine the presence of congenital anomalies or cannot reach a proper conclusion about the nature or the extent of an observed deformity. In some parts of the world, births may not be reported to any bureau of vital statistics; although failure to report does not account for the low incidence of clefts in black babies, it may explain some of the divergence in reported incidence. Birth certificates for thirty-three black babies with clefts of the prepalate, the palate, or both in a twelve-year period in one state, which had a total of more than one million births during that period of time, probably do not represent the true incidence of labial and palatal clefts among black children born in that state (Silberg, 1968).

Limitations of the sources from which information is obtained may decrease the reported incidence of congenital clefts of the prepalate and palate. One investigator (Milham, 1963) found that the total number of clefts in upstate New York was considerably higher when all sources of information were consulted than when only one was used. In Montana, 17 percent of the children born in a six-year period did not have their clefts listed on birth certificates (Bardanouve, 1969); and, in Pennsylvania during a four-year period, the total number of children born with clefts was 1,269 according to birth certificates but 1,592 when all sources were consulted (Ivy, 1957). Some of the variations in the reported incidence of congenital clefts may be the result of underreporting.

When a study of the incidence of clefts is restricted by uncontrollable conditions or by design, the findings may reflect the limitations. Most of the investigators whose findings are shown in Table 1-1 chose one geographical area or confined their search to the population of a specific country, city, county, or state. Some selected a particular age or age range for study. Other investigations, not included in Table 1-1, have been carried out in one or two hospitals, in a single school system, in one county, during a single year, or with a single racial group.

Whereas the first known reports of incidence of clefts of the prepalate or palate, as shown in Table 1-2, were from Russia and England, studies of this topic in more recent years have been undertaken in many parts of the world. Table 1-1 includes reports from large and small countries, and reports antedating 1960 came from many different lands. These geographic variations probably had some effect on the information provided.

Incidence figures are affected to a great extent also by the ways in which the data are reported. The tables show the incidence of clefts as one in a certain number of births, but several of the studies cited in the tables reported incidence in other ways. The figures in the tables were derived by converting the reports to one system of reporting that shows the ratio of babies with clefts to the number of babies born, with the first figure remaining constant and the second increasing as the incidence decreases. Thus, the statement that the incidence of clefts was one in 987 means that one baby with a cleft appeared in each 987 births; but such a statement refers to all types of clefts and does not specify whether the count was made from total births or live births.

Perhaps the greatest influence on data that show the incidence of clefts lies in the kinds of individuals who are included in the studies. What people made up the population from which the figures were derived? Were they babies who survived or died shortly after birth? Were they newborn infants, children admitted to hospitals for surgery, schoolchildren, adults? Did they have multiple handicaps, or was the cleft the only deformity? Were they members of one racial group or from several? Investigators who stated that the incidence of congenital clefts was one in 276 or one in 1,788 or one in 3,333 were reporting what they found through careful study, but their information could have been more meaningful if they had described the group from which they derived their data.

Eleven of the investigators whose reports were cited in Table 1-1 used information from records of live births to determine the incidence of clefts of the prepalate, palate, or both. Some used the total number of births for their computations. Others did not specify whether the records they studied included all births or only those who survived, and few reported the presence or absence of other anomalies in the babies they studied.

Differences in the apparent incidence of clefts may be the result of other kinds of variations in the people about whom information was collected. In Denmark, for example, some of the figures on incidence were computed from the number of children admitted for surgery at the one hospital in that country that provides surgical treatment for almost all the babies born with clefts (Fogh-Andersen, 1961). A report from New York City was based on a group made up of patients born in a hospital that served a high percentage of black citizens (Sesgin and Stark, 1961). Alan C. Stevenson and his colleagues (1966), in their work for the World Health Organization, depended on reports from twenty-four centers in sixteen countries and presented figures derived from 504 single births in which clefts were not associated with any other malformations.

Some investigations used still other kinds of groups. Children in one city school system were the population chosen for one study (Kessler, 1951). In others, only one national or racial group was considered, as in studies in Japan, Trinidad, and Turkey (Neel, 1958; E. L. S. Robertson, in Excerpta Medica Foundation, 1963; Borçbakan, 1969) and among North American Negroes (Altemus, 1966).

Among all the factors that seem to make for variation in the incidence of congenital clefts of the prepalate and palate, the effect of race is perhaps the best-demonstrated. Most general discussions of the incidence of clefts include the statement that those whose skins are black seem less susceptible to oral clefts than those whose skins are white, yellow, or red. Table 1-3 shows the results of studies in which race was considered. The low incidence of clefts among blacks, in comparison with the incidence in other groups, is shown clearly in this table. The data on North American Indians, although not entirely consistent, suggest that Indians in Montana and in British Columbia are more susceptible to clefts than non-Indians in these areas (Tretsven, 1963, 1965; International Medical Congress, 1964). In Hawaii, the admixture of races may obscure some of the figures on racial differences; but a study published in 1947 indicated that the incidence of clefts was highest in the Filipinos, Portuguese, and Japanese and lowest in the Chinese and Caucasians (Krantz and Henderson).

The incidence of congenital clefts of the prepalate and palate will vary with the race of the population studied, but the low incidence in the blacks will tend to decrease the incidence for any group that includes a large percentage of members of the Negro race. Thus, the range of incidence in a study published in 1965 (one cleft in each 624 births in Montana to one in each 1,681 in South Carolina) might be explained in part by the inclusion of figures from states with large black populations (Tennessee and South Carolina, for example). However, the report of one cleft in each 704 births in Missouri and the lower incidence of one in each 1,112 births in Oregon is difficult to understand on the basis of the distribution of blacks and whites in those states (Donahue, 1965).

A statement that one in each 770 or 876 or 1,000 children will be born with a cleft of the prepalate or palate or both is oversimplification. Clefts may be present in varying degrees, types, and combinations; and recent studies of incidence have considered these variations. Now, instead of using "cleft" in a general way, some reports include the percentage of clefts of the lip, of the palate, and of the lip and palate together. If "cleft lip" can be considered to correspond to "prepalatal cleft," then clefts involving both prepalate and palate appear more frequently than palatal or prepalatal

TABLE 1-3 INCIDENCE OF CLEFTS WHEN RACE IS A FACTOR

Incidence				
Whites	*Blacks*	*Others**	*Place*	*Investigator*
1:583	....	1:276	Montana	Tretsven, 1963
1:613	....	1:343	British Columbia	International Medical Congress, 1964
1:625	1:1,428	....	North Carolina	Richardson and Higgins, 1964
1:704	1:3,333	1:4,394	Brazil	International Medical Congress, 1964
1:724	1:2,013	....	Pennsylvania	Ivy, 1968
1:798	....	1:433	California	DeVoss, 1952
1:884	1:4,478	....	Missouri	Silberg, 1968
1:900	1:5,607	1:1,265	Wisconsin	Gilmore and Hofman, 1966
1:915	1:1,788	....	Baltimore	Davis, 1924
1:918	1:1,656	1:615	California	Loretz and others, 1961
1:929	1:2,415	....	Missouri	Olin, 1960
1:950	1:1,899	....	Brooklyn	Shapiro and others, 1958
1:1,000	1:1,400	1:1,800	California	Lutz and Moor, 1955
1:1,111	1:1,666†	1:1,428	New York	Erhardt and Nelson, 1964
1:1,336	1:4,097	....	Louisiana	Olin, 1960
1:1,939	....	1:283 1:408 1:600 1:1,332	Hawaii	Krantz and Henderson, 1947

* Indians in Montana, British Columbia, and Wisconsin; mulattoes in Brazil; unspecified in California (Loretz and others); Mexicans in California (Lutz and Moor); Puerto Ricans in New York; Filipinos (1:283), Portuguese (1:408), Japanese (1:600), and Chinese (1:1,332) in Hawaii.

† "Nonwhite"

clefts; and prepalatal clefts are lowest in frequency of occurrence. Table 1-4 shows that, although percentages differ, the average of fifteen studies confirms the statement that clefts involving both prepalate and palate will be more frequent than clefts of the palate by a ratio of 7:3 (Biggerstaff, 1969). The percentages in Table 1-4, derived from groups that contained more than 500 children and that represented widespread geographic locations, also support the ratio of 1:2:1 (clefts of the prepalate/clefts of both prepalate and palate/clefts of the palate) suggested by Fogh-Andersen (1942), although the percentage of prepalatal clefts (26 percent) was slightly lower than that of palatal clefts (28.1 percent).

Some relatively recent studies have reported the side on which the cleft occurs, confirming earlier statements that clefts of the lip appear with greater frequency on the left. In 850 consecutive cases at a large medical center between 1932 and 1965, for example, 55 percent of 211 clefts anterior

TABLE 1-4 INCIDENCE OF CLEFTS BY TYPE*

Percentage of clefts				
Lip	*Palate*	*Lip and palate*	*Investigator*	*Number in group*
22	26	52	Phair, 1947	1,134
22	34	43	Oldfield, 1959	1,041
23	24	53	Woolf and others, 1963	553
23	35	42	Oldfield and Tate, 1964	1,166
25	33	41	Silberg, 1968	1,149
25	34	41	Conway and others, 1968	850
26	26	48	Donahue, 1967	2,256
26	28	46	R. T. Millard, 1964	1,395
26	30	44	Gilmore and Hofman, 1966	2,162
27	19	53	Stevenson and others, 1966	504
27	29	44	Greene and others, 1964	4,451
27	31	42	Greene and others, 1965	2,162
28	21	51	Loretz and others, 1961	1,000
31	19	50	Hixon, 1951	695
32	33	35	Knox and Braithwaite, 1963	574

* The studies from which these data were obtained used "cleft lip" and "cleft palate" rather than "prepalatal cleft" and "palatal cleft."

to the incisive foramen were on the left side, 27 percent were on the right, and 11 percent were bilateral. The remaining 7 percent were classified as median or unknown (Conway and others, 1968). Information about the sidedness of palatal clefts is less clear. Some writers have considered that clefts posterior to the incisive foramen are central; others have said that the palatal cleft is on the right if the left palatal shelf is attached to the vomer; still others have identified the side of the defect only when both prepalate and palate were cleft.

The statement that individuals with clefts that involve both prepalate and palate will outnumber those with so-called "isolated clefts" of either is true, but it is also in need of qualification. The various types of clefts occur in varying percentages when the sex of the affected individual is considered. Evidence of the greater incidence of clefts in males than females is clear. However, when the specific type of cleft is a factor, the sex distributions change. Table 1-5 shows the results of nineteen studies that considered incidence by sex and by type of cleft. These figures demonstrate that, throughout a range of time and in many parts of the world, more males have clefts of the prepalatal area, more females have palatal clefts, and more males have complete clefts, those involving both areas.

Few reports on the incidence of clefts have included any information about bifid uvula, a type of palatal defect that is sometimes unrecognized because it does not have the adverse effects of other types of clefts. Examination of the mouth of a newborn child will not always reveal a small cleft in the uvula, but the presence of this anomaly in adults is surprisingly frequent. One series of examinations of 5,530 newborn infants found one labial cleft, two clefts of the lip and palate, three palatal clefts, and eleven malformations of the uvula (McIntosh and others, 1954). The incidence of uvular clefts noted in these infants, one in each 502 births, was very small in comparison with the incidence of one defect of the uvula in each 68 adults examined at the University of Minnesota (Meskin and others, 1964).

Another type of cleft that may be easily overlooked in the compilation of incidence figures is the submucosal or occult cleft. The covering of the structures by the intact mucous membrane conceals the incomplete bony or muscular development; and, unless acoustic manifestations or other circumstances bring about discovery through palpation or illumination, this kind of cleft may remain unidentified (Gylling and Soivio, 1965; Thaler and Smith, 1968). The number of individuals with such clefts has not been specifically determined, and one can only assume that many persons may

TABLE 1-5 INCIDENCE OF CLEFTS BY TYPE AND SEX AS SHOWN IN STUDIES CONDUCTED BETWEEN 1946 AND 1968*

Percentage of clefts							
Lip		*Palate*		*Both*			
M	*F*	*M*	*F*	*M*	*F*	*Place*	*Source*
63	37	37	63	69	31	Denmark	Fogh-Andersen, 1946
60	40	48	52	68	32	England	Oldfield, 1949
62	38	41	59	66	34	Germany	Kiskadden and others, 1949
79	21	29	71	80	20	Sweden	Böök, 1951
61	39	41	59	59	41	England	MacMahon and McKeown, 1953
63	37	43	57	67	33	Seattle	Beder and others, 1956
60	40	44	56	58	42	California	Loretz and others, 1961
70	30	27	73	45	55	New York City	Sesgin and Stark, 1961
63	37	47	53	73	27	Utah	Woolf and others, 1963
63	37	41	59	68	32	England	Knox and Braithwaite, 1963
65	35	41	59	66	34	Composite	Greene, 1963
61	39	41	59	70	30	England	Oldfield and Tate, 1964
63	36	43	56	66	34	Pennsylvania	R. T. Millard, 1964
63	37	47	52	65	35	Four states	Greene and others, 1964
62	38	43	57	67	33	Twenty-seven states	Greene and others, 1965
62	38	41	59	64	36	Sixteen countries	Stevenson and others, 1966
70	30	38	62	73	27	Scotland	Drillien and others, 1966
51	49	42	58	65	35	New York	Conway and others, 1968
61	39	38	62	69	31	Illinois	Meskin and others, 1968

* These incidence reports used the term "cleft lip." The incidence of clefts of the lip is higher in males than in females in all the reports cited. The incidence of clefts of the palate is higher in females than in males in all the reports cited. The incidence of clefts of both lip and palate is higher in males than in females in all but one of the reports cited.

go through life with submucosal clefts that are never detected and not counted in incidence figures.

Additional information has been gathered in the many attempts to find the incidence of prepalatal and palatal clefts. The place in birth order of the child with a cleft has been determined, as have the ages of the parents, season of birth, legitimacy, birth weight, and other factors relating to the pregnancy that resulted in a child with a cleft. Little agreement has been reached in reports on these matters. Studies of pregnancies resulting in babies with clefts have been more useful to those who seek the causes of clefts than to those who try to determine the incidence of these anomalies.

However, when he must provide information, what can the specialist report as the incidence of prepalatal and palatal clefts? Although he may need to qualify his statement in several ways, he can say, with some confidence, that one in approximately each 800 children born will have a cleft of the prepalate, the palate, or both. He may wish to modify that figure if he is speaking of special groups, stating that the incidence of congenital oral clefts is lower in some races than in others, that more boys than girls will have clefts, that girls will more often than boys present clefts of the palate. He may need to qualify his response in terms of the geographical location, the procedures used in determining incidence, the number of cases on which the figures are based, and the considerations made of locations of the clefts. His reply may be further influenced by his own findings or by those of a group with which he is associated. He will probably wish to add that improved methods of locating children and adults with these defects may increase the apparent incidence or that the number of babies born with these anomalies seems to be increasing. He may also conclude that other unknown factors, as well as the results of research on the causes of congenital anomalies, will undoubtedly influence the number of babies born with clefts of the prepalate or the palate during the twenty-first century.

CHAPTER TWO

Development and Function of the Prepalatal and Palatal Areas

UNDERSTANDING OF THE NORMAL GROWTH AND DEVELOPMENT OF STRUCTURES THAT WILL MAKE UP THE FACIAL AREA IS IMPORTANT TO THE SPEECH PATHOLOGIST WHO WILL PARTICIPATE IN THE MANAGEMENT OF THE CHILD WITH A CONGENITAL FACIAL ANOMALY AND ASSOCIATED DISORDERS OF COMMUNICATION.

The stages of embryonic and fetal development have been studied in detail by embryologists; and these specialists have provided descriptions of the series of prenatal events, examined certain aspects of normal embryos and fetuses, and sought evidence about developmental failures that result in abortions or congenital physical abnormalities.

Specialists who are not embryologists are often concerned with the facial areas, needing information about the period of prenatal development during which the head, face, lips, mouth, palate, and pharynx emerge. Speech pathologists, for example, should keep in mind certain concepts that will help them to understand the relationships between the structures for speech and those that develop concurrently with them, before and after birth. The considerations made by the speech pathologist may be practical, general, and specific.

If texts and articles on embryology are to be helpful to the speech pathologist, certain practical matters may need attention. The embryologist, like any other specialist, makes various approaches to his subject, reports size in terms that have special significance for him, and uses vocabulary that may not be entirely familiar to specialists from other fields.

Some texts on embryology approach the subject by using the development of each of the structures as their pattern of organization; others arrange their discussions in chronological order. Some describe the changes in the embryo in terms of its age; others relate changes to size. Some concentrate on the embryonic period; others cover both the embryonic and fetal stages. The complexity of the material and the simultaneity of many events make organization of such texts difficult, and some authors in the field of embryology combine a review of the general sequence of development with detailed discussions of the emergence of the various organs of the body. All use many drawings, diagrams, and photographs to supplement their texts; these illustrations can be very useful to the reader who views them with understanding of the relative size of the actual structure and the pictorial representation of it (Jordan and Kindred, 1942; Morris, 1953; Patten, 1953; Orban, 1957; Blechschmidt, 1961; Patten, in Pruzansky, 1961; Hamilton and others, 1962; Davies, 1963; Langman, 1963; Williams and others, 1966; Thomas, 1968; others).

The growth of the embryo and fetus, as reported by the embryologist, is often considered in terms of size. Pictures and diagrams, if they are to be clear, must enlarge and magnify the embryo and its parts. The inexperienced reader needs to note indications of magnification and to relate figures reporting size to measurements with which he is familiar if he does not know the metric system well. To facilitate such comparisons, Figure 2-1 shows the millimeter (0.03937 inch), the centimeter (10 millimeters), and the inch. In metric terms, 25.4 millimeters or 2.54 centimeters make up 1 inch.

For example, the first evidences of labial, palatal, and pharyngeal structures can often be detected in a normal embryo that is 7 to 8 millimeters in crown-rump length. This means that, in a line that represents the ultimate

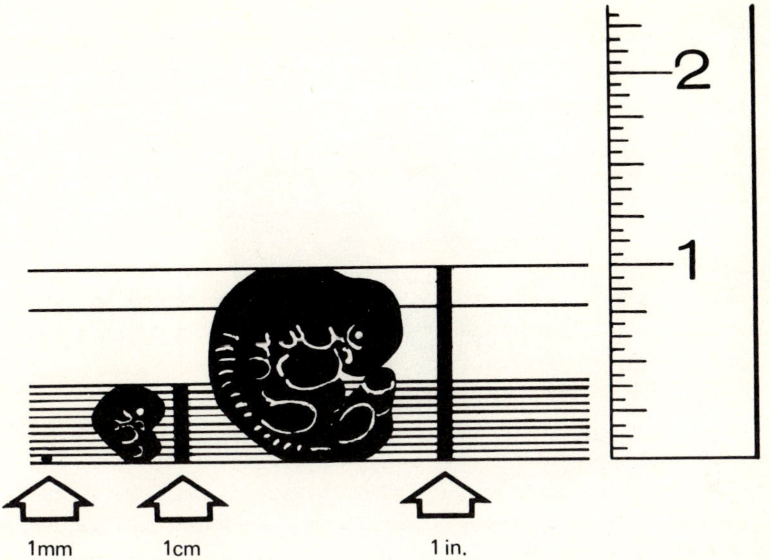

FIGURE 2-1 Comparison of millimeter, centimeter, and inch.

"sitting height," the embryo is less than ⅓ inch in length, 8 millimeters being 0.31496 inch. When an embryo of this size or smaller is enlarged in a drawing or photograph, as it must be for clarity, the reader must make some adjustments in his viewing; or he may be misled about the actual size of the embryo at that stage. In Figure 2-2, an embryo of 5 millimeters in crown-rump length is shown in its actual size and enlarged ten times to permit indication of the emerging structures of the total body.

Sometimes, in the earliest stages, the size of the embryo is reported in terms of the number of somites, or tiny masses of mesodermal cells, that appear along the neural tube. Until the embryo reaches a crown-rump length that can be measured with accuracy—at least 2 to 4 millimeters—the number of somites indicates its general size. Later, when the limbs have developed and the fetus has become more erect, the report of the crown-rump length (or sitting height) is supplemented with that of the crown-heel length (or standing height); and greater lengths are often reported in centimeters rather than in millimeters.

Another practical concern for the reader who is making the acquaintance of embryology but is not a specialist in that field is the matter of vocabulary. Some texts in embryology provide glossaries, and some explain terms when

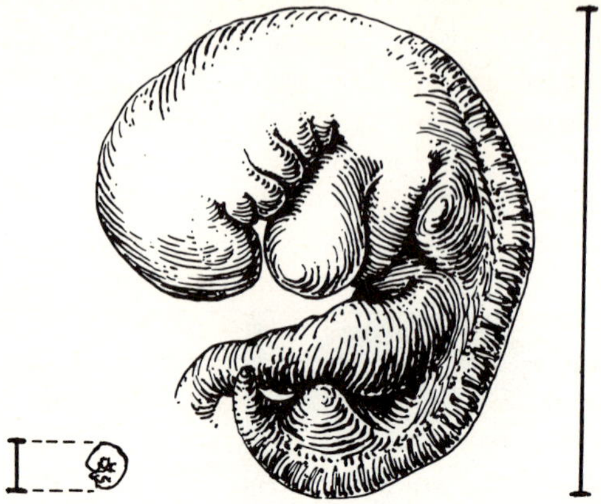

FIGURE 2-2 Embryo of 5 millimeters in crown-rump length, in actual size, and enlarged ten times.

they are first used. However, a basic vocabulary might well include some terms that are used to name the materials that make up the developing body, some that indicate procedures and results of development, and some that are used to indicate specific areas or places. These, together with more general terms, can assist the speech pathologist or audiologist who wishes to read texts or articles on embryology.

In the process of fertilization, germ cells from the parents unite; and the first material for the new organism is formed. Germ cells contain chromosomes, so named because they show as "colored bodies" when the cell is stained, that transmit the characteristics of the parents through the genes and determine the sex of the child.

As the cells in the fertilized ovum divide and increase in number, they become differentiated to perform certain functions. Three temporary layers of tissue form the beginnings of the structures of the body. These tissue layers are the ectoderm, or "outer skin," the mesoderm, or "middle skin," and the entoderm (sometimes endoderm), or "inner skin." The names of these three layers do not indicate their ultimate location, nor do the structures that eventually result from them necessarily correspond to the first positions of the layers. The ectodermal layer gives rise to the central nervous system, the peripheral nervous system, the epidermis and such related parts as the hair and nails and subcutaneous glands, the hypophysis or pituitary gland, the enamel organs of the teeth, and the epithelial lining (or covering layer) of a number of organs. The entodermal layer eventually becomes the epithelial lining of most of the respiratory tract, the tympanic cavity and Eustachian tube, most of the bladder and urethra, and the functional elements (parenchyma) of the thyroid, parathyroids, liver, and pancreas.

The mesodermal layer, which is of special interest to those who study the causal factors of clefts of the prepalate, gives rise to the important cardiovascular system; to connective tissue, cartilage, bone, joints, and skeletal muscles; to blood and lymph cells; to the walls of the heart and the blood and lymph vessels; and to the serous membranes, the kidneys and gonads, the spleen, and part of the suprarenal gland. The mesoderm is related to part of the early connective tissue, the mesenchyme, and also contributes to the earliest form of the embryo by making up the somites that appear as blocks of tissue along either side of the neural tube during the first month of embryonic life. The increase in amount of tissue that goes on through multiplication of cells during the prenatal period causes the mesoderm to expand and fill the spaces between the ectodermal and entodermal layers. These layers increase in area to maintain a cover for the mesoderm as it enlarges and becomes varied in shape. Ultimately, the three layers with which the body started become differentiated to form specific organs and tissues, bones and muscles, and nerves and glands, with epithelial coverings (the epidermis) and linings (the endothelial and mesothelial tissues or mucous membranes) outside and inside.

As the process of embryonic and fetal development takes place, the proliferation of the basic cells produces changes that, in turn, result in growth in many directions. The first hint of the parts that will eventually result from the growth is called a primordium or an anlage, which means "a laying on"; and subsequent growth results in modifications of shape that are variously named. Some of the names are self-explanatory—arch, bar, bud, cavity, fin, fold, groove, hillock, pit, pouch, pocket, plate, swelling, and wall. Others are perhaps less familiar—diverticulum, a pouch or pocket leading from a main cavity; duct, a tube or passage; foramen, a perforation; infundibulum, a funnel-shaped passage; lamina, a thin, flat plate; matrix, a mold in which something takes form or develops; pearl, a rounded mass of epithelial cells; process, a projection; prominence, another term for projection; raphe, a ridge or furrow at the line of union of two symmetrical parts; sinus, a hollow space; and sulcus, a groove or furrow.

Several of the primordial ("beginning") regions are of special interest to the speech pathologist or audiologist who traces the development of the facial area. Among these are the forebrain, the pericardial bulge, the stomodeum, and the branchial arches. Some of these emerging structures are shown in Figure 2-3, which includes an enlargement of ten times to permit differentiation and provide some detail. The forebrain, or prosencephalon, one of the three primary brain vesicles, develops into the cerebral hemispheres, the striate bodies, and the olfactory lobes. The forebrain occupies most of the head fold, which overhangs the pericardial bulge, in which the heart is developing; and, in the space between the head fold and the pericardium, the primitive mouth area, the stomodeum, appears. In the lateral areas of the head fold and the pericardial swelling, five arches begin to emerge in the pharyngeal area during the latter part of the first month of embryonic life. They eventually become the bones of the middle ear, the hyoid bone, and the cartilages of the larynx; and ventral expansions of the first arches,

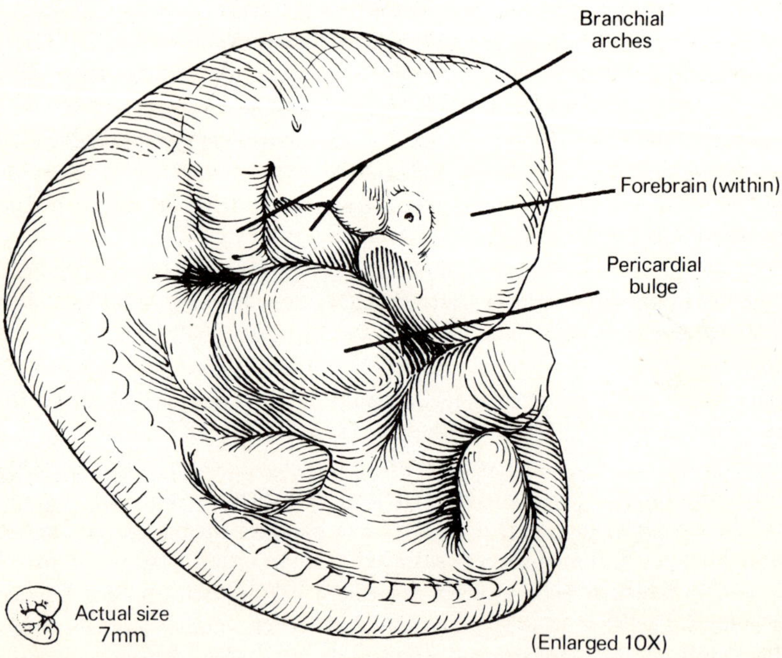

FIGURE 2-3 Embryo of 7 millimeters in crown-rump length, in actual size, and enlarged ten times to show emerging parts.

enlarged by mesoderm, form the paired swellings that increase to make up the bulk of the tongue.

The processes of growth during embryonic and fetal development are sometimes referred to as aggregation, massing together of materials; coalescence, fusion or blending of parts; chondrogenesis, formation of cartilage; differentiation, acquisition of distinguishing characteristics; formation, assuming a shape; fusion, "melting together" of parts; invagination, insertion or sheathing of one portion within another; migration, changing place; osteogenesis, formation of bone; penetration, entering deeply; and proliferation ("to bear offspring"), reproduction or multiplication of cells.

Armed with some practical concepts and some basic terminology, the speech pathologist or audiologist may review normal embryological development in order to have a better understanding of the abnormalities called clefts. In so doing, he needs to be aware of some general concepts that may help him as he studies the development of the facial area.

First, this development takes place in both the embryonic and the fetal stages of prenatal growth. In the early stages, the growing organism is called an embryo ("to grow from within"), although the first three weeks of the gestation period are sometimes termed the preembryonic stage. When the organism reaches the age of twenty-one days *in utero,* according to some (Williams and others, 1966), it enters the embryonic stage. One writer (Langman, 1963) considered the fourth to eighth weeks of development the embryonic period. Another (Davies, 1963) used the term "embryo" to indicate an age of twenty-one to twenty-three days, a size of 1.5 to 2.0 millimeters, and the presence of four to twelve paired somites.

However, Jack Davies pointed out that no definite point of transition from embryo to fetus can be stipulated, adding,

> The embryonic period is obviously one in which the essential external and internal structures characteristic of the adult are formed. In the present scheme this may be said to be achieved in embryos of about *30 mm* and at about the *seventh week of development.* The fetal period is characterized by the growth and elaboration of existing structures and, with possibly a few exceptions, by the formation of no new ones. [P. 43]*

James Blake Thomas (1968), in his chronological consideration of embryology, indicated the seventh week of development as the final stage of the embryonal period. He pointed out that, by the end of the seventh week, "differentiation and establishment of organs and organ systems are essentially

* Jack Davies, *Human Developmental Anatomy.* Copyright © 1963, The Ronald Press Company, New York.

complete with the remainder of prenatal development being concerned primarily with growth and physiological maturation" (p. 200). The embryo, at this stage, is still very small, having a crown-rump measurement of no more than 30 millimeters (1.18 inches) and weighing between 2 and 3 grams (about one-tenth of an ounce). In Figure 2-4, the actual size of the embryo at the beginning of the fetal period is contrasted with an enlargement that shows the structures that have become essentially complete.

Although P. L. Williams and his coauthors (1966) used the presence of somites as an indication of the beginning of the embryonic phase at the start of the fourth week, they stated that this stage lasted until the

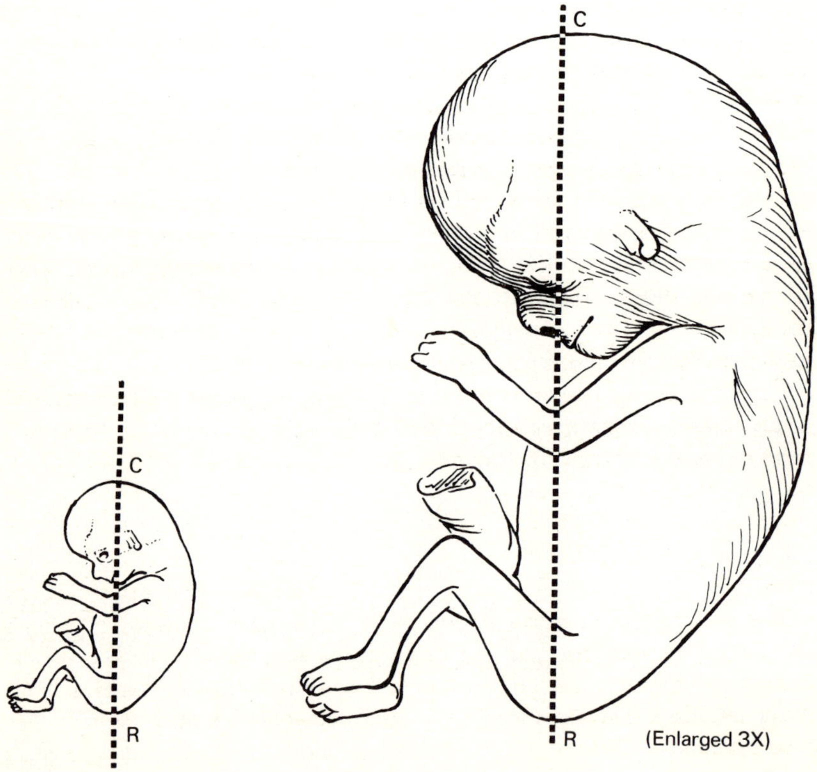

FIGURE 2-4 Embryo of 30 millimeters in crown-rump length, in actual size, and enlarged three times.

end of the eighth week and that the fetal stage was from eight weeks until term (the conclusion of the pregnancy, at which time delivery is expected); and many embryologists agree with this categorization by age. Some of the areas in the prepalate and palate, although formed by the end of the embryonic period, continue their development into the fetal stage; the special developmental steps for the prepalatal and palatal areas are described later in this chapter.

Another general point for the speech pathologist and audiologist to keep in mind is that the development of the human palate occurs as part of a complex process in which many events take place simultaneously. In presenting the rationale for his scheme of developmental horizons in human prenatal development, George L. Streeter (1942) said that he used the term "horizons" to emphasize the importance of thinking of the embryo as a living organism "which in its time takes on many guises, always progressing from the smaller and simpler to the larger and more complex" (p. 214). This progress includes all of the body and its various parts and appendages, with the emergence of many structures and systems during each stage or horizon. The concurrence of development of the many parts is difficult to describe, but some texts—that by E. Blechschmidt (1961), for example—show, through photographs and schematic representations, the various systems of the body at each of the stages of development. While concentrating his attention on the emergence of the lips, mouth, auditory mechanism, and pharynx, the speech pathologist or audiologist should not forget that those structures develop at the same time that many others are being formed.

The emphasis given by embryologists to the sequence of embryonic and fetal events, however, suggests that timing, as well as concurrence, is important to normal development in the prenatal period. A critical period for the emergence of the rudiments of future organs of the body is from the fourth to the sixth week; and, during that time, teratogenic agents can affect the developing structures. Jan Langman (1963) stressed the fact that most teratogenic agents are highly effective and produce numerous malformations during the phase of intensive differentiation. Each organ seems to go through its most susceptible stage early in its differentiation, the various body organs becoming susceptible one after another. When the embryo becomes a fetus, when differentiation gives way to growth, teratogenic agents seem to lose their effect.

The specialists interested in disorders of communication should recognize, additionally, that, even if the embryo becomes a fetus and the fetus comes to term and the newborn child is structurally normal, the baby is not a

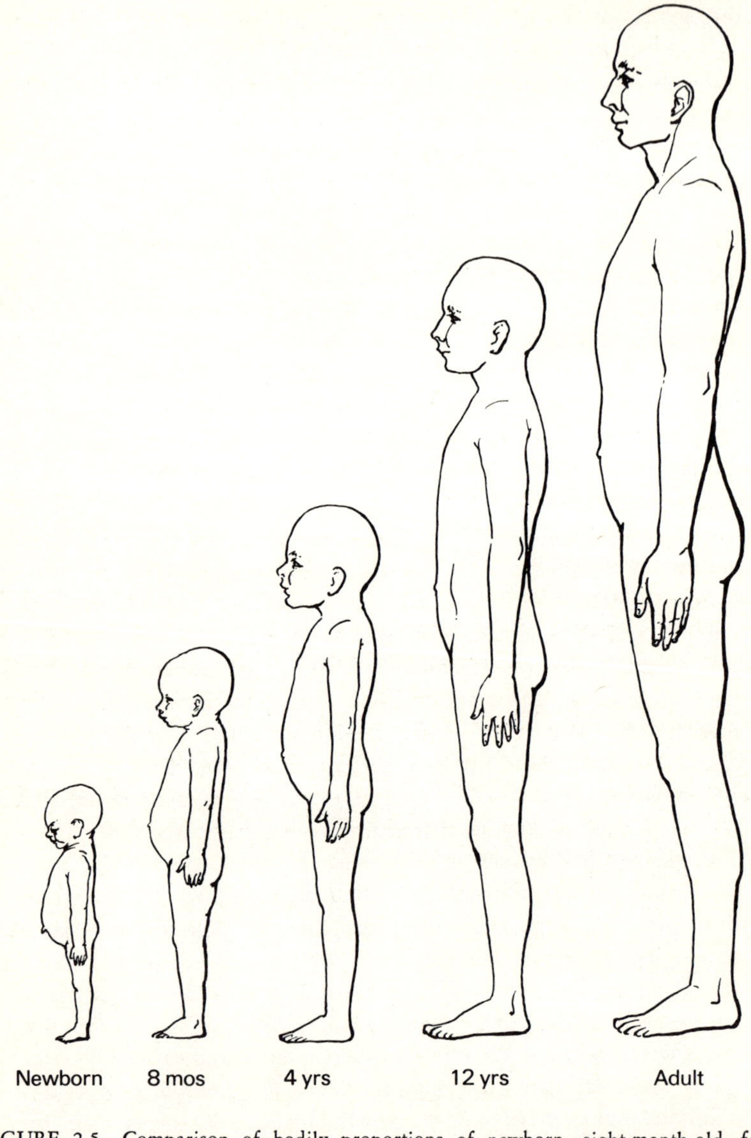

FIGURE 2-5 Comparison of bodily proportions of newborn, eight-month-old, four-year-old, twelve-year-old, and adult (*after Scammon, in Schaeffer, 1942*).

miniature replica of the adult. His head is proportionately much larger than it will be when he is grown, and his legs are short in comparison with the total length of his trunk. Figure 2-5 illustrates these differences in proportion.

The various tissues of the body, in postnatal life, will follow individual growth patterns that differ in rate, instead of following essentially the same pattern, as they did during fetal life. Many changes occur postnatally in the facial area, as the structures modify in both size and shape, as the stages of dentition occur, as the muscular influences of the masticatory facial skeleton show themselves, as the tissues grow, as the nose assumes its adult size and shape. Profiles of the adult and the child, shown in Figure 2-6, present some of the external differences that are accompanied by internal differences in size and shape and that change as the neonate becomes, progressively, the infant, the child, the adolescent, and the adult.

Although the structural principle of the adult, as Blechschmidt (1961) pointed out, may be evident in the first few weeks of intrauterine life, changes that occur in the normal facial area following birth are important in any study of congenital abnormalities of that area. James F. Bosma and Samuel G. Fletcher (1961–1962), in their review of the upper pharynx, traced the development of that area, saying that it enlarges in size, becomes progressively more mobile, modifies its spatial relationships to its extrinsic musculature, and changes the direction of its action during postnatal maturation. Other studies of normal pharyngeal size and function (J. Daniel Subtelny, 1955; Mazaheri, Nanda, and Sassouni, 1967) also have described the alterations that occur following birth. Modifications in dental structures have been traced in texts and articles from the dental profession (Graber, 1968; Savara and Singh, 1968; Scott, 1968; others); and Donald H. Enlow

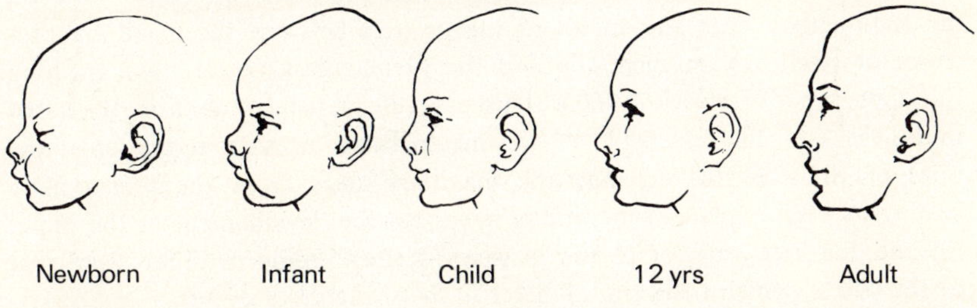

FIGURE 2-6 Comparison of profiles of newborn, infant, child, twelve-year-old, and adult (*after Scammon, in Schaeffer, 1942*).

(1968) stressed the fact that the entire face "undergoes progressive changes in which its configuration, proportions, and dimensions become markedly altered" after birth (p. 227).

Speech pathologists and audiologists may give specific consideration to the normal prenatal development of those parts of the body that are most responsible for the activities that result in oral communication. Those who are concerned with habilitation for persons born with prepalatal and palatal clefts may have special interest in the embryonic and fetal development of the facial area. They may be better able to understand the anomalies of that region and to explain them to others if they have some information about the way in which these structures come to normal completion.

Whether the term "process," as used by Wilhelm His (1880), a pioneer in embryology, is preferable to Streeter's terms, "swellings" or "ridges," the growth centers from which the face is derived can be discerned early in embryonic life. Around the stomodeum, the proliferation of ectoderm, mesoderm, and endoderm results in the formation of the frontonasal process, the mandibular process, the maxillary processes, the nasal pits, and a bilateral swelling called the globular process. Some of these rudimentary structures can be identified when the embryo is no more than 2 millimeters in length (approximately 0.08 inch), at about the same time that the heart begins to beat, between twenty-one and twenty-three days of embryonic life. Toward the end of the fifth week, the premaxillary, maxillary, and mandibular growth centers can be seen, although they must be enlarged for such an illustration as Figure 2-7. Increase in the size of the maxillary and mandibular areas narrows the mouth slit and widens the head, brings the eyes toward their ultimate position in the face, and causes the nasal folds to become more prominent.

Additional growth during the sixth and seventh weeks brings about the joining of the maxillary process with the lateral nasal processes to form the rudimentary nose and to fill in the grooves between the maxillary processes or swellings on each side and the premaxillary center, thus forming the upper lip (Warbrick, 1960). This point in prenatal growth is illustrated in Figure 2-8. The extension of the mesenchyme, or mesoderm, across the lines of division that separate the maxillary areas from the premaxillary center has been explained in various ways; but the development of the upper lip and the area anterior to the incisive foramen seems to differ from that of the palate, which fuses slightly later in the sequence of events.

Some writers (Chase, 1942; Davies, 1963; Fraser, 1967; Williams and others, 1966) used the term "fusion" to describe the joining of the maxillary and premaxillary areas; others (Langman, 1963; Patten, in Pruzansky, 1961)

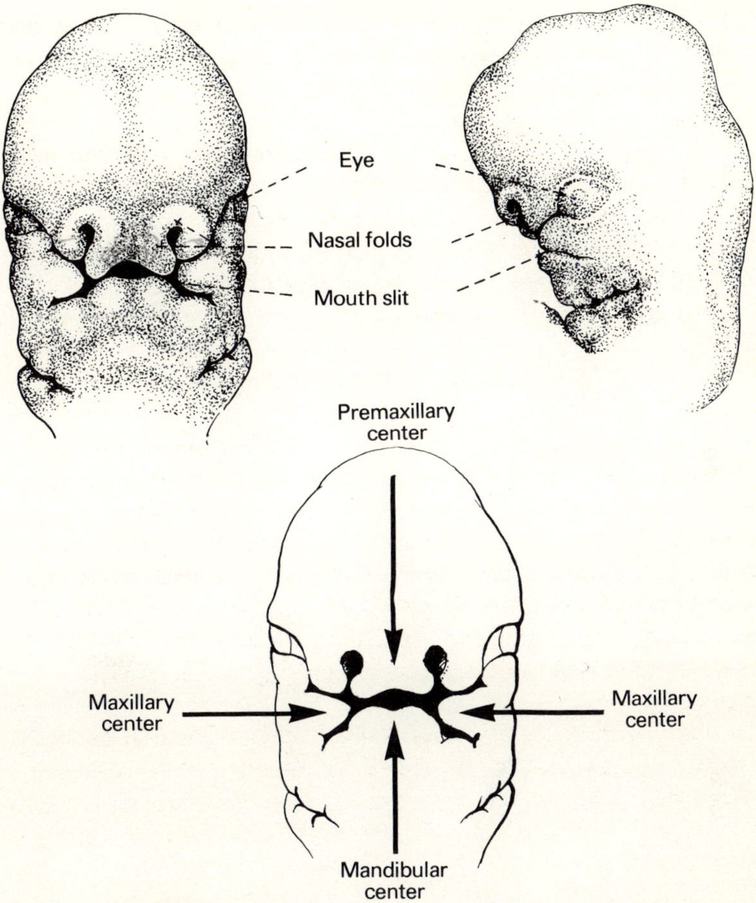

FIGURE 2-7 Premaxillary, maxillary, and mandibular centers and directions of growth in embryo of 12 to 14 millimeters, enlarged approximately twenty times (*after Patten, in Schaeffer, 1942*).

spoke of "merging" when they traced the development of the upper lip and the area sometimes called the premaxillary triangle. These differences in terminology may not express extreme differences of opinion, but the change from three parts—the two maxillary swellings and the premaxillary area—to one part—the intact upper lip—has been variously described and can be seen in Figures 2-7, 2-8, and 2-9.

M. Leon Canick (1954), discussing two schools of thought about the

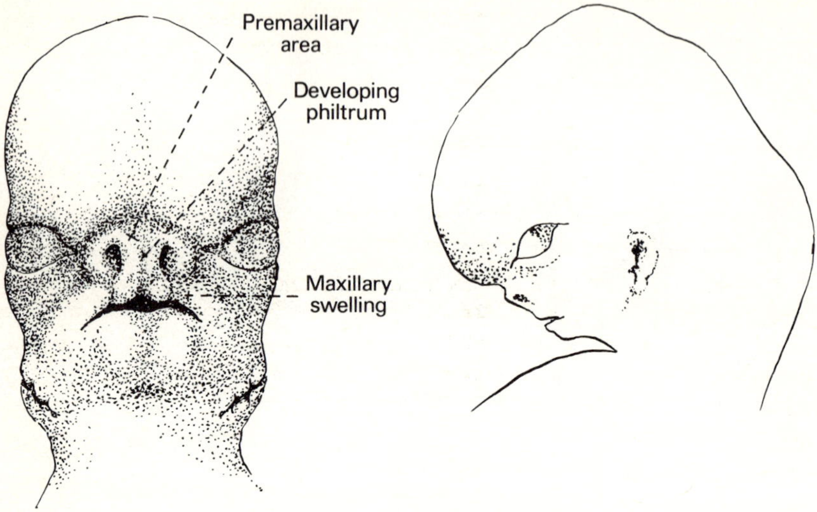

FIGURE 2-8 Formation of upper lip in embryo of 19 millimeters, enlarged approximately ten times (*after Patten, in Schaeffer, 1942*).

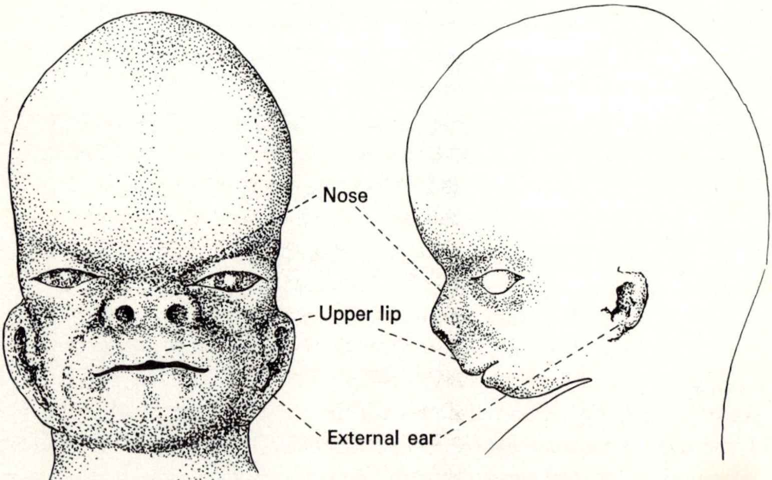

FIGURE 2-9 Upper lip in embryo of 27 to 30 millimeters, enlarged approximately ten times (*after Patten, in Schaeffer, 1942*).

development of the upper lip and the prepalate, cited the classic theory, which held that five major processes develop about the rim of the primitive oral cavity, grow together, and fuse to form the normal face; but he also pointed out that this point of view had been questioned by Victor Veau and others who believed that ectodermal tissues adjacent to the primitive nostrils are invaded by mesoderm from the edges of the oral cavity to form the upper lip, teeth, alveolus, and other parts in that area. Another comparison of points of view about the prenatal interrelationships between the maxillae and premaxilla was made by Bertram Kraus and Jay Decker in 1960. One concept, the fusion theory, they said, was that the premaxilla and the two maxillae unite by fusion at the ectofacial surface during the sixth to ninth weeks of embryonic life; the other, the overlap theory, was that the premaxilla is completely covered by prolongations of the frontal process of the maxillae between twelve and thirteen weeks of fetal life. These several explanations of the development of the normal upper lip were accepted until almost the middle of the twentieth century.

In 1936, Veau and Georges Politzer, setting the stage for subsequent work by Richard Stark and others, reported their findings from studies of 147 embryos in laboratories in Paris and Vienna. Veau had noted that the classic idea of fusion or coalescence did not agree with his clinical observations; and, although he respected the work done by zoologists, he felt that explanations of human development could not be based on studies of animals. Hence, he and Politzer described the successive stages of development in the primary palate of the normal human fetus, attributing the completion of the primary palate, or prepalate, to the extension of mesoderm through the epithelial wall that existed in an earlier stage. Stark's investigation (1954; Stark and Ehrmann, 1958), although it was concerned with embryos that showed clefts, supported this point of view. The studies of Veau, Politzer, Stark, Gian Töndury (in Pruzansky, 1961), and others have led some writers to use terms other than "fusion" or to point out that the classic theory has been questioned. These theories will be presented in more detail in Chapter Three, in their application to defective development. Regardless of the exact process, the upper lip and the other parts of the maxillary and premaxillary areas probably become complete in the normal embryo by the seventh week, toward the end of the embryonic period, before the embryo has reached a crown-rump length of 1 inch.

At first, the upper lip is smooth; but, later, a depression occurs in the center of the lip, underneath the columella of the nose, with a ridge on either side. This central depression, called the philtrum (Ivy, 1967), has been attributed to the persistence of the grooves between the globular elements of the frontonasal processes and to the heaping up of maxillary mesoderm on either side of the middle line; but some have maintained that the philtrum does not appear until several weeks after the upper lip is formed and all traces of the individual processes have disappeared (Monie and Cacciatore, 1962). In association with an increasing density of connective tissue in the median portion of the upper lip, the philtrum is usually apparent in the third or fourth month of fetal life. In Figure 2-10, the philtral ridges can be seen; the development of the philtrum is illustrated in Figures 2-7, 2-8, and 2-9.

In a process that is concurrent with the development of the upper lip, the vestibule of the mouth and the primary dental lamina in both jaws begin to form during the sixth week. By the end of the fourth month, the sulci that separate the lips from the alveolar ridges of the jaws have deepened, with only two attachments of tissue—the upper and lower labial frenula—remaining. The structures that will eventually be the teeth come from the posterior dental lamina; and, after changes in the fourth month,

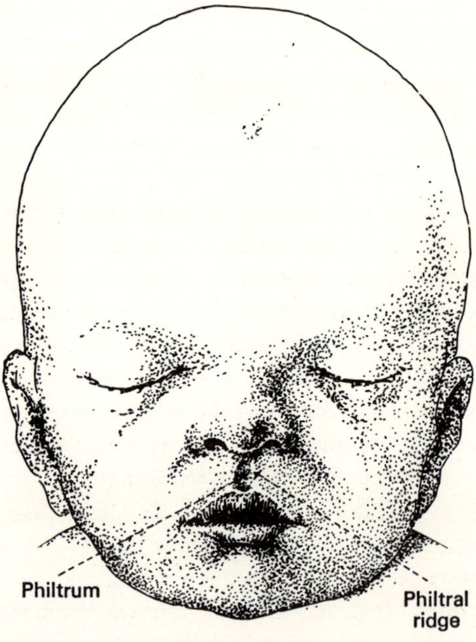

FIGURE 2-10 Development of philtral ridges in fetus of three to four months.

the enamel organs of the teeth are formed. At birth, the buds of the twenty deciduous teeth, the milk teeth, are present, with the germs of the permanent teeth and the rudiments of four additional second teeth, the permanent first molars, also being present.

The upper lip, the conjoined maxillae and premaxilla, and the alveolar areas as far posterior as the incisive foramen form the prepalate as the term is used here. This area is usually complete, in the normally developing organism, before the transition from embryo to fetus. However, the palatal area, although it starts its development during the embryonic period, probably does not complete it until almost the end of the twelfth week, the conclusion of the first trimester of pregnancy.

The way in which the normal palate develops and fuses is not often disputed. The palatal shelves of the maxilla appear in the thirty-five-day embryo; but they remain in an almost vertical plane, protruding downward into the spaces (the paralingual sulci) at the sides of the developing tongue for several weeks. The position of the shelves in the paralingual sulci is shown in Figure 2-11.

As the tongue moves away from the nasal septum and shifts downward, the palatal shelves move upward until they lie in a horizontal plane. According to a recent investigation (Humphrey, 1969), mouth-opening reflexes in the fetus draw the tongue from between the palatal shelves as a result of mandibular depression; and differences in pressure between the closed nasal area and the oral region when the tongue is withdrawn create an upward pull on the palatal shelves. At about the ninth week, now in the fetal period, the palatine processes move together and fuse at the midline with each other and with the front part of the nasal septum that lies above them (Kraus, 1960; Ewers, 1968; Moss and others, 1968). The closure of the gap between the shelves probably proceeds from front to back, as shown in Figure 2-12, the bony part of the palate fusing first and the soft tissues growing together last, all the way to the projecting uvula. However, some writers have suggested that palatal fusion begins near the midpoint and spreads both anteriorly and posteriorly (Fischel, in Wood and Kraus, 1962) or follows a pattern in which closure starts near the anterior end and proceeds to the middle half of the palate and then to the anterior fourth and the posterior fourth (Hochstetter, in Fulton, 1957).

This process of closure, shown by line drawings and some photographs in many texts, was studied in detail by Kraus, Hironori Kitamura, and Ralph A. Latham (1966). By means of sections (thin slices) taken through the heads of forty-seven normal embryos and fetuses, they showed the stages

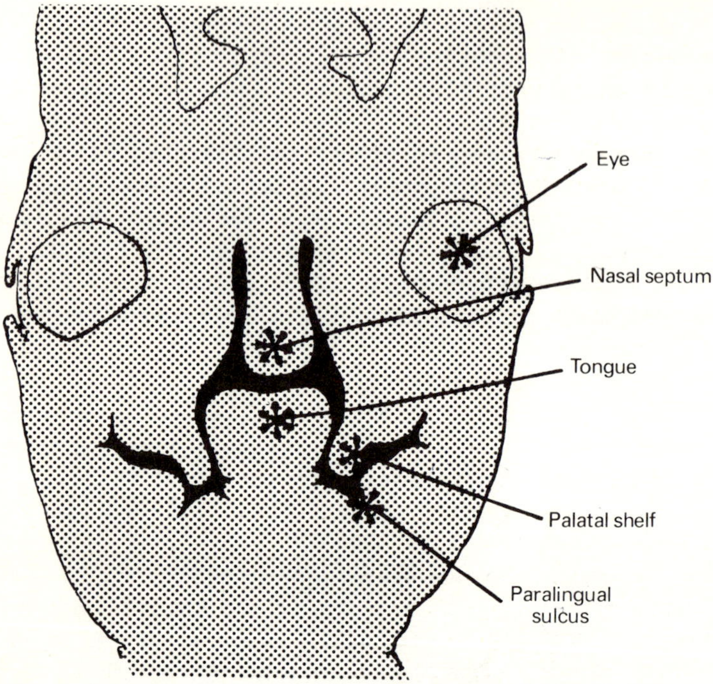

FIGURE 2-11 Positions of palatal shelves in paralingual sulci in embryo of forty-five days, enlarged fifteen times (*after Kraus, Kitamura, and Latham, 1966*).

of development of the palate from thirty-five days to birth; and the positional changes and ultimate fusion of the palatal shelves were illustrated in their *Atlas of Developmental Anatomy of the Face.* The photographs showed that, if the progressive fusion of the palatal shelves proceeds normally, the division between the oral and nasal cavities is complete by the twelfth week, when the fetus has reached a crown-heel (standing) length of approximately 7 centimeters (2.75 inches). Observations of other human embryos at various stages from seven to twelve weeks of prenatal age confirmed the sequence of closure of the palate from front to back but suggested that the soft palate develops by means of mesenchymal merging rather than by epithelial fusion of the entire palatal process (Burdi and Faist, 1967).

Kitamura (1966) provided a description of the normal development of the palate, showing, in tabular form and in drawings, the typical chronology of this development from thirty-three to sixty days of "ovulation age," with crown-rump lengths from 8 to 47 millimeters. By the thirty-fifth day, according to his schedule, the primordial palatal shelves begin to form a processlike projection; and, in the succeeding six days, "remarkable development of the palatal shelf occurs" (p. 242). By the forty-seventh day, the palatal shelves, vertically located at first, elevate to a horizontal position and fuse in the area of the hard palate. During the seventh week, fusion is completed; and mesenchymal penetration starts. By the sixtieth day, mesenchymal penetration is complete.

The bony palate continues its growth throughout the remaining prenatal months, increasing in width at a greater rate than in length. At birth, there-

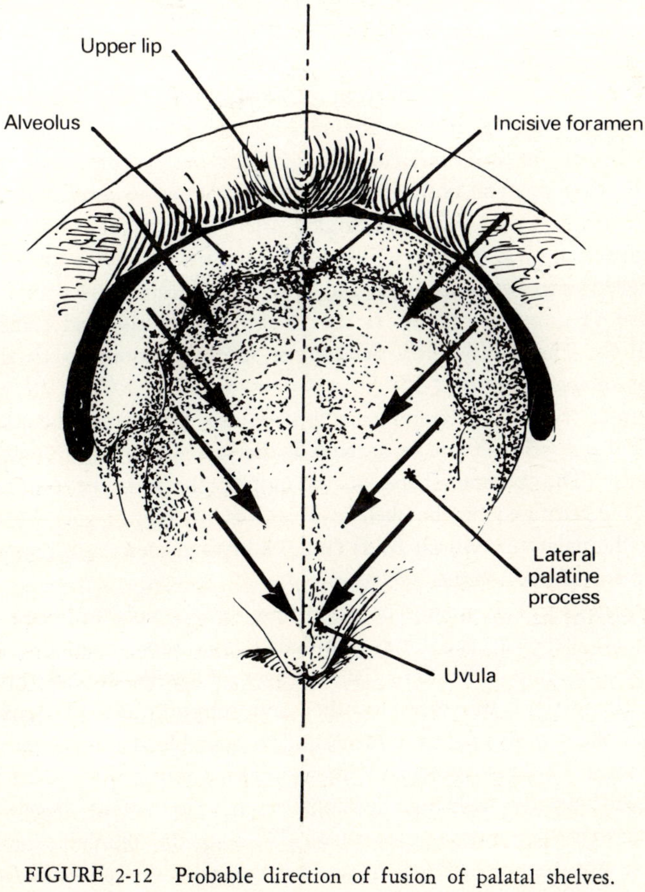

FIGURE 2-12 Probable direction of fusion of palatal shelves.

fore, the palate is broad; but the growth activity continues because of appositional growth at the tuberosities until, in the adult, palatal length is greater than palatal width (Ewers, 1968).

Other processes, accompanying the growth of the prepalate and palate, result in the development of additional structures that are of interest to the speech pathologist and audiologist—the jaws, the ears, the tongue, and the pharynx. These are derived directly or indirectly from the pharyngeal arches that can be seen very early in embryonic life and that enlarge and modify to form the larynx and ear, the hyoid bone, and the maxilla and mandible. In the first of these pharyngeal arches, called the mandibular arch, the formation of cartilage and the change of cartilage to bone result in the malleus and incus. The stapes is formed from part of the second pharyngeal arch, and the hyoid bone and the cartilages of the larynx are formed from this and the other pharyngeal arches.

From the floor of the embryonic pharynx, where the portions of the first pharyngeal arches nearest the midline come together, two swellings emerge, increase in size, and fuse to form the major portion of the front part of the tongue. The posterior third of the tongue is derived from mesodermal increase in the third pharyngeal arch. The tongue lies high in the mouth cavity at first and is in close approximation to, if not in contact with, the down-growing nasal septum. The tongue then moves, or is pulled, downward (Humphrey, 1969) as the palatal shelves rise and come toward the midline. The position of the tongue in its relationship to the nasal septum is shown in Figure 2-11.

The anterior and posterior faucial pillars also come from the pharyngeal arches, and the palatine tonsils develop at the location of the second pharyngeal pouch. The general shape of the upper pharynx, the oropharyngeal region, is determined by the skeletal aspects of the fetus; and the development of the palatopharyngeal folds from embryonal mesoderm resembles the development of the tongue.

The tissues formed in embryonic and fetal development and present in the normal body are of several kinds—epithelial, connective, muscular, and nervous. These develop and differentiate to cover or line the surfaces or cavities, to bind the various structures together and support them, to move them, to provide the stimulus for movement, and to carry blood and lymph throughout the body. The development of these tissues goes on during the prenatal period, concurrently with the development of the various clearly defined structures that they compose or serve. Without the muscular or nervous tissue, the lips, tongue, soft palate, and pharyngeal walls could not be moved by the infant or the adult; and the organs used for the production, direction, resonation, and modification of the airstream from the lungs and larynx could not perform their functions adequately.

The speech pathologist and audiologist, in their concern for information on the normal development of the prepalate and palate in the human, should not lose sight of the extensive amount of research on prenatal development in animals that has served as a preface and a supplement to studies of human embryology. In the past, embryologists studied many types of animals, large and small, similar to humans and different from them, in their attempts to determine the complex sequence of events during the prenatal period. Reports from such research are extensive. Reports from investigations of human embryos and fetuses are more recent; and, even today, some of the information on human development is postulated on studies of animals. Some texts on embryology, in fact, refer to specific embryos in certain collections in a manner that suggests that studies of the human embryo have been restricted by the limited number of specimens obtainable. Streeter (1942) commented that His and his contemporaries were limited by "scarce and poor material"; and Streeter's own descriptions were drawn from a study of thirty-eight embryos, some collected as early as 1893. Veau and Politzer (1936) felt that the 147 embryos they examined represented an unusually large number of specimens, and Stark's (1954) elaboration of the Veau and Politzer study reported findings from six human fetal specimens with clefts. However, recent accumulations of specimens in modern research centers provided a total of 25,000 aborted fetuses and embryos gathered during twelve years by 250 hospitals, from which Kraus and his colleagues drew the thirty-five cleft and and forty-seven noncleft heads they used in their 1966 study.

As additional research, facilitated by constantly improving techniques and tools, can be undertaken with increasing numbers of human specimens, the information about prenatal development will increase; and the speech pathologist and audiologist will need to be alert to new theories and new findings on the formation of the prepalate and palate, a development that requires "the delicate integration of many processes" and that involves "synchronized interactions of shelf, tongue, jaw, and head" (Fraser, 1967, pp. 1603, 1606,; 1968, pp. 189, 194).

In attempting to illustrate prenatal growth, some writers of texts on embryology have presented, diagrammatically, in actual size, the developmental levels of the human embryo from fertilization to eight or nine weeks (Arey, 1965; Williams and others, 1966). A tiny dot has been used to represent the ovum, from which the human develops; and the progressive growth, differentiation, and specialization of the structures of the human body can be appreciated when the newborn infant is compared with that dot. Then, when the adult, with all of his mature capacities, is contrasted to the neonate, the complexities of human structures and functions become all the more apparent. Complete understanding of these structures and of their functions is not possible, but some comprehension of the processes that produce normal human beings is important to the study of deviations from normal.

MOST CHILDREN BORN WITH NORMALLY DEVELOPED STRUCTURES WILL ACQUIRE SKILL IN USING THE VARIOUS PARTS OF THE BODY IN THE COMPLICATED PROCESS OF SPEECH.

From the outset, the tongue and the lips are used in the process of nursing and eating. An intact hard palate provides a firm surface against which the infant can press the nipple, and the normal division between the oral cavity and the nasal cavities helps to direct the milk and the food properly as the lateral and posterior pharyngeal walls participate with the tongue and palate in the process of swallowing.

With the development of language, the laryngeal structures used for crying, gurgling, babbling, and other expressive activities produce and modify the vocal tone or permit the stream of air to pass through the larynx without causing audible vibrations. Each part of the total muscular activity that results in spoken language, from respiration to phonation to resonation and articulation, requires fine coordination and control of structures with which the speech pathologist is familiar. The normal activities of the muscles of inhalation and exhalation, of the larynx and tongue, and of the face and lips, with the innervation for these actions, have been described in general and in detail in many texts and articles. The structures and the functions of the velopharyngeal valving mechanism, similarly, have been studied extensively.

RESEARCH WORKERS FROM VARIOUS FIELDS HAVE REPORTED ON THE SIZE OF THE VARIOUS PARTS OF THE VELOPHARYNGEAL VALVING MECHANISM AND ON THE MUSCULATURE OF NORMAL VELOPHARYNGEAL CLOSURE.

Some reports have described the pharyngeal area in detail (Bosma and Fletcher, 1961–1962); some have considered the configurations of the pharynx and the ways in which the parts of the upper vocal tract are coupled in normal speech (Huntington, in Spriestersbach and Sherman, 1968). Measurements of the nasopharynx and soft palate by several investigators have provided data that are fairly consistent. The depth of the nasopharynx, for example, was found to be 20, 25, and from 23.5 to 31.8 millimeters in three different studies (Ricketts, 1954; Mazaheri and others, 1964; Yules, Northway, and Chase, 1968). This depth of the pharyngeal airspace seemed to increase with age, at least in the upper and middle pharyngeal portions, until the children in one experimental group reached twelve years (Chierici, 1967). The thickness of the soft palate, which apparently is established by the time a child reaches the age of five, was 6.5 to 13 millimeters, 8.5 millimeters, 8 to 9 millimeters, and 9.5 millimeters in four groups of normal subjects (Ricketts, 1954; J. Daniel Subtelny, 1957; Mazaheri and others, 1964; Yules, Northway, and Chase, 1968). The length of the soft palate was reported as ranging from 31 to 39.5 millimeters and as averaging 27.13 millimeters in two groups of normal subjects (Mazaheri and others, 1964; Yules, Northway, and Chase, 1968). These and other reports have provided information to supplement previous studies of the pharyngeal area by anatomists and physiologists.

Evidence from cineradiographic studies has led some writers to increase the number of muscles usually listed as being responsible for the closure of the pharyngonasal passageway. Although many texts consider the musculature of the palate separately from the musculature of the pharynx, the aggregation of muscles, working in concert, is responsible for the reduction or elimination of the space between the posterior part of the soft palate and the walls of the pharynx. Anteroposterior views of the valving action indicate that the lift-and-retract action of the palate may be supplemented by some movement of the lateral walls of the pharynx toward the midline and even, in some instances, by forward movement of the posterior pharyngeal wall at or near the level of Passavant's pad. The muscular activities that result in the closure of the passageway from the oropharynx to the posterior nasal cavity may vary with individuals; and the amount of closure or opening required for nonnasal or nasal speech sounds may also be an individual matter, with resonance factors from the oral cavity contributing to the presence or absence of "perceived nasality."

In general, and with many individual exceptions, the vowel sounds and most of the consonant sounds of American English reach the open air and the ear of the listener by passing through the oral cavity. The three nasal consonant sounds go through the nasal cavities, although they also require resonance from the oral cavity or the oropharynx to make each different from the others. Velopharyngeal valving for the sounds of American English speech requires the opening as well as the closing of the passageway from the back of the mouth to the nose, although closure occurs more frequently than patency.

Direct observation of the soft palate is sometimes possible when, following surgery, a patient has a wide opening in the lateral wall of the cheek. The movements that can be seen directly may be affected by several factors, such as the disturbance to muscle balance by surgery, the lack of a closed oral cavity, and changes in pressure patterns; however, some descriptions of the action of the soft palate, tongue, and pharynx have been made from these observations. One observer (Bloomer, 1953) commented that the complexity of valve patterning and its variability in the two patients he studied and the differences within each suggest the need for "a much more individualized consideration of muscle structures and actions than has generally been suggested by other observers" (p. 246). Another (Calnan, 1953) reported, from his direct observation, that

> the palate tensed in preparation and then made a tentative half-hearted elevation. As soon as speech started, the palate elevated, the circular ring mechanism contracted, and the mucosa bunched up: this condition was maintained with very slight alteration of the velum, which acted purely as a valve: the tongue, on the other hand, was seen dancing about below and apparently doing all the work. [P. 290]

The sphincteric action of the pharynx and the elevation of the middle third of the velum resulted in closure at a point well above the arch of the atlas and above the level of Passavant's pad, according to this report; and the description of the musculature involved, in spite of the abnormalities of the structures, was in general agreement with descriptions from studies in which direct observation was not possible.

At least five sets of muscles seem to contribute to closure of the passage from the oropharynx to the nasal cavities (Fritzell, 1969b). Each has a special name and a major function. The tensor veli palatini probably depresses the anterior part of the velum. The levator veli palatini, considered to be the most important of the muscles accomplishing velopharyngeal closure in speech, moves the midportion of the soft palate upward and backward. The palatoglossus muscle, sometimes referred to as the glossopalatinus, is the antagonist to the levator. The palatopharyngeus, sometimes called the pharyngopalatinus, pulls the soft palate in a dorsocaudal direction, stretches and adducts the posterior faucial pillars, moves the lateral walls of the upper pharynx in a medial direction, and elevates the pharyngeal walls. The superior constrictor of the pharynx narrows the upper pharynx and may also cause forward bulging of the posterior pharyngeal wall. The stylopharyngeus muscle may contribute to the total of velopharyngeal closure, while the presence of adenoidal tissue may reduce the dimensions of the pharynx at or above the level of the lift-and-bulge. The muscles of the uvula shorten the uvula when they contract, but no information is available on their possible participation in speech.

The muscles that contribute to velopharyngeal closure are set in a kind of circle around the passageway and coordinate in rapid movement to close and open the passage. Summarizing his description of this circular set of muscles, J. Whillis (1930) said:

> It would appear that there is a constant band of muscle fibers passing from the superior constrictor into the palate, and that these fibers are on a level with the ridge of Passavant. It is suggested that they play an important part in shutting off the naso-pharynx, and that the name of palatopharyngeal sphincter should be given to them. [P. 95]

The so-called ring of Whillis includes the muscles that have been named; and the term "sphincter" has been accepted by a number of writers who have discussed velopharyngeal closure since Whillis investigated the musculature of the nasopharynx (Van Gelder, 1965).

> Currently, it is thought that in addition to upward and backward movement of the soft palate, there is also significant medial movement of the lateral walls of the nasopharynx. In other words, velopharyngeal closure is thought to be somewhat akin to a sphincter-like action. [Zemlin, 1968, p. 309]

THE VELOPHARYNGEAL VALVE HAS AT LEAST TWO MAJOR FUNCTIONS FOR SPEECH: IT CONTROLS THE DIRECTION OF THE STREAM OF SOUND ORIGINATED AT THE LARYNX, AND IT PROVIDES FOR THE PRESSURE THAT IS REQUIRED AS THE VOICED OR VOICELESS STREAM OF AIR GOES THROUGH THE MOUTH IN THE PRODUCTION OF PLOSIVE AND FRICATIVE SOUNDS.

Whether the velopharyngeal valve is considered as part of the resonating mechanism or as part of the articulatory mechanism, it participates in the direction of the airstream and in the building up of mouth pressure. In fact, one may not wish to separate resonance from articulation except for convenience in considering each in its turn, then recombining them.

The velopharyngeal valve, in controlling the direction of the airstream, is involved in the resonance phenomenon known as nasality. If the passageway to the nasal cavities remains open enough to permit vocal tone to go into the nose as well as into the mouth, the resulting sound will have nasal as well as oral resonance. The size and shape of the mouth cavity for vowel sounds, for instance, may determine the phoneme that is perceived; but the addition of nasal resonance will change the sound in such a manner that, although it is recognized, it may be said to be nasalized. However, James F. Curtis (1969) pointed out that speech nasalization is not a simple acoustical phenomenon that can be described in terms of the amount of nasal resonance. Rather, he said, variations in nasal coupling produce complex effects on the spectrum of the speech signal and affect the intensity of the output and the phonatory function. In addition, factors that are not phonetic may influence the position of the velum in its participation in closure. With increased vocal effort, for example, the velum assumes a higher position; and with increased vocal frequency, the velum is lower (Platt and Noll, 1969). Hence, one can find no simple explanation of the function of the velopharyngeal valve in the modification of resonance; but the opening and closing of the velopharyngeal passageway undoubtedly contribute to the presence or absence of nasal resonance.

The velopharyngeal valve also participates in the establishment of pressure used for various articulatory activities. In this aspect of its function, the velopharyngeal sphincter might be considered part of the articulatory mechanism, because many of the consonant sounds of American English, whether they are voiced or voiceless, require pressure for plosion, as in /b/ or /d/, or for friction, as in /s/ or /v/.

If air, with or without vocal tone, is to be directed through the mouth cavity, so that it may be impeded or stopped by the action of the various articulators, the velopharyngeal passage must be closed to an extent that will permit the building up of air pressure in the mouth. In speech produced with normal structures, the closure and opening of the velopharyngeal passageway occur rapidly and accurately. The normal speaker changes from /s/ to /n/ to /i/ to /z/ for the word "sneeze" without being aware of the adjustments he is making at the velopharyngeal isthmus. He goes through a sequence, in saying "pins," from /p/ to /ɪ/ to /n/ to /z/ without any specific awareness of opening and closing the velopharyngeal passageway as he produces and combines a plosive, a vowel, a nasal, and a fricative in rapid succession, probably within the framework of a much longer utterance. In these articulatory adjustments, he uses the velopharyngeal valve to enable him to add the element of pressure that makes the plosive and fricative sounds conform to the pattern of the language he is speaking.

In its function as an articulator, the pharynx seems to resemble the other articulators, which vary in the sequence of articulation for one phoneme to that for the next (Kelsey and others, n.d., probably 1968). The velopharyngeal valve thus becomes subject to the effects of physiological coarticulation, the overlapping of the "physiological gestures" during speech production. However, these coarticulations, as well as the many other physiological gestures that take place during connected speech, occur without specific or conscious direction from the speaker if the end result of these activities is acceptable to him and to his listeners.

The normal functioning of the velopharyngeal valve, even if it is carried out without conscious effort by the speaker, is a complicated process that has been the subject of much investigation. For many years, velopharyngeal closure during speech was described as a simple action to which the soft palate made the greatest contribution; but modern research has demonstrated that velopharyngeal closure involves a complex set of muscles, nerves, and tissues and a complex set of activities in which they participate.

When Philippus Gustavus Passavant (1869) published his observations on velopharyngeal closure during speech, he was describing patients with palatal clefts. Although he did not investigate this closure in individuals with normal structures, Passavant suggested that the protruding ridge that he noted in his patients was part of the mechanism for closure in all speakers. His article included illustrations of the area that came to be known as Passavant's bar, ridge, or pad; Figure 2-13 has been adapted from these illustrations.

Passavant believed that the bulging of the superior constrictor on the posterior pharyngeal wall at the level of the base of the uvula, accompanied by the raising and pushing back of the velum, caused closure of the passageway from the oropharynx to the nasopharynx; but more recent investigations have suggested that the act of velopharyngeal closure, or valving, is more complex. The velopharyngeal mechanism does not function as a simple sphincter but includes anterior and mesial movement of the lateral and posterior pharyngeal walls as well as elevation of the velum (Harrington, 1944). Five components may be needed for closure of the nasopharyngeal isthmus: the side-to-side narrowing of the oropharynx by contraction of the fauces, the approximation of the lateral walls of the oropharynx by contraction of the superior constrictor muscles of the pharynx, the elevation of the soft palate by the levator palati muscles, the movements of the tongue, and "perhaps some forward advancement of the posterior pharyngeal wall" (Green, 1959).

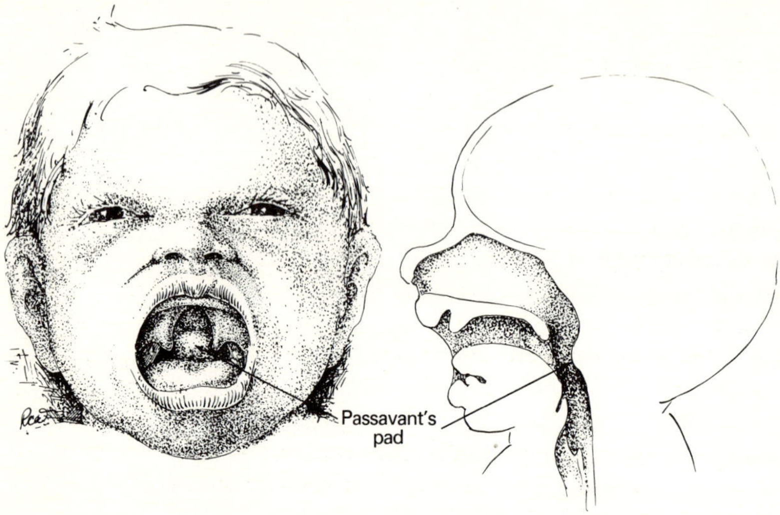

FIGURE 2-13 Location of Passavant's pad.

James Calnan (1954a), questioning Passavant's theory, concluded that Passavant's pad can and does occur in association with cleft palate but is not a factor in normal speech. Clinical observations of patients with palatal clefts have confirmed the first part of Calnan's statement (Carpenter and Morris, 1968); and some modern speech scientists have agreed with the second part, describing velopharyngeal action in speakers with normal structures in terms of a sphincterlike action that takes place without assistance from the ridge that Passavant described.

That velopharyngeal activities vary with the task in which the palatopharyngeal sphincter is involved was confirmed by Kenneth Moll's study (1965) of velopharyngeal function in individuals with normal structures and normal speech. However, Moll pointed out that, "even on tasks in which velopharyngeal closure may be achieved, such as swallowing, blowing, and gagging, observations concerning velar and pharyngeal movements may not accurately reflect the situation during speech production" (p. 120). Additional complicating factors, such as the durational characteristics of speech sounds and the position of the tongue in speech activities, were discussed by Moll and Thomas Shriner (1967), James Lubker (1968), Kenneth Bzoch (1968), and others.

Veau said that the belief that the pharynx operated like a sphincter was *une erreur, une grosse erreur;* and his illustrations of normal pharyngeal closure showed the soft palate as a valve (*un clapet*) that raised and lowered to control the passageway between the oropharynx and the nasal cavities (Veau and Borel-Maisonny, 1943). However, the use of the terms "valve" and "valving" by modern writers suggests that they consider that velopharyngeal closure may take place by means of sphincteric action. D. C. Spriestersbach, for example (in Olin, 1960), spoke of "leakage through the velopharyngeal valve" (p. 72); and Bosma and Fletcher (1961–1962) used "pharyngeal valving" as a term to signify the division of the oropharynx from the nasal cavities by means of muscular activity. In 1953, Calnan stated that nasopharyngeal closure was the result of a compound action of a sphincter and a flap valve, the sphincter being the lateral pharyngeal closure and the valve being the elevated velum. However, three years later, Calnan described palatopharyngeal incompetence in a way that suggested that he did not believe that the closure of the palatopharyngeal passageway was sphincterlike.

Certainly, the closure of the pharyngeal passageway is not achieved by any single action, such as the gatelike swinging of the soft palate or the simple forward protrusion of the posterior pharyngeal wall. Rather, this closure for speech, in an individual with normal structures and function, is the result of finely timed and coordinated activities of several sets of muscles. W. G. Holdsworth (1963) emphasized this concept when he said,

> The various sounds which comprise speech require different settings of the palatopharyngeal aperture, so that in speaking, as sound succeeds sound, the orifice must be altered, and the palate moved, at great speed. Unless there is complete control of the air stream into the nose there can be no distinctness of speech. [P. 8]

The "different settings of the palatopharyngeal aperture" have been discussed by many writers, some of whom use such terms as "palatopharyngeal orifice," "pharyngeal isthmus," "nasopharyngeal isthmus," "nasopharyngeal port," and "palatopharyngeal sphincter" to indicate the area extending from behind the oral cavity to the posterior part of the nasal cavity. The need for modifying this passageway "at great speed" is apparent when one considers the brief space of time required to say, for example, "Come here now, Mary," in which the palatopharyngeal aperture is modified at least six times if it closes for the consonant sounds requiring mouth pressure and for the vowel sounds and opens for the nasal consonants. Investigations of the way in which the palatal "valve" or "sphincter" moves during speech have provided evidence of differing activities in the levator and tensor muscles in the production of nasal and nonnasal sounds (Fritzell, 1963, 1969a) and showed that the palate prepared for velopharyngeal closure "before words were actually spoken" (Calnan, 1953, p. 290). The rate at which the movements of the velopharyngeal closure mechanism occurs is difficult to specify for speakers with normal structure because of individual variations, the different frequency with which nasal and nonnasal sounds appear in various contexts, and problems of electromyographic measurement. However, the acoustic evidence of shifts from nasal to nonnasal sounds is relatively clear, even if different listeners report different degrees of nasality or lack of nasality when they evaluate the same speaker.

Holdsworth's term "complete control" may not mean "complete closure." Some writers have suggested that normal speakers show complete velopharyngeal "closure" or "seal" (Hagerty and others, 1958; Bzoch and others, 1959). However, others have stated that complete closure is not essential in the production of speech that is perceived as normal (Bosma and Fletcher, 1961–1962; Subtelny and others, 1961; Moll, 1962; Mazaheri and others, 1964; Shelton and others, 1965; Warren, 1965; Massengill and Bryson, 1967).

Many attempts have been made to measure normal velopharyngeal closure, however it occurs. As instrumentation improved, the rubber bags and carnival blowers previously used to evaluate velopharyngeal closure were replaced by radiographic films and other measuring devices; films are now used extensively in studies of the structures that modify the size and shape of the pharyngonasal isthmus.

Radiographic films progressed from "still" or static roentgenographic pictures to "moving" or cineradiographic pictures to "sound movies" (Miller, 1959; O'Hara, 1963). Lateral views of the pharynx, obtained with roentgenographic or cinefluorographic techniques, can show the positions and movements of the tongue and soft palate in their relationships to the posterior pharyngeal wall during speech. With simultaneous recordings of the sound signals, such pictures can help the speech scientist or other investigator to determine the extent of closure at the midline during the production of speech sounds, singly or in sequence. Permanent recordings on various kinds of film and television tape allow detailed study and measurement of the rapid and frequent changes that occur in the pharyngeal area during speech.

An early description of procedures for studying connected speech from roentgen cinefilms and sound spectrograms predicted that combinations of "tomographic and cineradiographic methods" would provide "great possibilities for continuous studies of the physiological changes in the speech organs in relation to the connected speech produced" (Björk, 1961, p. 92). Such studies have been conducted and have provided information about speakers with normal structures that can be projected to studies of individuals with congenital palatal clefts (Kirkpatrick and Olmsted, 1959; Björk and Nylén, 1961; Warren and Hofmann, 1961; Morris and Smith, 1962; McWilliams and Girdany, 1964; Mazaheri and others, 1964; Shelton and others, 1964; Sloan and others, 1964; Massengill and Bryson, 1967; Peat, 1968; Yules, Northway, and Chase, 1968; Mazaheri and Sahni, 1969; others). As views can be obtained in an anteroposterior direction and as the interference posed by the bony structures is eliminated (T. H. Johnson and others, 1967; Griffith and others, 1968), the contribution of the lateral walls of the pharynx to velopharyngeal valving can be more clearly defined.

Other methods of studying velopharyngeal activity have been devised in recent years. Measurements of airflow and intraoral pressure, electromyography, and studies using ultrasound, cited in Chapter Six, have contributed to the understanding of the way in which the pharynx functions in altering the direction of the stream of air and in providing closure for the establishment of pressure through the mouth.

The effectiveness of palatopharyngeal closure cannot always be judged, however, from visual evidence of the apertures that remain or are obliterated by muscular activity. The audible signals generated and modified by a speaker are evaluated by a listener, and "nasality" in speech is often based on auditory perception rather than on measurement of an aperture or area. The sensitivity of the auditor may be an important factor in the evaluation he makes of the output of the speaker; and listeners do not always agree on the presence, absence, or amount of nasality in the wide range of normal speech. The final evaluation, clinically at least, may be the prerogative of the listener, who tends to react to what he perceives regardless of the physical structures of the speaker (Ritter, 1962); and the listener's cultural and experiential background may be as important as the speaker's oral-pharyngeal-nasal tract resonance system in nasality as it is perceived.

Speakers with normal structures show individual variations spectrographically, cinefluorographically, and acoustically (Dickson, 1962, 1969) that appear also in speakers with congenital palatal clefts. Continued research with present and future instrumentation may eventually permit the establishment of measures that can be used as referents. At the present time, however, the problems of comparing data are compounded by "the lack of any single set of parameters accepted as standard for measuring the nasal and oral pharynx" (Yules, Northway, and Chase, 1968).

CHAPTER THREE

Causes of Clefts of the Prepalate and Palate

WHEN THE PARENTS OF A CHILD BORN WITH A CLEFT OF THE PREPALATE OR PALATE SEE THE CHILD OR ARE TOLD OF HIS MALFORMATION, THEIR REACTIONS OFTEN INCLUDE, IN ADDITION TO VARIED EXPRESSIONS OF EMOTIONAL DISTURBANCE, AN INQUIRY ABOUT THE CAUSE OF THE ANOMALY.

They want to know why their child was born with such a defect, how this event could have happened in their family, what factors were responsible for the advent of a child with a deformity. Although they need some explanation as soon as they discover that the child has an oral cleft, they may not be able to accept or understand explanations of the several theories on the etiology of prepalatal and palatal clefts. The parent, in time of stress, may be a poor listener or may seek only reassurance that the child's malformation was not his or her fault. Presentation of appropriate information about the cause of clefts is a difficult task for any specialist, and a statement that the specific cause is unknown may be the best brief reply to make to the disturbed parent. Detailed explanations, if they are needed or appropriate, may be postponed until more effective communication is possible.

Specialists in the field of speech pathology have some need for knowledge about the various theories on the etiology of malformations of the lip, alveolus, and palate. They need such information for their own understanding of the complexities of the problem as well as for explanations they may make at some time to parents or others who inquire about the cause of these congenital anomalies.

The search for causes of physical defects present at birth has been a long and continuing process. In a discussion of epidemiologic aspects of the problem of congenital malformations, W. P. Kennedy (1967) commented: "From the earliest times the problems of congenital defects have puzzled and troubled man, first because of magic and theologic ideas, then from the practical difficulties of affected survivors and the distress and often guilt feelings of the parents" (p. 1). In attempts to solve the puzzle and meet the practical difficulties for a particular group of parents and children, many investigators have sought the etiological factors of oral clefts. In spite of the continuously growing number of research studies, the cause of these anomalies is still elusive; and the questions resulting from the research are often more numerous than the answers. Nevertheless, attempts to find the cause or causes of congenital clefts have resulted in the refutation of many superstitions, in the evolution of theories that can be tested, and in the presentation of points of view that can be respected even by those who cannot agree with them.

LONG BEFORE THE TWENTIETH CENTURY, SOME SUPERSTITIONS, THEORIES, AND POINTS OF VIEW WERE PROPOSED AND DEFENDED BY OBSERVERS WHO TRIED TO DETERMINE THE CAUSE OF CONGENITAL ANOMALIES OF THE PREPALATE AND PALATE.

Their methods were not those of modern research, but their findings indicated that the two basic theories most frequently postulated today are not entirely new. Environment and heredity were cited as possible causes for oral clefts even during the time that superstition wielded the greatest influence.

Environmental factors were considered by some early writers. In the eighteenth century, William Hunter asked women who were about to deliver their children whether anything had especially affected their minds during the pregnancy. In no instance, he reported, could a coincidence be detected between the woman's answer and any abnormality present in her child when it was born. However, the woman who had a child with congenital anomalies would frequently recall, after the child was born, some event that might have caused the defect (Warkany and Kalter, 1962).

John Keating's *Cyclopedia of the Diseases of Children,* published in 1890, listed twenty-one reports, published in medical and psychological journals between 1868 and 1886, citing maternal impressions during the first three or four months of pregnancies that resulted in clefts. In most instances, the deformity in the child was like the deformity that had frightened or disturbed the mother. The author of the chapter did not accept the theory of maternal impressions without question; but he did suggest that every physician should warn his pregnant patients "of the necessity for avoiding powerful emotions of every kind, and especially those which are of a distressing character" (p. 216).

Although one of the nineteenth-century writers on dentistry (Kingsley, 1880) could not identify the causes of the arrest of development, he attributed the origin of cleft palate to such an arrest and added that the large majority of cases came "from the lower walks of life, from the poorly nourished and physically depraved" (p. 207), suggesting that he considered environment a possible causal factor in palatal clefts.

Studies on heredity as a factor in clefts of the prepalate and palate also antedate the modern era. According to Poul Fogh-Andersen (1942), articles published in the eighteenth century and in the first half of the nineteenth reported evidence of familial incidence of clefts. Some of the early studies cited incidence without elaborating their findings; others pointed out heredity as a cause in all cases in which several members of a family had "the affection"; still others described families in which clefts of various kinds appeared through several generations. Fogh-Andersen did not believe that the early reports permitted any conclusions, and he had more confidence in investigations in the first half of the twentieth century that were based on large numbers of cases rather than on single families.

Some of the early writers accepted the possibility of multiple causes for congenital clefts. Francis Mason (1877), for example, expressed the belief that clefts were caused by shock or impression on the mother or by heredity. Truman Brophy (1923) cited heredity, prenatal impressions, and imperfect nutrition as causes for clefts. He also noted that the appearance of a cleft in only one of a set of twins provided refutation of maternal impressions, and he discussed the fissures of the lower lip described by Sir Arthur Keith (1940) and others that now constitute part of Van der Woude's syndrome (1954). Others considered shock, mechanical trauma, the mother's health and nutrition, intrauterine factors, supernumerary teeth, and local abnormalities as possible combined causes of clefts.

The forward-looking writers of the eighteenth and nineteenth centuries could do little to overcome the superstitions that have surrounded the presence of physical differences. In medieval times, congenital anomalies were considered acts of God; and, even in the present century, the parent with feelings of guilt sometimes attributes the malformation in his child to some factor that minimizes his responsibility for an offspring with a physical defect.

These ideas about the occurrence of congenital anomalies are understandable in the light of man's belief in the supernatural; for centuries, psychic shocks or mechanical traumas during pregnancy were thought to cause cleft malformations. Mason (1877) provided examples of superstition about the appearance of cleft palate from a period in which such beliefs were very common. He described two cases:

> . . . in one case now under my observation the mother attributes the deformity to the fact that when she was pregnant one of her other children fell on a walking stick and split open the soft palate. In another, the mother said it was due, she believed, to her having longed for some particular fish which had a huge mouth. What the fish was I could not understand. She assured me that this occurred at about the sixth week of gestation. [P. 65]

Many scientists attempted to combat these ideas. Leslie B. Arey, for example, in the fifth edition (1946) of his textbook of developmental anatomy, said firmly: "It should be sufficient merely to state that the worldwide superstition that fright or accident to a pregnant mother can 'mark' her unborn babe in a correlated way is not even a possibility" (p. 174); and his refutation of superstition is typical of other similar statements. However, even today, almost anyone who has conferred with parents or grandparents of children born with clefts has heard such explanations as:

> I knew that the baby might have something wrong with him because I got so scared the day the horse fell in the well.
>
> I was on my way to the mailbox when up out of the bush at the side of the path jumped this big rabbit. I got so scared I almost fainted; so, when the baby came two weeks later, I really wasn't surprised he had a harelip.

> I told my daughter-in-law she shouldn't have taken care of that neighbor child with a cleft palate when she was pregnant. Oh, he's a sweet little boy; but she should have known she might have one of her own with a split palate—as she did, you know—if she was with one of that kind so often.

In many instances, the incident to which the defect has been attributed took place long after the deficiency in the lip or palate was already present. Perhaps the term "split palate" suggested that a normally developed structure was torn open by some traumatic episode, or perhaps the parent's lack of information about normal prenatal development contributed to his acceptance of a well-remembered incident as the cause of the congenital cleft. Josef Warkany (1959) pointed out that the history of teratology "does not teach us much about the origin, prevention, or treatment of congenital malformations; but it tells us a great deal about the human mind and its reactions to unexplained phenomena" (p. 94). His comment that "ancient beliefs often plague the parents even today" was quite appropriate.

AS MEN FOUND WAYS TO GATHER INFORMATION UNDER CONTROLLED CONDITIONS AND AS STATISTICAL TREATMENT OF DATA BECAME POSSIBLE, THE SEARCH FOR THE POSSIBLE CAUSE OR CAUSES OF CONGENITAL CLEFTS OF THE PREPALATE AND PALATE SETTLED ON TWO QUESTIONS: WHY DO SUCH CLEFTS OCCUR DURING THE EMBRYONIC PERIOD, AND HOW DO THEY HAPPEN?

Investigators gave their attention to one or both of these questions; and, as a result of many recent studies on the etiology (the "why") and the pathogenesis (the "how") of congenital facial clefts, the specialist may be a bit closer to a reply that he can give with confidence to the parent who asks, "But why did this happen to us?"

The investigator who studies the "why" and "how" of clefts of the prepalate and palate faces multiple problems. As the descriptive epidemiology of these anomalies emerges "out of a potpourri of theory, belief, and fact" (Greene, 1963, p. 599), those who look for reasons and those who study developmental processes that turn out to be unsuccessful have expressed their concern for the many barriers to research on "a struggle that goes on in the darkness of the uterus" (Warkany, in Pruzansky, 1961, p. 206). Some of the restrictions to research in this darkness are typical of most investigations that involve humans as subjects, but some are peculiar to the study of congenital clefts.

Intentional induction of congenital anomalies by means of certain agents thought to be teratogenic must be confined to animals. Experimental procedures that include modification of nutrition, use of radiation, deprivation of oxygen, administration of drugs, and introduction of stress and shock can provide information about the reactions of mice and rats and swine; but humans cannot be used as subjects for such studies, and the experimental animals differ from the human in many ways. In this limitation, research on clefts is similar to research on other congenital anomalies.

In another general way, research findings from experimental work are limited. Speaking of nutritional experiments, Warkany (1958) reminded research workers that, in the application of animal experiments to questions of congenital malformations in man, "great care must be exercised, since the animals are subjected to artificial environmental conditions which are not likely to occur in human beings" (p. 2023). In another context (1957), he said, "But, although much can be learned of the pathogenic pathways of the condition from animal experimentation, it would be premature and dangerous to infer that parallels exist between the etiologies of the experimental and human abnormalities" (p. 9). Conversely, human embryos may encounter prenatal environmental conditions that do not occur in experimental laboratories and that sometimes cannot be identified or isolated.

Even carefully designed experiments that are acceptable in their use of human subjects encounter some problems. The human subject, regardless of his willingness to cooperate, cannot remain in a completely controlled environment. The experimenter who uses humans as subjects cannot be sure of the effect of attitudes, introspections, emotional responses, or situational factors on the behavior of the subject.

The difficulties that beset the investigator who seeks answers to questions about humans are increased when the research is focused on the prenatal period and on anomalies present at birth. The defect being studied cannot be identified until the child is born; the individuals who present anomalies of the prepalate and palate at birth are widely scattered geographically and relatively few in number; and, even if the teratologist could know in advance that a certain pregnancy would terminate in the birth of a child with a prepalatal or palatal cleft, he would have difficulties in observing the development of the child in fetal and embryonic life to note the stages of pathomorphology.

Studies in prospect and in retrospect also pose problems to the investigator. In some instances, identification of families in which instances of congenital anomalies can be anticipated will permit prospective studies. The mother of one child with a palatal cleft may be observed during a subsequent pregnancy that might be expected to produce a second child with such a congenital anomaly. However, the length of the human gestation period, the possibility that the expected child will have no physical abnormality, and the difficulty of thorough study of the pregnancy can complicate such experimentation. Information obtained in retrospect is often biased by the emotional reaction of the parent to the birth of a child with a physical malformation. The necessity for depending on reports of events during the early part of the pregnancy, events that took place months before the interview, also raises questions about the usefulness of such information. The structure of the interview, the intellectual and emotional status of the informant, and the time lag can affect the findings in retrospective studies.

Another barrier to the accumulation of data is that certain remedial measures, which are designed to minimize the congenital defect, must begin as soon as the defect is noted. Hence, the answers to some questions about clefts of the prepalate or palate may be obscured by the treatment for these clefts; and some kinds of tests that might be used to determine the possible etiology of the cleft would interfere with therapeutic measures that should be instituted. Careful evaluation of the premature baby, for example, may be restricted by the need for maintaining life in the child; and necessary early surgical treatment may cause the removal of the child from the hospital of his birth and from the investigator who had hoped to learn as much as possible about him and his family.

Karl Erhardt, in his introductory address to the First International Conference on Congenital Malformations (in Fishbein, 1961), cited additional factors that make for difficulties in research on defects that are present at birth, saying:

> The pathogenic course in teratology from inciting event to observed defect follows many pathways. The same inciting event may result in quite different defects; yet similar defects may derive from various etiologic factors. A given factor does not invariably produce the effect that might have been expected. Some embryos affected by a specific type of insult may die and be aborted, while others proceed to a term delivery despite a serious malformation. Simple relations obviously are not to be anticipated in research relating to the etiology of congenital malformations. [P. 25]

In spite of the difficulties in research designed to discover the causes and the developmental phases of clefts, many investigators have undertaken studies to determine the reasons for the defective end products of some pregnancies and the elements that enter into the deviant developmental patterns. Most of the research is designed to answer one or both of the basic questions that have been asked so often: Why is a child born with a cleft, and how does the cleft occur during the prenatal period?

UNTIL VERY RECENTLY, ONE WAS FORCED TO ANSWER THE FIRST OF THESE QUESTIONS—WHAT CAUSES CLEFTS OF THE LIP, ALVEOLUS, AND PALATE?—WITH AN HONEST ACKNOWLEDGMENT OF IGNORANCE. NOW, HOWEVER, THE ACCUMULATION OF INFORMATION AND OPINION PERMITS, BUT COMPLICATES, A REPLY.

When superstitious explanations were ruled out, two major points of view were expressed: one stated that congenital clefts of the prepalate and palate were the result of genetic, or endogenous, factors; the other declared that they resulted from factors in the uterine environment, from exogenous factors. Each of these theories had its proponents; but, at the present time, a single explanation that combines these two is being accepted by more and more investigators. The theory of multiple causation, considered later in this chapter, was summarized by F. Clarke Fraser (1959) when he said that "most congenital malformations are the result of complex interactions between multifactorial genetic and environmental systems" (p. 100). Nevertheless, each of the two theories has had its proponents and its opponents.

Attention to the genetic basis for congenital clefts was stimulated by Fogh-Andersen's work in Denmark, reported in 1942. His study had several purposes:

> To make an investigation into the average frequency of the malformation . . . to investigate into the occurrence of the malformation among the relatives of a number of patients . . . to demonstrate whether heredity should be regarded as an etiological factor for all forms of harelip and cleft palate . . . to set up some applicable empirical figures of genetic prognosis . . . to advance a theory as to the manner of inheritance . . . and finally on the basis of these investigations to give expression to contingent eugenic considerations. [P. 14]

Although he classified clefts as harelip alone, harelip plus cleft palate, and cleft palate alone, Fogh-Andersen (1942) presented his conclusions in terms of "two different malformations with no genetic connection" (p. 250), harelip with or without associated cleft palate and isolated cleft palate. His findings were based on a study of 703 patients and their families, and he drew a number of conclusions. He found that, for patients with clefts in both the prepalate and palate, similar defects were presented by about 2 percent of the children of these patients, by about 4.4 percent of the patients' siblings when the parents were normal, and by about 14 percent of the siblings when one parent had clefts in both areas. For those of his patients with "isolated cleft palate," the frequency of a similar anomaly was about 7 percent among their children, about 12 percent among their siblings when the parents were normal and a hereditary disposition could be determined, about 1.8 percent among the siblings when the parents were normal and no hereditary disposition could be assumed, and about 17 percent among the siblings if one parent had cleft palate. Fogh-Andersen summarized thus:

> The figures exceed by far the average frequency figures for the [general] population (ha.(+cl.pa.): 0.11 per cent and cl.pa.: 0.04 per cent), and thus it has been proved that heredity is an etiological factor both of ha.(+cl.pa.) and of isolated cl.pa. [P. 251]

Fogh-Andersen reported cases in which heredity did not seem to be the etiological factor, but he was consistent in maintaining his theory about the inheritance of clefts. In 1957, he stated:

> The question of the etiology of harelip and cleft palate, being of great theoretical as well as practical eugenic interest, is still a partially unsolved problem. Until recently works on the etiology have been published which apparently might support the assumption of exogenic factors such as nutritional deficiencies, infections, or intoxications during pregnancy.
>
> There is still no doubt, however, that the most important etiological factor is that of heredity. . . . Two different cleft formations exist with no genetic connection and with a different manner of inheritance, viz: (1) harelip with or without associated cleft palate, occurring most often in males, and mostly inherited as a recessive character (so-called "conditioned dominance"), and (2) cleft palate alone, most frequently found in females, only inherited in a smaller number of cases and then as a dominant character with failing manifestation. [In Skoog and Ivy, 1957, p. 159]

Later, Fogh-Andersen reported that, although he still believed that heredity was the main etiological factor in the formation of facial clefts, he recognized that at least three-fifths of the patients with clefts of the prepalate with or without palatal clefts and four-fifths of those with cleft palate were what he termed "solitary" cases, in which hereditary factors could not be clearly demonstrated (in Schuchardt, 1966).

Fogh-Andersen's work had a strong influence on other investigators. His two categories—clefts of the prepalate with or without clefts of the palate and isolated palatal clefts—were used in other research projects, and reports from those studies are sometimes difficult to compare with information based on three categories—clefts of the prepalate, clefts of the palate, and clefts involving both areas. The effects of these differences in categorization will be evident in later considerations in this chapter and again in the discussion of types of clefts in Chapter Four.

Many investigators have agreed with Fogh-Andersen's theory of the genetic basis for congenital clefts. Strong evidence for hereditary factors was found, for example, in a small village in Sweden in which the incidence of clefts of the prepalate, palate, or both was one in each one hundred births, suggesting that "out of every 5 inhabitants of X, one had the hereditary factor" (Sanders, 1934, p. 495). Other data (Mather and Philip, 1940) showed that at least two genes, one an autosomal recessive and the other a sex-linked recessive, govern the inheritance of clefts, at least in the three ethnically close human populations studied. Another report (Murphy, 1947) indicated that congenital malformations, in general, were usually the result of factors in the male or female germ cells prior to fertilization; and forty individuals with facial clefts were among the 935 cases investigated. A familial disposition of as much as 40 percent was one of several genetic factors cited in a review of the etiology of clefts (Canick, 1954). Fraser (1955), after pointing out that no clear-cut environmental agent had been found to cause cleft palate, added:

> The excellent study of Fogh-Andersen has shown that, in most cases, clefts of the lip and/or palate are caused by a genetic predisposition, probably multifactorial, interacting with undefined environmental circumstances. [P. 362]

Others (MacMahon and McKeown, 1953; Stiegler and Berry, 1958; Stark, in Levin, 1962; Woolf and others, 1963; Fukuhara, 1965; Coccia and others, 1969) supported Fogh-Andersen's genetic theory.

Some have questioned Fogh-Andersen's defense of his theory. They suggested that he did not take into account the children who were stillborn or who died before the time of operation (Drillien and others, 1966), that his explanation did not apply to all of the children born with clefts, and that environmental factors have been clearly demonstrated to be the cause of orofacial clefts. Several reports showed familial incidence of prepalatal and palatal clefts to be lower than Fogh-Andersen indicated (Birch-Jensen, 1949;

Lutz and Moor, 1955; Peer, Strean, and others, 1958; Oldfield and Tate, 1964). Inheritance in Fogh-Andersen's patients was a demonstrable factor in 37 percent of the cases of prepalatal cleft with or without cleft palate and in 19 percent of the cases of isolated cleft palate, and figures similar to those obtained from the research in Denmark were reported from a study of 169 families in Scotland (Drillien and others, 1966). One-third of the children in the group in Scotland had relatives who also had clefts, although the investigators were unable to report general agreement about the mechanisms involved in hereditary predisposition to clefts. However, two-thirds of the group were born with clefts that must have resulted from environmental factors or from genetic factors that could not be identified. Joachim Gabka put the question bluntly to a conference of plastic surgeons:

> To-day the most well-known factor of the aetiology of clefts is inheritance, although we only find 25–30 per cent. hereditary conditions in our fissure patients. How are we able to explain the remaining 75 per cent.? [In Wallace, 1960, p. 7]

The cause of congenital facial clefts cannot be limited to heredity, and most writers seem to be willing to grant that this is the case.

With the specification of the number of human chromosomes at the beginning of the second half of the twentieth century, the attention of investigators turned to the study of congenital anomalies brought about by chromosomal aberrations. Trisomic mongolism was described in 1959 (Lejeune and others), and the identification of the anomaly of chromosomes thought to be responsible for mongolism led to some investigation of the possibility that prepalatal and palatal clefts might be the result of some deviant chromosomal factor. In one group of thirty-seven selected cases, chromosomal aberrations were found in two boys and two girls with palatal clefts, other physical anomalies, and mental retardation (Drillien and others, 1966). Another study, in which eleven patients with clefts were evaluated (Šubrt and others, 1966), found deviations in the number or size of chromosomes in only one, a child with Down's syndrome (mongolism). More than thirty investigations since 1960 have shown that the search for genetic factors responsible for clefts has not overlooked cytogenetics, the study of the origin and development of cells (Wolstenholme and Porter, 1967).

The presence of a cleft in only one of a pair of identical, or monozygotic, twins has posed some problems to both the geneticists and the environmentalists, although chiefly to the former. If both twins in a monozygotic pair have clefts, then genetic factors would seem to be involved; but one investigation (Metrakos and others, 1958) found no concordance (appearance of the same defect in both twins) in the two sets of monozygotic twins studied, although a concordance percentage of 31 for eighteen sets of monozygotic twins has been reported in the literature. For dizygotic twins, those who are fraternal but not identical and who may differ in sex, concordance of clefts, which was 6.3 percent for a total of sixty-six sets reported in the literature, was not found. Another charting (Drillien and others, 1966) of findings from studies of twins showed that 41.7 percent of the monozygotic pairs showed concordance for cleft lip with or without cleft palate and that 8.3 percent showed concordance for cleft palate alone. These figures were higher than those reported for the dizygotic pairs, in which concordances of 7.0 and 7.7 percent, respectively, were found for prepalatal and palatal clefts in combination and for palatal clefts alone. Others (Brophy, 1923; Stark, in Levin, 1962; Palmer and Machida, 1964) provided further information about the incidence of clefts in identical twins, reporting cases of identical twins with clefts of the prepalate and palate and fifteen cases of identical twins with clefts, with discordance in nine and concordance in six pairs.

The summary of twin studies in a review of the epidemiology of clefts (Greene, 1963) was necessarily brief:

> The available data on the concordance of monozygotic and dizygotic twins, at least one of whom has a facial cleft, strongly indicates—despite the small numbers in the studies and the difficulties in determining zygosity—that genetic factors play a significant role in the etiology of clefts of the lip and palate. At the same time, it is quite apparent that there are other forces which impede or aid these genetic influences or independently produce phenocopies. [P. 596]

Although some congenital clefts of the lip and palate are the result of genetic factors already identified or yet to be found, individuals who do not demonstrate endogenous causes for their labial and palatal clefts must have been subjected to some kind of environmental influence that brought about the congenital anomaly. These many exogenous factors have been studied extensively in animals; the results of some of this research may be applicable to humans, if proper precautions are taken in the interpretation of the findings.

Some of the factors that have been investigated in human subjects have more direct effects than others on embryological development. Such influences as parental age, birth order, season of birth, geographical location, and race are not intrauterine; and only one of these seems to be closely related to the appearance of congenital clefts. Questions about these influences have been answered in a variety of ways.

Does parental age affect the incidence of clefts of the prepalate and palate? Negative answers were given by some (Fogh-Andersen, 1942; McEvitt, 1952; Lutz and Moor, 1955). Others (Phair, 1947; MacMahon and McKeown, 1953; Mazaheri, 1958; Loretz and others, 1961; Greene and others, 1964; Hay, 1967) found some relationship between parents' ages and the appearance of clefts in their children. The incidence of combined clefts seemed to be greater in children of older parents, but clefts in only one area were apparently not related to parental age. A study in Britain (MacMahon and McKeown, 1953) indicated that the incidence of palatal clefts was independent of the mother's age, and an investigation in the United States (Hay, 1967) showed that increased parental age did not bring about an increase in prepalatal clefts.

Is the child who appears early in the birth order in a family more likely to have a cleft than one who is second-, third-, or later-born; or is the risk of cleft greater in a child born even later in a sequence of children? A first-born with a cleft may have no siblings because of parental fear that other children might have the same defect as the first; and the appearance of a child with a cleft, at any point, may reduce the probability of additional children. The information provided by research is not conclusive. In one group of patients, children with clefts of the prepalate and palate were among the later-born (Mazaheri, 1958). One of the conclusions from a study in Japan was that "cleft lips and cleft palates are significantly increased in the 5th or later births" (Fujino and others, 1963, p. 330). Analysis of data obtained in Germany did not reveal a relationship between clefts and the place in the birth order (Bethmann, 1969).

Does the season in which the child is born—or, perhaps more logically, in which he was conceived and spent his first three embryonic months—have any effect on the incidence of clefts? Investigations of season of birth are related to intrauterine factors more than to those of general environment, because certain viral infections, such as influenza, tend to be more common at certain times of the year. However, little evidence has been presented to demonstrate a relationship between the incidence of clefts and the season of birth (Fraser and Calnan, 1961). Studies that have found such a relationship have not agreed on the season that showed the greatest incidence. In California, more babies with clefts were born in June, July, and August

(Lutz and Moor, 1955). In Czechoslovakia, March, April, and May were the months in which greater numbers of children were born with clefts (Červenka and others, 1969). In Japan, those same three months seemed to be the ones in which more combined clefts appeared; but the seasonal incidence of palatal clefts was not clearly apparent (Fujino and others, 1963).

Does the geographical location affect the possibility of producing a child with a cleft of the prepalate or palate? One unusual report suggested that congenital malformations, clefts among them, were influenced by the cyclonic circulation of air and atmospheric changes; and the writer (Peterson, 1934) cited reports from examinations of draftees in World War I to show that men from Maine and Vermont had more clefts than men from the southwestern states. More conventional studies have indicated that geography plays little part in the incidence of clefts, except that certain racial groups constitute a fairly large percentage of the population in certain geographical areas (Krantz and Henderson, 1947; Schwartz, 1954; Donahue, 1965).

The effects of geology rather than geography were investigated in two studies. One found that the glaciated area of New Jersey produced fewer children with clefts than the driftless area of Wisconsin (Brown, 1939). The other determined the incidence of clefts in two geologically different parts of New York following an observation that the number of congenital malformations of all kinds seemed unusally high in a certain area that had extensive rock formations with relatively high concentrations of radioactive elements (Gentry and others, 1959). Although they pointed out that some other agent might be responsible for the differences they found, the investigators suggested that radiation might be a primary etiological agent in the occurrence of clefts. This same possibility had been explored in a study of the potential effects of the atomic bombs that fell on Hiroshima (Plummer, 1952), but no clefts appeared in the children of eleven mothers who were in the first trimester of pregnancy and close to the center of greatest exposure at the time of the blast. Conclusions cannot be drawn with confidence, but those who seek the cause of congenital clefts of the prepalate and palate may find further study of such factors as radiation more fruitful than investigations of geographical locations in general.

Does race affect the incidence of clefts? The answer to this question is clear. Figures in Chapter One show that congenital clefts are less frequent in the Negro and more frequent in the Japanese than in the Caucasian. Most of the studies that have considered the influence of race have determined the racial background of only the mothers of children with clefts, and future studies of this topic may be influenced by information about the fathers and by the mixture of races resulting from sociological changes in the twentieth century.

Except for race, then, the effect of factors in the environment, but not in the intrauterine environment, seems to be negligible. Research on parental age, birth order, season of birth, and geographical location will probably not be pursued with great diligence in the future, even though such investigations can be more readily undertaken with human subjects than the research on teratogenic agents and other endogenous factors that have a direct effect on the embryo within the uterus.

The study of the effect of teratogens on humans is relatively recent. James Neel, speaking of congenital malformations in general, said:

> The very high frequency of serious disorders of development, only a fraction of which survive to the late stages of pregnancy and then are labeled congenital defects, has long been recognized for many mammals, but only recently documented in man. [In Fishbein, 1961, p. 67]

Several reasons for the lack of investigations involving human subjects have been recounted. However, as causes for human deformities are sought intramaternally and as drugs, viral infections, and nutrition are demonstrated to affect the fetus as well as, or even rather than, the mother, studies of humans will replace those of animals in attempts to find the reasons for congenital clefts that appear in one of each 800 human babies born throughout the world today.

Richard Stark and others (1962) listed more than twenty complications during early pregnancy reported by mothers of seventy-nine children with facial clefts; and Richard Donahue (1967) obtained, from birth records of five states, a list of thirteen such factors. Stress and radiation appeared in both lists; and ten or more of Stark's informants cited miscarriage, vomiting, infertility, and vaginal bleeding as factors in their pregnancies. M. Leon Canick's extensive list of factors that have been studied as possible causes of clefts (1954) also included radiation but added such other major categories as maternal impressions, deficiencies of vitamins, excesses of insulin and cortisone, administration of chemicals, lack of oxygen, infections, maternal age and birth order, biochemical changes, deficiencies in nutrition, and circulatory embarrassment. More than sixty methods exist for the experimental production of congenital malformations in animals (Wilson, in Fishbein, 1961); but Fraser (1959) suggested that only five environmental agents were causes of congenital malformations in human beings—radiation, rubella, toxoplasma organism, folic acid deficiency, and progestins.

The effects of nutrition, drugs, radiation, viral infections, pressure changes, and stress on the embryo in animals and humans have been subjected to many investigations; and the findings from these studies, although they have not given any one answer that can be accepted without qualification, shed some light on the effect of the environment on the incidence of clefts (Wilson, 1959). The possible impacts of such other factors as hyperthermia, cysts, serum proteins and protein synthesis, synostosis of the cervical vertebrae (Ross and Lindsay, 1965), head size, diabetes, toxoplasmosis (Erdélyi, 1957), negative or positive rhesus states, uterine position, thalidomide (Fogh-Andersen, 1966), flexure of the cranial base (Moss, 1956), insulin antagonism in the mother (Vallance-Owen and others, 1967), and a maternal history of previous miscarriages have also been reported. In this ever-increasing amount of information, certain consistencies appear; but the differences in opinions still seem to outweigh the agreements.

Nutritional deficiencies may affect the embryo if their influence occurs at certain points in the prenatal developmental time schedule. Investigations of the effects of nutritional variations have both supported and denied the value of vitamin supplements to lessen the chance of clefts of the prepalate and palate. On the basis of a study of 164 children with clefts attending a special training program, two investigators (Stiegler and Berry, 1958) concluded that nutrition was a precipitating factor in the appearance of clefts. Evidence from animal experiments led to a decision, following another study, to give vitamins to mothers who had children with clefts if these mothers had subsequent pregnancies (Conway, 1958). In a total of 137 subsequent pregnancies, the fifty-nine infants born to mothers who received vitamin therapy during the first trimester had no clefts; among the seventy-eight children born to mothers who did not receive vitamin therapy, four had clefts of the prepalate, palate, or both. In 400 pregnancies resulting in the births of children with clefts, 306 of the children came from families with no history of clefting; and, of these, 275 were born to mothers who took vitamins irregularly, late in the pregnancies, or not at all (Peer, Strean, and others, 1958). However, other investigators (Fraser and Warburton, 1964), after administering vitamins to women who had previously had children with clefts, concluded that the subsequent pregnancies were not affected by the dietary supplement. Prenatal administration of vitamins, according to this research, is acceptable if it is not in excess; but such vitamin therapy will not prevent the occurrence of malformations.

Interest in the effects of vitamin deficiencies on the incidence of congenital anomalies, clefts among them, was fostered by Warkany's studies on animals as early as 1940. Describing his early experiments, Warkany (1958) said:

> Extensive studies in small laboratory animals were made possible when my associates and I found that a syndrome of skeletal malformations could be induced in rats by maternal riboflavin deficiency. . . . Cleft palate was present in about one-half of the abnormal young. . . . The studies demonstrated that a high incidence of posterior cleft palate (without harelip), an internal skeletal malformation, can be induced by a chemical deficiency in stocks of rats that were free of the anomaly. . . . [P. 2020]

In interpreting his experiments, Warkany stated that the results found from studies of animals

> do not prove that congenital malformations in man are due to maternal dietary deficiencies. . . . The fact that a teratogenic method produces a certain malformation in rats does not permit the conclusion that it will be equally effective in mice. How much more hazardous is it then to equate such animal experiments with human conditions. [P. 2022]

Birth deformities, including clefts, in animals have been induced by deprivation of vitamins and nucleic acids and by administration of an excess of certain vitamins (Excerpta Medica Foundation, 1963). However, the time factor is important in the results of such experimental work; and the importance of certain days following impregnation of rats and mice has been recognized by investigators who have attempted to induce or prevent congenital defects of the palate in the offspring of these "small laboratory animals." Identification of the time schedule in humans is more difficult, and control of the administration or restriction of certain nutritional elements in the first trimester of human pregnancies may be almost impossible unless the pregnancy is recognized quickly and the mother is under care before the eighth or ninth week.

The effects of various drugs on the outcome of pregnancies in humans and animals have been reported by many investigators. However, the major amount of work in this field has concentrated on the administration of cortisone, which is produced by the body as a normal hormone to regulate carbohydrate balance. Although thyroxine, Prelabon, trypan blue, and other drugs have been considered, the work of Fraser and of Lyndon Peer and his associates focused attention on cortisone as a possible teratogenic agent for animals, particularly mice.

Prior to Fraser's description of the ways in which cortisone affected his experimental animals, an article in *Lancet* reported a case in which a woman received cortisone therapy for persistent problems with diarrhea and anemia. When the cessation of menstruation noted before and during the time that she was taking cortisone was identified as the result of pregnancy, cortisone treatment was discontinued at about the eighteenth week after the conception of a child who was stillborn with a large postalveolar palatal cleft and other anomalies. The reporters felt that they had no justification for attributing the cleft palate to the administration of cortisone to the mother during her early pregnancy, but they advised that the possibility of early pregnancy should be excluded before the administration of cortisone to women of child-bearing age (Harris and Ross, 1956). A response to this report cited two cases. In the first, a mother was given cortisone in early pregnancy and had a male child, thought to be premature, who had a cleft palate involving the soft tissues. In the second, a mother who had received cortisone daily during the first twelve weeks of pregnancy had a child who was born four weeks prematurely but had no congenital anomalies (Doig and Coltman, 1956). Other studies have attributed the occurrence of cleft palate in some infants to treatment of the mother with high doses of cortisone during pregnancy (International Medical Congress, 1964). The effects of cortisone on humans, however, have not been as clearly demonstrated as on animals.

Fraser's reports (1955, 1960; in Pruzansky, 1961; in Fishbein, 1961) on his production of clefts in mice by administration of cortisone, which apparently delays the movement of the palatal shelves to the horizontal position, illustrated both the specificity and the variability of the findings from such experimental work. Using a single agent, cortisone, in a standard treatment daily for four days, in a single kind of experimental animal, the mouse, he found a single teratogenic effect, cleft of the palate. This encouraging specificity, however, was partially negated by the variabilities that were noted. If the treatment began after the palate normally closed, it had no effect. When the treatment began eleven days after insemination, it produced cleft palate in virtually all embryos of one particular strain of mice, the A/Jax, but in only 17 percent of another, the C57BL/6. Results of crossbreeding, which reduced the incidence of cleft palates in both hybrid groups, suggested that the probability that an embryo will have a cleft palate following maternal cortisone treatment "depends on the maternal, as well as the foetal, genotype" (Fraser, in Pruzansky, 1961, p. 190). When the difference between the time schedules in the two strains was weighed and the earlier closing of palates in the resistant mice was determined, the evidence led to the conclusion that "the embryos in which palate closure normally occurs earlier have the lower frequencies of cleft palate following treatment with cortisone" (Fraser in Pruzansky, 1961, p. 192). One more variation that required consideration was that, although most of the babies born to mothers in the cleft-resistant strain of mice after the standard treatment with cortisone had no palatal clefts, some of the baby mice with identical genetic backgrounds and identical environments, littermates of those without clefts, were born with cleft palates. Fraser considered this variable the most puzzling and perhaps the most important of all but had to report that he and his colleagues had not been able to identify positively "any intra-uterine variable associated more often with embryos that have a cleft palate following cortisone treatment than with their genetically similar littermates that do not" (in Pruzansky, 1961, p. 193).

Investigating the effect of other elements, Lyndon Peer, Walter H. Bryan, and their colleagues (1958) used saline solution alone, added it to cortisone, substituted vitamin B_6 and folic acid for saline solution in the combinations, and administered the standard treatment of cortisone to one strain of mice. In 127 offspring whose mothers were given cortisone daily during the period thought to be critical, 109 had palatal clefts. Untreated control groups and groups given injections of saline solution produced no babies with clefts; and the incidence of clefts was reduced when vitamin B_6, folic acid, or both were combined with the cortisone.

Radiation, sometimes cited as a factor in the incidence of clefts in animals, has not been shown to have significant effects on humans. A. Berndorfer (in Schuchardt, 1966) reported that 20 percent of the mothers of 1,500 children with congenital anomalies, including 220 with clefts, had been exposed to roentgen radiation during pregnancy; but he did not specify whether or not such exposure occurred during the early months. One study (Murphy, 1947) suggested that therapeutic pelvic irradiation during pregnancy could cause malformation but did not find that clefts resulted from such exposure. Only indeterminate results of radiation were reported in a discussion (Sayegh, 1964) of congenital malformations in general. However, internal radiation of animals, by injection, produced twenty-four mice with clefts, mostly clefts of the palate, in a total of forty-nine fetuses when the radiated dose was administered during the fourteenth day of the pregnancy, whereas only eleven of 129 control fetuses had clefts (Goljan, 1968). Lack of extensive evidence suggests that radiation, unless internal, is probably not a teratogenic agent for clefts or that research on this topic has been insufficient.

The human placenta is not a highly effective barrier against infection (Eichenwald, 1965), and viruses and bacteria can cross from the maternal side to the fetal circulation. Among the possible results of maternal infection during pregnancy is that of teratogenesis, in which the fetus does not abort but survives to show the effect of the mother's disease. Reports (Gregg, 1942, 1945) on the coincidence of an epidemic of German measles (rubella) in New South Wales and the appearance, a few months later, of children with deformities led to further investigation of the results of mothers' infections on their children. Rubella results in anomalies of the eye, ear, and heart most frequently; but it is a teratogenic agent in only one-third to one-fifth of the cases and only if the mother has it during the first two to ten weeks of gestation. Even then, the effects on the embryo do not always parallel the intensity of the maternal disease; and rubella does not seem to cause clefts. An oral cleft appeared in only one of forty-nine children studied following the epidemic of German measles and may have been coincidental in that case and in others that have been reported infrequently.

If rubella is not an important factor, do other viral infections influence the incidence of clefts? Mumps and influenza are among those infectious diseases suspected of an association with clefts, but neither of them has been shown to be significant. However, a report that the incidence of clefts was higher in urban than in rural areas in England led to the recommendation that the effect of infections in more densely populated areas should be studied (Woolf and others, 1963).

Another infectious disease, toxoplasmosis, was found in 11.8 percent of mothers whose children had clefts and in only 4.5 percent of the general population (Erdélyi, 1957). In additional investigations of this same problem, positive test results for toxoplasmosis were obtained in 6.4 percent of sixty-one mothers whose children had "fissure anomalies" and in 3 percent of the general population. The investigator believed that toxoplasmosis may, in some cases, produce congenital anomalies, the embryo being affected by the diaplacental route. However, he warned, toxoplasmosis should be regarded as only one of many exogenous causes of such anomalies and not as an essential etiological factor.

At least one other investigator (Gabka, in Wallace, 1960) reported "special connections between the origin of the cleft formations and the toxoplasmosis" (pp. 7–8); and this reporter also indicated that "toxoplasmosis is one of the many exogenous factors, which also has a primary influence on the origin of the foetal clefts" (p. 8). The observation that children of farm laborers had more clefts than children whose fathers had any other occupation (Greene and others, 1964), in combination with the note that women in contact with domestic animals are more likely to contract toxoplasmosis than men (Erdélyi, 1957), may stimulate further investigation.

Changes in conditions of pressure within the amniotic sac have been thought to bring about deformities when the fetal environment is modified by the puncture of the sac walls or by oxygen deprivation. Some research has indicated that puncture of the amniotic sac brings about malformations in mice but not in humans; however, a group at McGill University (Trasler and others, 1956) cautioned that withdrawal of amniotic fluid to determine the sex of a child might induce cleft palate. In 115 malformed and 190 normal children, anomalies in the amniotic fluid were significantly higher in the defective group, which included children with defects other than clefts (Sayegh, 1964). Fraser (1955) described an interference to shelf force resulting from puncture of the amniotic sac in mice for the injection of cortisone just before palatal closure. The heads of the mice pressed down on their chests; and the pressure of the tongue seemed too great for the palatine shelves, which could not force the tongue down and continue their movement toward the midline and fusion. Similar observations were made on the development of fetal mice following withdrawal of amniotic fluid just prior to the time of normal palatal closure (Walker, 1959).

Reduction of atmospheric pressure or limitation of oxygen (hypoxia) can cause anomalies, including clefts, in animals if such deprivation occurs at the critical point in prenatal development (Warkany and Kalter, 1957; Ingalls and Philbrook, 1958). Dysplastic lesions of the facial and oral tissues as a result of local necroses, probably due to a circulatory failure that might be placental in nature, also were cited as causes of palatal clefts. According to this point of view, the palate is vulnerable to such circulatory failures because of its bilateral origin and because of the marginal areas where capillaries are formed during approximation and fusion of the palatine processes (Keith, 1940).

Investigators of such relatively specific factors as nutrition, drugs, and radiation, although they encountered many difficulties, did not have the problems of those who tried to find whether or not emotional stress contributed to the incidence of clefts in animals and humans. The maternal memory bias mentioned by Fraser (1959) undoubtedly affected the findings in retrospective studies, and the differences in findings may have resulted from acceptance or rejection of reports made by mothers who had traumatic and emotional episodes during the first trimesters of pregnancies that resulted in children with clefts.

In one investigation (Strean and Peer, 1956), 228 mothers of children with clefts, 221 white and 7 black, were asked to list any emotional disturbances they experienced during the first trimester of the pregnancy being studied. Fifty-two of these mothers reported disease or trauma in the eighth to tenth week; and 155 cited deaths in the family, loss of employment, incompatibility, concern over a previous miscarriage, and other emotional factors during the first three months. Using the same group as a control, the investigators found that few of the mothers had similar disturbances during pregnancies with their other children and that 10 percent refrained from becoming pregnant again after the birth of a child with a cleft. The conclusion drawn was:

> There must be a threshold of stress tolerance (for physiologic as well as psychologic stress) below which normal children result. This threshold may vary with different individuals and also with the same woman, depending upon the factors operating at the specific time. [P. 4]

In another report, one of the investigators (Peer, in Wallace, 1960) defined stress as any factor occurring during pregnancy which may adversely affect the development of an embryo; and the stress factor, as he used it at that time, included vitamin deficiency, cortisone intoxication, oxygen deprivation, exposure to x-ray, and virus infections as well as psychological stress. He stated:

> It is possible that some pregnant women, as a result of stress in the early months of pregnancy, secrete cortisone in sufficient amounts to inhibit palatal fusion in the embryo, even though they are receiving B_6 and folic acid in their diets. [P. 18]

The explanation that stress resulted in the catabolic effect of an abundance of cortisone was in agreement with that made by Warkany, from his experimentations with animals. Speaking of the old theory of maternal impressions, Warkany (1959) said, "Since fright can cause a release of adrenal hormones and since cortisone can induce cleft palate in certain strains of mice, a new mechanism has been found for those who want to believe in the ancient theory" (pp. 89–90).

Others (Fraser and Warburton, 1964), feeling that the maternal memory bias might have influenced conclusions, reviewed data from earlier studies and showed that stress was a factor during the first trimester of pregnancy for 18.2 percent of children born with clefts of the prepalate and palate, for 15.3 percent of those born with palatal clefts, and for 14.4 percent of the controls. The investigators conceded that the mothers reported emotional upsets more often in the pregnancies that led to the birth of the affected children than in those of their siblings, but they believed that the difference represented the tendency of the mother or the interviewer to look harder for relevant prenatal events when a child was defective. Stark and his colleagues (1962) advised that maternal stress should be largely discounted "since it cannot be properly evaluated"; they added that stress "may well have assumed the role of the twentieth century 'maternal impressions' " (p. 552).

To determine the effects of stress on animals, an experimenter subjected pregnant mice to noise, jets of air, shaking in buckets, noise of high intensity, restraint, and deprivation of food and water. The incidence of clefts in the offspring of these animals was low in comparison with that produced by cortisone, and the study offered little evidence that stress alone is teratogenic for mice (Rosenzweig, 1966).

Other psychological factors also have been investigated. Of three mothers who were institutionalized during the first trimester of pregnancy for acute depression and had five to seven applications of electroshock therapy, one had a male child with labiopalatine cleft. The defect in this child might have been present even if his mother had not received electroshock but had been emotionally disturbed, or it might have occurred quite coincidentally (Viparelli and Mastrangelo, 1964). In another study (Sayegh, 1964), psychic traumas, such as emotional shock, terror, and chronic anxiety, were significantly greater among mothers in the group whose children had malformations, not necessarily clefts. Mothers who had previous miscarriages might well be considered to experience some stress during a pregnancy, and twenty of seventy-nine informants reported miscarriage before the birth of a child with a cleft of the palate or of both prepalate and palate to Stark and his colleagues (1962); but none reported this experience prior to the birth of a child with a prepalatal cleft.

WHEN THE EVIDENCE FROM PROPONENTS OF GENETIC FACTORS AND FROM THOSE WHO ATTRIBUTE CONGENITAL CLEFTS TO ENVIRONMENTAL FACTORS HAS BEEN ASSEMBLED AND REVIEWED, ONE MAJOR AREA OF AGREEMENT IS EVIDENT. ALMOST WITHOUT EXCEPTION, THOSE WHO SUPPORT THE GENETIC THEORY CONCEDE THAT ENVIRONMENTAL FACTORS HAVE SOME EFFECT; AND, ALMOST WITHOUT EXCEPTION, THOSE WHO BELIEVE THAT ENVIRONMENT IS MORE IMPORTANT THAN INHERITANCE AS A CAUSE OF CLEFTS ACCEPT THE FACT THAT INHERITANCE CAN HAVE SOME EFFECT.

As a result of this agreement, theories that combine the major reasons for the appearance of clefts have been proposed by current writers, with varying emphases. The following statements illustrate this point:

> It seems reasonable to suppose that, where there exists a predisposition to abnormal development, additional factors may seal the fate of a developing part by exerting their influences during the early stages of intra-uterine life. [McNeil, 1954, pp. 99–100]

> From era to era the favor has swung from the devil to heredity to the environment to variations on these themes. . . . Hence, in animal experiments it seems that a complex interplay of genetic and environmental factors is responsible for the appearance of cleft palate. [Warkany and Kalter, 1957, p. 9]

> . . . the genetic predisposition may make the embryo react in a particular way to rather minor environmental difference. . . . Any single clinical entity is likely to include a variety of etiologically different types. [Fraser, 1959, p. 100; 1960, p. 155]

> The preceding century presented a very great number of different experiences regarding the causative factors, but in recent years most of these aetiological elements have proved to be more or less important, and gradually all investigators have adopted the view that endogenic factors such as the inheritance as well as exogenic factors such as the environmental agents must be an important causative element. [Gabka, in Wallace, 1960, p. 7]

> A reasonable assumption would seem to be that, in the 75 per cent. of patients with a negative family history, two factors may be required to result in cleft palate or cleft lip offspring—the genetic racial tendency for cleft palate or lip deformity strengthened or enforced by a stress factor during the mother's pregnancy. [Peer, in Wallace, 1960, p. 16]

> The germ plasm may be susceptible hereditarily to teratogenic insults otherwise innocuous. . . . [Stark and others, 1962, p. 552]

> Though there is strong evidence that both genetic and environmental forces are involved in cleft formation, the genetic mechanism has not been described adequately nor have specific environmental forces been identified. Theories based on environment alone or on genetics alone cannot fully explain the data in the literature. [Greene, 1963, p. 599]

> Sporadic case families and multiple case families occur at a frequency in the population supporting the hypothesis that congenital clefts of the lip and palate are etiologically heterogeneous. [Woolf and others, 1963, p. 214]

> Over the last 10 years, their etiology [clefts of the lip, palate, and jaw] has been studied but, similar to other investigators, we have failed to establish

> whether the malformation and its causes could be traced back to some external influence (during the intrauterine development of the fetus), or are of purely genetic nature. [Hollmann, 1969, p. 167]

Fraser's statement in 1955, although it antedates some of the above, could serve as a summary of these opinions:

> . . . it is clear that palate closure is a complicated event, involving several delicately integrated processes. Presumably each of these processes is influenced by many genetic and environmental factors. It is useless, therefore, to think of cleft palate as a single entity, or to argue about whether it is hereditary or environmental in origin. [P. 360]

The theory of single cause sufficed when knowledge of congenital anomalies and of oral clefts was limited. Superstition was often comforting because it required only acceptance, not complete understanding, and because it tended to place responsibility on the uncontrollable, not on the decisions, choices, or actions of man. Attributing clefts to inheritance brought some responsibility; and eugenic advice, which might be followed or not, became available to those who would take advantage of it. Evidence that clefts can result from environmental factors, not all of which can be controlled, confused the issue and distributed the responsibility among physicians, parents, and fate. The combination of theories of inheritance and environment seems to provide the best solution to the question of the cause of clefts of the prepalate and palate. These anomalies probably result from an unfortuitous combination of circumstances, genetic and environmental, temporal and spatial, controllable and beyond control, physical and psychological.

Many questions about the etiology of clefts remain unanswered, in spite of the diligence with which the causes of these congenital anomalies have been sought. Studies of familial incidence, race, types and locations of clefts, sex differences, the effects of teratogenic agents, and other factors have not explained all the inconsistencies and contradictions that remain.

If one accepts the fact that congenital anomalies of the prepalate and palate appear with more frequency in some families than in the general population, what accounts for the appearance, in these same families, of many members who do not have clefts? What is the explanation for the large percentage of children with clefts whose families show no previous incidence of this physical anomaly or others?

How does race affect the incidence of clefts? The evidence of differences is clear, but what factors in certain races cause a higher incidence? Fraser

(1959), pointing out that clefts associated with multiple defects were more common in the Japanese than in Caucasians, added:

> It is as if the Japanese had a lower threshold of abnormality for harelip than the Caucasians, so that a developmental disturbance causing a central nervous system malformation would be more likely to push a Japanese than a Caucasian over the harelip threshold as well. [P. 105]

This evidence of the susceptibility to clefts in one of the Oriental races also mentioned in other reports (Krantz and Henderson, 1947; Neel, 1958) is not confirmed by data on incidence in the Chinese in Hawaii, who seemed more resistant to clefts than the Japanese. Perhaps the consistently low incidence of clefts in some races can be explained by eugenic practices that resulted in the death of malformed infants in some primitive tribes; but why do American Indians, who also may have used these practices, have a high incidence of clefts? If heredity is a major factor in the incidence of clefts, did intermarriage among American Indians in the past (Tretsven, 1965) contribute to the high incidence of clefts in this group today? In such a case, should not the modern custom of marriage outside the tribe have reduced the incidence? Other questions on racial variations are similar (Carter, 1963). Would the low incidence of facial clefts in nonwhites in the United States and Europe be found also in natives of West Africa? One report (Millard and McNeill, 1965) provided an example of a geographically separate area with a preponderantly black population that had a low incidence of clefts, but the question of incidence in more isolated parts of the world still remains. Would Japanese who had been in the United States for two or three generations have the same high incidence of clefts as those who had not left their native country? If skin color affects the resistance to clefts, then the lower incidence in Negroes, mulattoes, and Puerto Ricans and the higher incidence in countries such as Finland and Denmark might support this idea. According to Mason (1877), "Mr. Ramsey, who read a paper at the Odontological Society in 1865, stated . . . that he had never seen a case of cleft palate in which the patient's complexion was dark" (p. 65). Considering this point, Mason was inclined to think that most of the patients he had seen had a somewhat nervous temperament and that many, perhaps the majority, had fair complexions. If skin color is the important factor, do peoples with certain complexions reside in areas that affect the incidence of clefts; or do groups with certain skin colors experience nutritional deprivations or excesses that may account for the differences?

How do theories on cause account for the types and locations of clefts? If, as evidence in Chapter One suggests, unilateral clefts appear more often on the left than on the right, is this the result of fetal position, of the possibility that the left side of the body is less completely developed, of the sex of the child, or of some other factor? What defends the right side? What makes the left more vulnerable?

Why are the prepalate and the palate, as separate entities, less susceptible to anomaly than the combination of the two? The distribution of cleft types, shown in Chapter One, shows that this is the case. Can questions on incidence of isolated and combined clefts be answered by findings from studies that differentiate the developmental patterns of the prepalatal area from those of the palate, as Chapter Two indicated?

Do factors that determine the sex of the child also reduce the resistance of the male, who is apparently more susceptible to congenital anomalies; or do they increase the resistance of the female? Does the female, in spite of her resistance to clefts in general, have a special weakness that results in the appearance of more palatal clefts? The more frequent occurrence of prepalatal clefts in the male and of palatal clefts in the female, as cited in Chapter One, needs explanation. What is the significance of the statement (Meskin and others, 1968) that, independent of major cleft type, the female with a facial cleft appears to have a greater likelihood of demonstrating a complete cleft than does her male counterpart?

If one monozygotic twin has a cleft and the other does not, what environmental influences affect one fetus and not the other? Does one crowd the other and bring about positional impediments to the moving palatal shelves, thus producing a condition that interferes with fusion? Are some twin pairs thought to be monozygotic really dizygotic and hence independently vulnerable or resistant to clefts? Why does twinning seem to predispose to clefts, and why does this predisposition differ in its effects?

Teratogenic agents of various kinds have produced clefts in experimental animals, but their variant effectiveness gives rise to other questions. Why did one strain of mice produce so many babies with cleft palates while another did not? What made cortisone the effective agent it was for the susceptible strain? Why did some animals react to riboflavin deficiency by producing young with posterior cleft palates but not anterior clefts? In the human, what limits the effect of rubella on the lip and palate while permitting it to affect the eye and ear?

What relationships exist between clefts of the facial area and other congenital anomalies? Do the clefts, in the absence of other deformities, bring about abortions in which the presence of clefts is not detected? The multiply deformed fetus may abort and die before term, but does the singly deformed fetus with a cleft of the prepalate or palate do so? According to one report (Drillien and others, 1966), 8.47 percent of babies with clefts in the group studied were stillborn or died soon after birth; and data from a study of death certificates (Murphy, 1947) showed that 4 percent of 935 malformed babies who died had clefts. When cleft of the prepalate or palate was the only anomaly, 88 percent of children in another study (McKeown and Record, in Wolstenholme and O'Connor, 1960) survived during the five years in which records were kept; but none of those with multiple anomalies reached the age of five. The appearance of absence deformities, congenital defects in which the upper extremities are missing or only partly formed, was accompanied by a high incidence of clefts of the prepalate and palate, according to Arne Birch-Jensen (1949). However, among the relatives of those with deformities of absence, the number of oral clefts did not exceed that in the general population. Why are some malformations accompanied by clefts while others are not? What influences that produce the Pierre Robin syndrome (micrognathia) sometimes bring about clefts as part of the anomaly? One hypothesis (Latham, 1966) was that the palatal cleft commonly associated with the Pierre Robin syndrome is a developmental defect resulting from obstruction by the tongue. Does this condition prevent the movements of the palatal shelves?

What is the significance of microforms of clefts? Do such anomalies as congenitally missing or displaced incisor teeth and pits in the lower lip represent minor deviations that could be classified as near misses, in which, under other circumstances, a cleft of the prepalate, palate, or both might have occurred? If incisor anomalies are not microforms of cleft palate (Woolf and others, 1965), is the bifid uvula, which has a higher incidence than clefts in anterior areas, a microform? What accounts for its frequency of occurrence? Can the submucosal cleft be considered a microform?

Investigation of these and many other possible inquiries about the presence of clefts in some children and the absence of them in others, about the variations in the clefts themselves, and about the factors that make for susceptibility or resistance will continue to challenge scientists for many years. Eventually, perhaps, answers to old and new questions will be seen in such perspective and relationship that the etiology of labial and palatal clefts will be more clearly understood. In the meantime, one can only echo Fraser's exclamation: "Perhaps the surprising thing is that the palate manages to close successfully so often!" (1960, p. 154).

A CLEFT INVOLVING THE LIP, THE ALVEOLAR RIDGE, THE HARD PALATE, THE SOFT PALATE, OR ALL OF THESE PARTS WAS ONCE EXPLAINED AS FAILURE OF FUSION. MORE RECENT INFORMATION HAS SHOWN THAT THE ANSWER TO "HOW DOES A CLEFT OCCUR?" MUST BE MORE ELABORATE.

Is a congenital cleft brought about by something that happens or by something that fails to happen? If the phrase "failure of fusion" can explain how clefts occur in some parts of the face, what explanation can be given for those that appear in other parts? Consideration of pathogenesis, the development of a morbid condition, as well as of etiology, the reasons for the defect, can facilitate the management of many diseases and can also increase understanding of physical abnormalities that are present at birth.

Until the middle of the twentieth century, most discussions of congenital clefts stated or implied that they resulted from the failure of the parts to come together and fuse. The descriptions in texts and articles were very similar. The following examples, although they range in time from 1799 to 1966, differ in terminology and style but not in basic information:

> . . . if a rosebud is blighted, some leaves curl up and the flower is ill-shaped, or perhaps only a few leaves appear, the rest being never completely formed or unfolded. Hence, the hare lip; the two sides of the face, which are said to be formed separately, being hereby prevented from growing together. [Underwood, 1799, in Mettler, 1947, p. 734]

> Harelip is a congenital malformation, arising from an arrest of development of the foetal structures. [In cleft palate] . . . various degrees of fissure, either of the hard or soft palate, will result from non-union. [Mason, 1877, pp. 2, 60]

> The various forms of harelip and cleft palate arise from failure of union of the separate processes which enter into the formation of the mouth and lip, the degree of the deformity depending on the incompleteness of the fusion of the individual segments. [Berry and Legg, 1912, p. 8]

> Cleft lip is nearly always due to failure of union of well developed tissues . . . . cleft palate is a fissure, a non-union of well developed parts, not, with rare exceptions, the result of arrested development nor failure of a normal quantity of tissue to enter into its structure. [Brophy, 1923, pp. 1, 73]

> It is evident that the normal development of the face is a very complicated process, involving the orderly conduct on the part of at least five pairs of primordia, and depending upon a regular and precise plan of fusion,

which neither halts prematurely nor continues excessively. [Jordan and Kindred, 1942, p. 113]

Hare-lip—a congenital malformation of the upper lip due to failure of fusion of the maxillary processes with the frontonasal process, frequently associated with cleft palate. [MacNalty, *British Medical Dictionary,* 1961, p. 656]

When the human body is formed before birth, the lips sometimes fail to grow together as they should. The result of such a failure is called harelip. In the more severe cases the palate also fails to grow together, so that harelip is combined with cleft palate. [Fishbein, *An Illustrated Medical and Health Encyclopedia,* 1963, p. 1351]

Cleft lip—a congenital facial deformity of the lip (usually the upper lip) characterized by nonfusion or malfusion of one or more of the three embryologic processes that form the upper lip. [*Stedman's Medical Dictionary,* 1966, p. 914]

As early as 1910, experiments with cat embryos led investigators to suspect that the failure in development responsible for labial clefts was not the same as the failure of fusion of the palatal shelves. Later work led to the hypothesis that, as Victor Veau explained it, a cleft in the palate is the arrest of the disappearance of the epithelial membrane, which remains intact, not penetrated by the adjacent mesoderm (Converse, 1962).

Veau was certainly aware of the theories on embryological development, although his interest in that field developed after he was sixty years old. In his text on cleft palate (1931), he omitted any discussion of embryology, saying that he hoped to undertake a study of that topic some day. Within a few years, he had done so, in collaboration with Georges Politzer of Vienna (1936). Their conclusions about the pathogenesis of bilateral, unilateral, and simple unilateral cleft lip were as follows:

Even if we disregard the difference in dynamic force in the borders of the [epithelial] wall, we find a fundamental element of unity in cleft lip. In essence, the malformation is a reduction in the dynamic force of the mesodermic masses separated at the outset by the epithelial wall. If the diminution of that force is considerable, the wall remains intact. The conjoining of its epithelial elements, which is normal, will automatically produce the cleft by preventing the union of the edges. In this case, cleft lip is total. If the diminution is less, the wall disappears only partially. This results in cleft lip with a bridge. If the lessening of force is very slight, the mesenchyme has lost its power when it invades the epithelial wall and does not have enough energy to form a completely normal lip. The result is simple cleft lip. [P. 325]

The article by Veau and Politzer, published in a French journal, did not seem to have great influence in the United States, where many writers continued, for a number of years, to follow the classical point of view. However, in 1954, Stark differentiated between the pathogenic factors responsible for prepalatal clefts and those that brought about clefts of the palate. Using the terms "primary palate," which he defined as the prolabium, the premaxilla, and the cartilaginous septum, and "secondary palate," the hard and soft palates posterior to the incisive foramen, Stark questioned the theory of the early German anatomists. This theory had proposed that the central third of the face develops from a series of facial processes, mesodermal projections covered with ectoderm, that grow together and fuse. Stark felt that, because the studies that resulted in this classic theory had used animal specimens and had been limited by less efficient instruments and techniques than those available by 1950, he should reexamine the pathogenesis of facial clefts.

In the areas of the hard and soft palate, the secondary palate, in the embryos he examined, Stark found no evidence to refute the classical theory. However, in the primary palate, the areas of the prolabium and premaxilla, he noted an absence of mesoderm at the points at which clefts occurred. In early stages of development, Stark reported, the lip and premaxilla exist as an epithelial wall in which three masses of mesoderm are normally present. If these masses grow and unite, they form the normal upper lip and premaxilla. If, however, the mesoderm is inadequate, it will not penetrate the epithelial structure; and the results of this lack of mesodermal penetration are defects of prolabial musculature and cartilage and of premaxillary teeth and bone.

In an additional report on this topic (in Schuchardt, 1966), Stark stated:

> We concluded that in all probability the primary palate exists *de novo* as an epithelial structure, and that three areas of mesodermal reinforcement are needed if this area is to develop normally. If one or two of these mesodermal masses are absent or deficient, a cleft or clefts will ensue, and the cleft or clefts will be complete or incompete, depending upon the degree of mesodermal deficiency. [P. 221]

This theory provided explanations for some anomalies—Simonart's bands and medial clefts of the lip, for example—that could not be reconciled to the classic theory of failure of fusion as the cause for clefts in the prepalatal area.

In palatal clefts, however, failure of fusion continues to be accepted as the pathogenic factor. Whether the term "palatal" refers to the area posterior to the alveolar ridge or to the incisive foramen, certain barriers to the fusion of the outgrowing palatine shelves can result in a cleft.

The shelves, which must reach midline and fuse to form an intact palate, hang down at first, with the tongue between them, as illustrated in Figure 2-11. As they move upward to a horizontal position and move toward each other, they displace the tongue and occupy the space it previously filled. In this process, the impetus given to the shelves, known as shelf force, may help to overcome the resistance of the tongue. At the same time, growth of the posterior pharyngeal wall, the mandible, and head becomes part of a complex sequence of events that is susceptible to interruption or delay. A pattern of slowness in the horizontal positioning of the shelves in female embryos (Burdi and Silvey, 1969) may help to explain the greater incidence of palatal clefts to which the female seems susceptible. Fraser (1967), theorizing about both sexes, suggested that cleft palate could occur as a result of

> . . . delay in shelf movement, due to increased shelf force, or increased tongue resistance, or other obstruction to the shelf; an abnormal shelf, which may be too narrow, or pathologically incapable of movement; failure of shelf fusion; abnormal head width; or post-closure opening. [P. 1605]

Thus, the ultimate failure of fusion, commonly accepted as the cause of palatal clefts, may be the result of events that take place before the shelves come into contact and have the opportunity to fuse or after contact has been established.

The possibility of rupture of already-fused palatal shelves, mentioned by Fraser, was confirmed in experimentation with animals in a report (Angelici, 1968) of the reopening of fused epithelial surfaces in the palatal shelves of two A/Jax mouse embryos. In describing epithelial remnants and epithelial pearls, another investigator (Kitamura, 1966) interpreted these clumps of epithelial tissue as evidence that most palatal clefts in humans are the result of postfusion rupture that results from some embryopathic condition. Although many writers have seemed to believe that, once the mesenchymal fusion takes place, a cleft cannot occur, the statement that epithelial pearls or remnants are the site of original fusion, followed by rupture, presented a scientific point of view that supported early beliefs that a cleft was a split or rupture of a completely formed structure.

THE DIFFERENCES BETWEEN CLEFTS OF THE PREPALATE AND THOSE OF THE PALATE SUGGEST THAT THESE ARE TWO QUITE DISPARATE PHENOMENA GENETICALLY, ENVIRONMENTALLY, AND PATHOMORPHOLOGICALLY.

Clefts of the prepalate and palate differ in a number of ways. Classifications of clefts have recognized these differences, as discussions in Chapter Four will indicate. The genetic point of view, with its distinction between the terms "harelip with or without cleft palate" and "cleft palate," also differentiated the prepalatal from the palatal area, although not in the same way that research on morphology tended to separate the two kinds of clefts. The preponderance of palatal clefts in fetuses of experimental animals subjected to environmental teratogenic agents also emphasized the difference between clefts of the palate and those of the prepalate. The times at which growth of the two areas takes place also differ, as the descriptions in Chapter Two pointed out. One failure may even lead to the other, and

> . . . disturbances of growth leading to the cleft of lip and alveolar process may disturb the further changes to such a degree that, secondarily, failure of formation of the primary palate may prevent the normal formation of the secondary palate. [Orban, 1957, p. 18]

Differentiation of the processes of growth of the prepalate and palate and of interruptions to these processes may facilitate research on the incidence, types, and causes of clefts. Recognition of the differences between prepalatal and palatal clefts may bring a desirable consistency in terminology to laboratories and clinics, to journals and texts, to study and teaching, and to specialists' discussions of congenital orofacial anomalies. Furthermore, recognition of the effects of the two kinds of clefts on appearance and on speech may lead to modification and improvement in management of the children who present these problems.

However, the fact that clefts of the prepalate and palate do not always occur separately, even though they may have differing morphologies, often necessitates joint consideration of the two anomalies. If, as incidence figures in Chapter One indicated, clefts of both the prepalate and the palate occur in approximately half of the children who present clefts, those concerned with habilitation must be prepared to provide management for the three major types of congenital orofacial malformations; the considerations in succeeding chapters will recognize this fact, in spite of the advantages of separating prepalatal from palatal clefts in the search for causal factors.

CHAPTER FOUR

Types and Effects of Clefts

THE STRUCTURAL VARIATIONS IN THE NEWBORN WHO PRESENT CONGENITAL ANOMALIES OF THE FACIAL AREA HAVE BEEN CLASSIFIED IN MANY WAYS.

The embryologist, looking at developing structures, chooses his classifications on the basis of his particular interest. The surgeon, concerned with the observable postnatal manifestations of embryological malfunction, classifies clefts in terms of his reparative techniques. The dentist establishes classifications that apply to his specific concerns. The geneticist may classify in conformance to principles that have been shown to affect the inheritance of the malformation. The speech pathologist may be influenced by the relationships of the clefts to speech behavior. Regardless of their specialties, those who are concerned with the prevention or management of clefts of the prepalate and palate recognize that various classifications have been established to distinguish the type, severity, and location of the structural defects; and they may find that adoption of a mutually acceptable system of classification will facilitate interdisciplinary communication.

No single system of classification of clefts has been adopted, although many have been proposed. Some of the plans have been complex; others have used relatively simple terminology but complicated subcategories; still others have been so simplified that they could not be accepted by members of all the disciplines concerned. Prior to 1958, many individuals proposed classifications for such clefts, each choosing the types and combinations that seemed appropriate to him.

Truman Brophy, for example, based his surgical procedures on the type of cleft and described sixteen different types, picturing fifteen of them in the text he published in 1923. Werner Birkenfeld (1926) listed four types of clefts—cleft lip, cleft of the hard palate, cleft of the soft palate, and cleft lip in conjunction with cleft palate. J. Sanders's report (1934) on the incidence of clefts in Holland used the term "harelip" to mean cleft lip with or without cleft palate and included "cleft hard palate" and "cleft soft palate" as additional classifications. Poul Fogh-Andersen stated (1942) that the Scandinavians distinguished simply among "harelip," "harelip plus cleft palate," and "cleft palate"; but he reported on only two categories in his discussion of the inheritance of clefts. George Dorrance and J. W. Bransfield used six classes in a discussion in 1946; and C. Kerr McNeil, in a publication in 1954, presented a four-class system that was applicable to the dental operator and that was based on the degree of severity of the palatal deformity. Others cited, as the three major categories of clefts, those of the lip, of the lip and palate and velum, and of the palate and velum; and they added the category of an insufficient palate that might affect speech (Pruzansky, 1953; Koepp-Baker, in Travis, 1957).

Among the early classifications that have endured are those proposed by John Staige Davis and Harry Ritchie (1922) and by Victor Veau (1931). These two systems were based on similar concepts. The classifications made by Davis and Ritchie were derived from the proposition that the alveolar process was the logical foundation for a surgical grouping of clefts, and Veau's classifications were also "essentially surgical."

Davis and Ritchie categorized clefts in three groups: (1) those of the prealveolar process, in which the lip was cleft unilaterally or bilaterally or even medially, the alveolar process was normal, and a palatal cleft might be present; (2) those of the postalveolar process, in which the alveolar process was normal but the soft palate, hard palate, and perhaps the lip were affected; and (3) those of the alveolar process, with which clefts of the lip and palate were usually associated.

Veau described the following types of palatal clefts: (1) simple divisions of the soft palate; (2) divisions of the soft palate and of the hard palate without cleft lip; (3) unilateral clefts, in which the alveolar ridge was involved, the cleft being between the premaxilla and maxilla; and (4) bilateral clefts, in which the premaxilla was completely isolated, with accompanying total bilateral labial clefts. In describing prepalatal clefts, Veau (1938) used another fourfold grouping: simple unilateral cleft of the lip, total unilateral, simple bilateral, and complete bilateral. Veau stipulated that palatal clefts did not accompany the simple unilateral form of cleft lip. He divided the simple bilateral form into two subclasses, symmetrical and asymmetrical; and he made three divisions in the total bilateral form, two accompanied by cleft palate and one without palatal cleft.

Although Veau's classification of prepalatal clefts did not achieve great popularity, his system of categorizing clefts of the palate became the classic description and has persisted to the present. Reference to a "Type I cleft" or a "Type III cleft" was convenient; the use of a posterior-to-anterior sequence seemed logical; and Veau was held in high regard by members of the several disciplines that needed to report clefts by type.

Until 1958, most descriptions of clefts followed Veau's plan or the one proposed by Davis and Ritchie. Since 1958, changes in classifications of clefts have been recommended by several writers; and a new system of categorization has been adopted by the American Cleft Palate Association.

Some modifications of Veau's classifications were introduced in centers in the United States (Bzoch, 1960; Olin, 1960). A system of categorization used in Spain (Vilar-Sancho, 1962) identified the four anatomic elements that can be affected by latinized initial letters of Greek words. "K" indicated a cleft of the lip, "G" a cleft of the alveolar process, "U" a cleft of the hard palate, and "S" a cleft of the soft palate. A complete bilateral cleft of both prepalate and palate, in this system, would be designated as "K2 G2 U2 S Sk." The Hamburg system, based on embryonic aspects (Pfeifer, in Schuchardt, 1966), used a schematic representation of the affected areas, with the different types of clefts being shown by darkening or shading areas on the drawings. Procedures for coding classifications of clefts were recommended (McCabe, 1966; Santiago, 1969) to permit specific description and to facilitate data retrieval for research purposes. These proposals appeared in the literature from several disciplines after the American Cleft Palate Association had accepted the plan presented by its Nomenclature Committee, but none has been widely adopted.

In 1958, Desmond Kernahan and Richard Stark had proposed that the incisive foramen, representing the junction between the "primary" and "secondary" palates, was a more suitable point on which to base a classification than was the alveolus, the basis of Davis and Ritchie's groupings. They pointed out:

> At the time of the original presentation of Davis and Ritchie's anatomical classification, Blair commented that, "with future development in cleft lip and cleft palate surgery, the alveolar division might come to be disregarded and one would have a classification based upon an anatomical concept which had not stood the test of time." This statement has proved prophetic in light of subsequent advances in embryology, with doubt being cast upon the classical concept of fusion of facial processes by the newer theory of mesodermal penetration, and in the light of surgical advance which closes the lip and anterior palate as the first operation on the deformed child in most clinics. [Stark and Kernahan, 1959, p. 45]

The categories of clefts that Stark and Kernahan (1959) proposed were:

> *Clefts of primary palate:* Clefts lying anterior to the incisive foramen, clefts occurring in the "primary palate" as a result of failure of proper mesodermal penetration. Thus this group would include defects from minor notches of the lip to encircling defects of the premaxilla.
>
> *Clefts of secondary palate:* Clefts lying posterior to the incisive foramen, those due to a failure of the fusion of the two palatal processes which should form the secondary palate.
>
> *Clefts of primary and secondary palate:* Clefts which combine these two important embryological events, failure of normal development of both the "primary" and the "secondary" palates which implies prolonged, continuing insult to developing germ plasm. [P. 46]

The Nomenclature Committee of the American Cleft Palate Association recommended that the association adopt a morphological classification of congenital clefts based on the categories suggested by Kernahan and Stark. In its reports (Harkins and others, 1960, 1962), the committee designated the incisive foramen as the point of division but changed the terms "primary palate" and "secondary palate" to "prepalate" and "palate." Illustrations accompanying that report have been adapted for the following figures, which show some of the various types of prepalatal and palatal clefts.

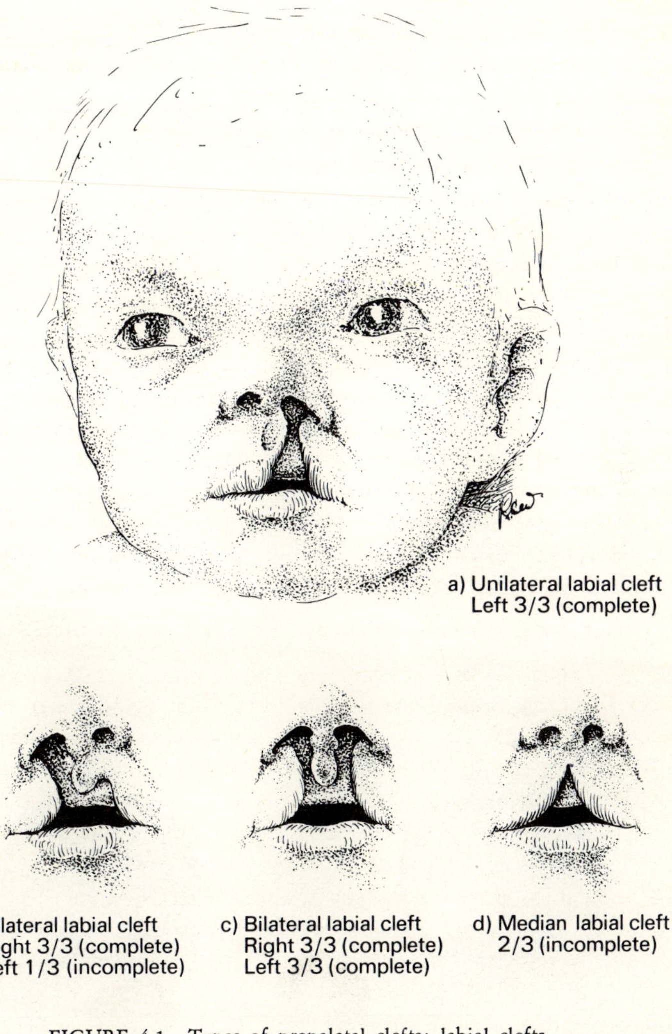

FIGURE 4-1 Types of prepalatal clefts: labial clefts.

In the plan adopted by the American Cleft Palate Association in 1960, a labial cleft may be unilateral, bilateral, or median; the side on which a unilateral cleft appears is stated; and the extent of a labial cleft, from the vermilion border of the lip toward the nostril, is indicated in thirds. Figure 4-1 shows some of the types of labial clefts, including a median cleft of the lip, a classification that has been questioned by those who believe that the so-called median cleft is really unilateral. However, the anomaly, though rare, has been reported by some investigators (Ecker, 1958; Fogh-Andersen, 1965; Baibak and Bromberg, 1966; Gier and Fast, 1967) and has been described (Millard and Williams, 1968) as any congenital, vertical cleft through the center of the upper lip, with no vestige of the prolabium present.

A cleft of the alveolar process, in the plan accepted by the American Cleft Palate Association, is also described in terms of location and extent, with submucous clefts in the alveolar area being included in this category. Some examples of alveolar clefts are shown in Figure 4-2.

A prepalatal cleft, one that involves both the lip and the alveolus, is described by side and extent; protrusion of the prepalate is designated as none, slight, moderate, or marked; and rotation of the prepalate is reported in these same terms. In Figure 4-3, some typical prepalatal clefts are illustrated; Figure 4-4 shows the protruding premaxilla and prolabium.

A cleft of the soft palate, in this classification system, is described by its posteroanterior extent in thirds and by its maximum width in millimeters; and palatal shortness or a submucous cleft in the area of the soft palate

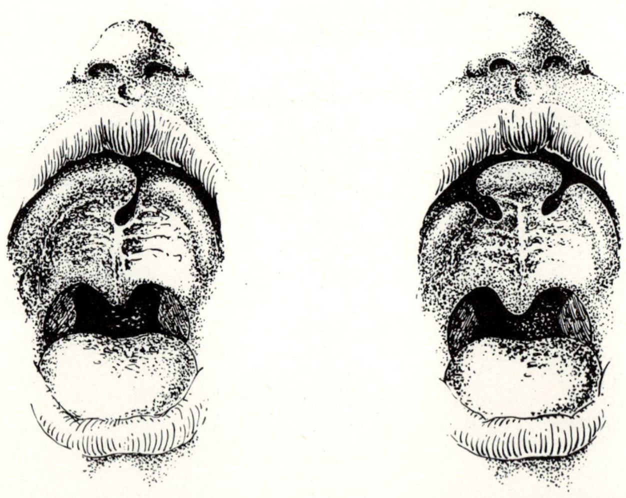

a) Unilateral alveolar cleft
Left 3/3 (complete)

b) Bilateral alveolar cleft
Right 3/3 (complete)
Left 3/3 (complete)

FIGURE 4-2 Types of prepalatal clefts: alveolar clefts.

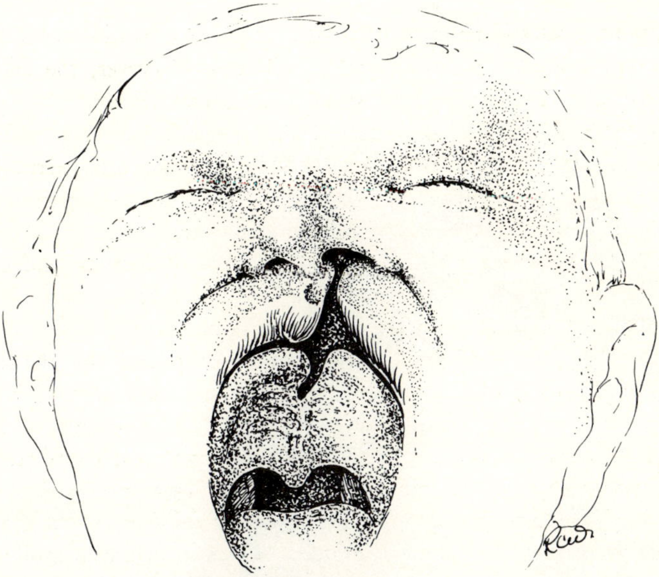

a) Unilateral clefts of lip and alveolar process (prepalate)
Left lip 3/3 (complete)
Left alv. process 3/3 (complete)

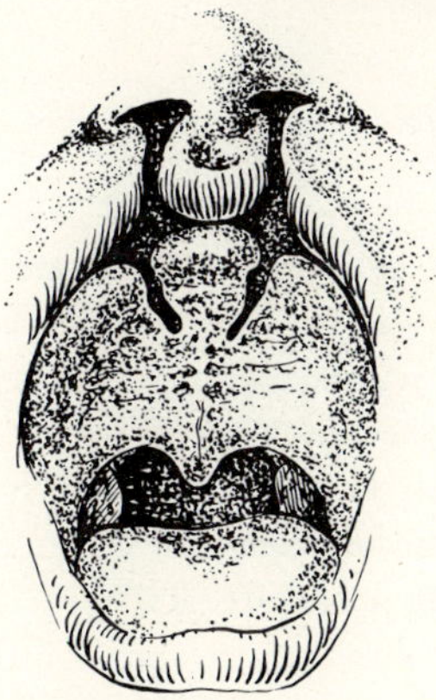

b) Bilateral clefts
Right 3/3 (complete)
Left 3/3 (complete)

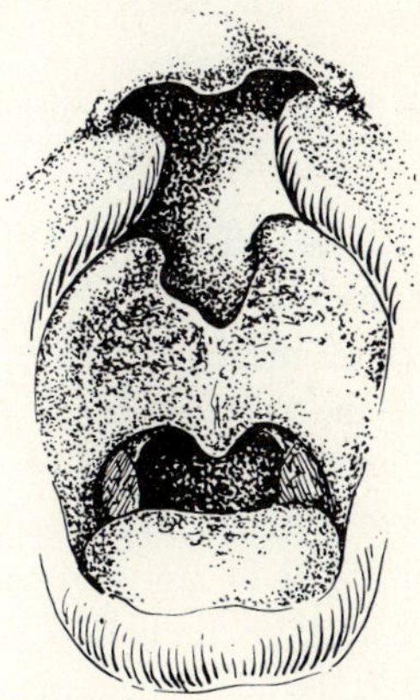

c) Median cleft of lip and alveolar process
Premaxilla and overlying lip absent

FIGURE 4-3 Types of prepalatal clefts: labial and alveolar clefts.

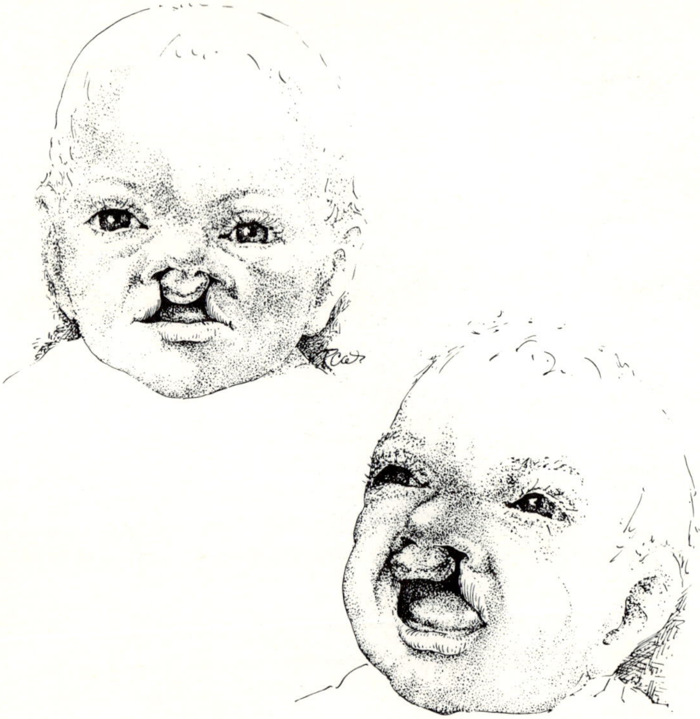

FIGURE 4-4 Types of prepalatal clefts: protrusion of premaxilla and prolabium.

can be reported. These variations in clefts of the soft palate are shown in Figure 4-5.

A cleft of the hard palate, if one exists without being combined with a cleft of the soft palate, is reported in posteroanterior extent by thirds, in width, in the attachment of one palatal shelf to the vomer if such attachment is observed, and in the extent of any submucous cleft that be present.

Combinations of clefts of the hard and soft palate are described in terms used for a cleft of the palatal area. These combinations are shown in Figures 4-6 and 4-7, the attachment of one palatal shelf to the vomer being illustrated in Figure 4-7.

An additional category provided by the Nomenclature Committee included rare or atypical clefts, such as those of the mandibular process (Monroe, 1966), those that are nasoocular in direction, and those that are oroocular. This fourth classification might well include, also, several other kinds of

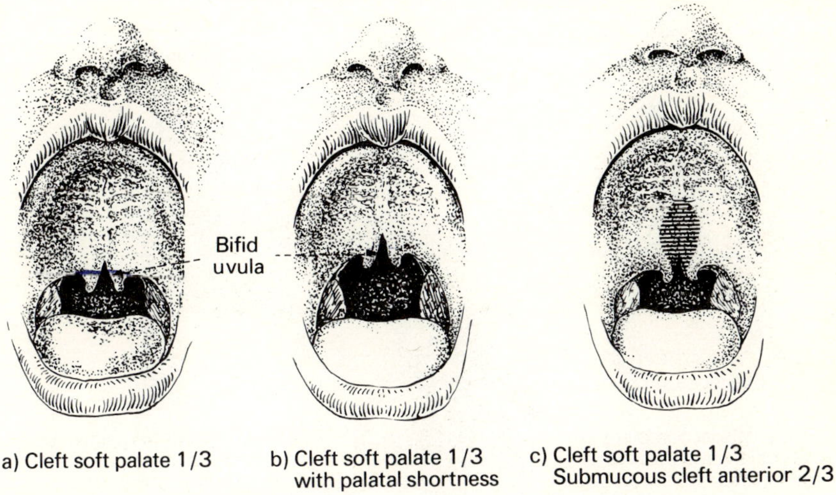

FIGURE 4-5 Types of palatal clefts: clefts of the soft palate.

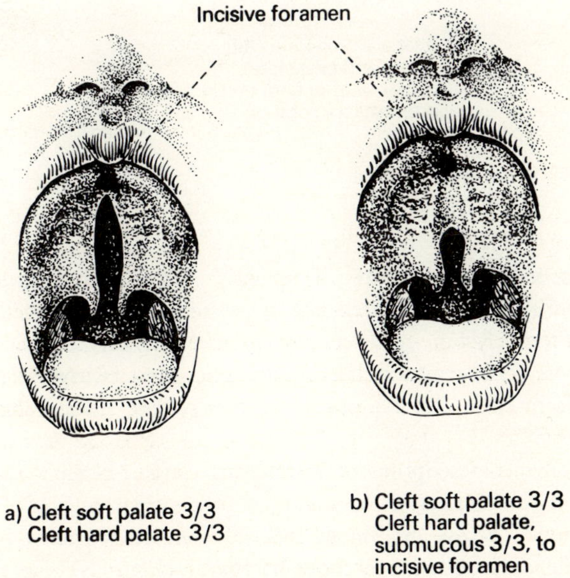

FIGURE 4-6 Types of palatal clefts: clefts of the hard palate.

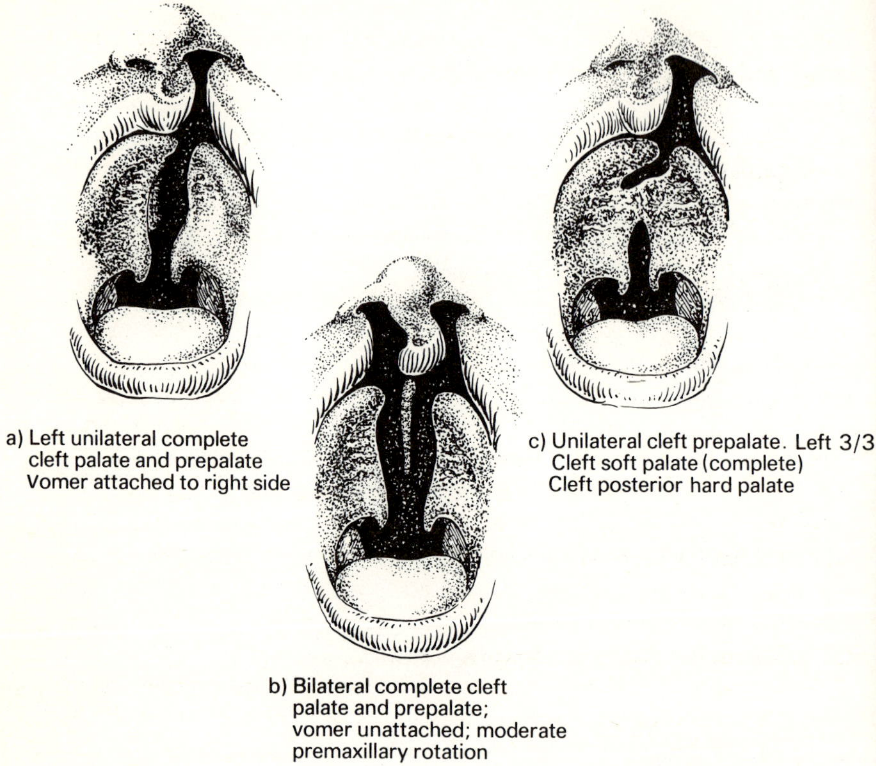

FIGURE 4-7 Types of palatal clefts: clefts of the hard and soft palates.

orofacial anomalies that appear infrequently: submucous clefts that are not associated with clefts of the prepalate or palate, clefts that sometimes accompany the Pierre Robin syndrome, congenital pits in the lower lip, the "cleft lip nose," congenital palatal insufficiency, and transverse facial clefts. These malformations can be placed in the general classification of "rare clefts."

James Calnan's description of submucous clefts (1954b) included considerations of the diagnostic signs and symptoms characteristic of the failure of muscle union across the velum that is often accompanied by shortness of the palate and incompetent velopharyngeal closure. These defects may not be visible, and their presence may not be detected until their influence on speech can be noted. Occult, or hidden, clefts of the hard palate also may occur, the bony palate being incomplete but covered with mucous membrane; and such clefts are not readily discerned by observation. However, abnormal patterns of swallowing, a short palate, a large oropharyngeal isthmus, and evidence from transillumination may indicate the presence of a submucous cleft in the region of the soft or the hard palate, although the mucous membrane covering of the prepalate and palate is intact.

Described in detail by Pierre Robin, the syndrome that bears his name sometimes combines an incomplete cleft of the palate with micrognathia and glossoptosis. The baby born with a small jaw and abnormal backward positioning of the tongue presents problems in respiration and feeding; and, if a palatal cleft is also present, the difficulties are increased, although probably not to the extent suggested by Robin. Studies of this syndrome (Randall and others, 1965; Cocke, 1966; Latham, 1966; McEvitt, 1968) indicated that the palatal clefts often associated with the syndrome are secondary to the mandibular retrognathia, that the fusion of the palate may have been prevented by the retropositioning of the tongue, that the etiology of the syndrome has not been clearly established, and that the normal growth potential noted in some Pierre Robin patients does not exist in all of them. Although Robin stated that this condition occurs in three out of five babies, the syndrome is relatively infrequent (Randall and others, 1965).

The appearance of clefts in conjunction with pits in the lower lip, referred to as Van der Woude's syndrome, constitutes another type of defect that could be called atypical. Congenital mandibular lip pits are rare, only 200 being reported between 1835 and 1967; the association of clefts of the prepalate or palate with these defects has been variously reported. Anne Van der Woude (1954) found that 80 percent of the cases with "fistula labii inferioris congenita" had clefts of the prepalate, palate, or both. Others (Coccia and Bixler, 1967) stated that almost one-third of those born with pits in the lower lip are free from clefts. In sixty-six cases with these labial defects, the tendency was toward clefts of both prepalate and palate, according to other investigators (Červenka and others, 1967). Van der Woude pointed out that the effects of the syndrome may vary and that it occurs infrequently.

The defect called "cleft lip nose," in which a nasal deformity resembling those that occur with labial clefts appears as an isolated anomaly, is also rare. Reports of a small number of cases (Boo-Chai and Tange, 1968; Tulenko, 1968) indicated that the defect may result from a mild mesodermal deficiency and that it may occur in conjunction with congenital labial scars or minimal labial clefts as well as alone.

Various degrees of palatal insufficiency have been noted in individuals whose palates are intact. In some instances, the shortness of the soft palate is the deviation from normal. In others, the palate has adequate length; but the oropharynx is so deep that velopharyngeal valving cannot be accomplished successfully. These conditions of congenital palatopharyngeal inadequacy have been observed as accompaniments to prepalatal clefts and in conjunction with anomalies of the cervical area. Roentgencephalometric review of a large number of cases (Osborne and Pruzansky, 1968) showed greater prevalence of cervical anomalies in patients with "congenital palatopharyngeal incompetence," the term used to describe nasality without overt palatal cleft, than in those with clefts of the prepalate or palate. Another study (Mason and Hoster, 1968) referred to congenital pharyngeal incompetence as a "cleft subtype" and reported eleven cases with congenital palatopharyngeal incompetence and labial clefts. The presence of a short palate, an abnormally deep nasopharynx, or a combination of the two, can be considered in the category of atypical conditions of the orofacial area.

Another rare type of anomaly is the congenital transverse facial cleft, an unusual condition that results from failure of embryonic mandibular and maxillary processes to fuse and form the corners of the mouth (Powell and Jenkins, 1968; Boo-Chai, 1969). In a period of thirty years, one observer (Fogh-Andersen, 1965) found only twelve such malformations in a total of almost 4,000 patients with facial clefts. This type of anomaly will be seen rarely and, with the even less frequent oblique cleft (Sakurai and others, 1966), can logically be placed in the category of atypical orofacial defects.

With appropriate provision for thorough description, therefore, the types of clefts can be put into four major classes: clefts of the prepalate, clefts of the palate, clefts of both prepalate and palate, and atypical defects. This system of classification seems to meet the requirements set by the Nomenclature Committee of the American Cleft Palate Association. It contains concise but clear definitions of terms, it is convenient to use, and it can stimulate research by providing common terminology for the exchange of information. Although "prepalatal" may be a controversial term (Ivy, 1962a), "primary" and "secondary" seem less desirable because of the use made of these terms in describing surgical procedures. Even if the prepalate is of "primary" order in prenatal development, the terms "prepalatal" and "palatal" are convenient to use as modifiers of "cleft" and can be changed readily to noun forms.

The consistency and relative simplicity of the system of classification just described in some detail could make it useful to all the disciplines concerned with congenital anomalies of the facial area. Records could include classifications that would be clear to all who read them, and the four major types of clefts could be numbered if numerical indication proved to be a convenience. However, the subclassifications of the system defended here are important to clarity of description; and the statement that a child has "a labial cleft, right, two-thirds" might be more specific than the statement that he has "a cleft lip." Similarly, "prepalatal cleft, bilateral, one-third" might be more meaningful than "a cleft of both the lip and the alveolar process, each of which is incompletely affected." Surely, "bilateral prepalatal cleft and palatal cleft, both three-thirds, with protrusion and rotation to the left of the prepalate" would be more specific than "complete cleft of the lip and palate." Perhaps no one system of classifying congenital clefts will ever be adopted. The plan presented here has not been used widely (McCabe, 1966); but it seems to have many advantages for those concerned with individuals with clefts, whether that concern is with management or with research.

JUST AS DIFFERENT COMBINATIONS OF CIRCUMSTANCES RESULT IN VARIOUS TYPES OF CONGENITAL CLEFTS, SO THESE CLEFTS AFFECT CHILDREN IN VARIOUS WAYS.

No single or simple description of the effects of clefts is possible, although the typical speech and typical personality of the cleft palate child have been described.

One child may have speech that is like that of many others born with the same general physical malformations; another may speak well, with or without special training. Some may have hearing losses; others will escape the involvements of defective hearing. Some children with severely deforming clefts may be accepted by their families; others, whose congenital facial anomalies are minimal, may be rejected. One child born with a cleft of the prepalate or palate may use his limited intellectual capacities maximally; another may have normal or better-than-normal intelligence but fail to achieve academically and socially. The child with a repaired cleft may present problems in social adjustment that lessen as he becomes an adult; or he may seem well-adjusted until he reaches adolescence and then present some deviations in personality. He may, throughout his life, be far more like others than different from them; or he may, almost from the outset, present multiple problems in adjustment, learning, and communication. Some of the individual differences of the child born with a cleft may be the result of his physical anomalies; other differences may have little relationship to his physical deviations but may stem from traits that would have been present if the child had been born with no physical malformation.

The effects of a congenital cleft of the prepalate, palate, or both will vary with the type and extent of the anomaly, the age of the individual, his hearing, his environment, his intelligence, his personal characteristics, the management provided for him, and the combinations of circumstances that influence any individual. Edward Lis (in Irwin, 1965) stressed these variations when he pointed out that the child with a cleft is like all other children in some ways, like other children with clefts in his susceptibility to all the complications known to the cleft palate group, and like no other children in his own unique combination of problems and health needs.

The presence of a congenital cleft can affect the community as well as the family and the individual. If one in each 800 children is born with this anomaly, communities in which 1,000 children are born each year might anticipate one with a cleft. In a school population of 10,000, approximately ten children with clefts might be enrolled. In a state with an annual birth rate of 100,000, more than 100 children with clefts could be born each year. Each community will vary, and these figures are only possibilities; but they point up the fact that communities may be faced with the need for providing attention to such problems. Most of the children born with clefts will survive, and most of their families will need financial assistance from state or local agencies for the care the children will require over a long period of time. Nathaniel Levin (1962) pointed out that a cleft palate individual is more fortunate than other crippled children, "for when given skilled attention and with good results, the facial appearance and speech can approximate the normal" (p. 761); but he might have added that the skilled attention is a long-term process that will involve greater costs than most families can bear and that the community, whether local or statewide, will need to assist the family by providing and financing, wholly or partially, the many services that will be needed.

In most instances, the child whose congenital cleft has been adequately treated will be able to succeed in the classroom; but the local community will be expected to provide some remedial services for him. Children in remote areas are no less liable to clefts than those in the cities, and provision of multiple services often involves transportation to nearby or distant centers or residence in an intensive remedial program. The birth of a child with a cleft thus presents the community with some special and long-term problems. Many of these can be managed through state or private agencies for crippled children, through local medical or dental or educational services, through college or university clinics, and through other facilities at the state or local level. Some of the cooperative approaches to management for children with congenital clefts, to be considered in Chapter Five, are relatively recent developments that can do a great deal to assist the community, the child, and the family.

The families into which children with prepalatal and palatal clefts are born seem to represent wide ranges of social, educational, and economic status. More than half will be families in which no similar congenital anomaly has been known and to which the birth of a child with a cleft can be particularly devastating because it presents the parents with a problem about which they have little or no information (McWilliams, 1956). In the group of children studied by Fogh-Andersen (1942), 67 percent came from families with no known disposition to clefts; Levin (1962) reported that about 80 percent of children with cleft palate are born to families which have no previous record of such a defect; and Ralph Schwartz (1954) found that 85 percent of the cases he investigated came from families with no history of clefts.

No clear evidence has been presented to show that the families of children born with clefts are necessarily at low socioeconomic levels. Children who are receiving services from state agencies are frequently used as subjects in studies on clefts because they are readily available to the research worker, and this unavoidable bias in selection of subjects may lead to the general impression that children with clefts appear more often in families with low incomes. The children from high-income families may receive care on a private basis and thus be excluded from groups used to determine the typical characteristics of individuals with congenital clefts.

Clinical observations of the reactions of the family of a child born with a cleft have included such descriptions as "silent accusations leading to friction between the father and mother" (Van Riper, 1963, p. 420); "problems . . . of feeding" (Olin, 1960, p. 28); "fear, pity, worry or revulsion" (Levin, 1962, p. 761); and "it is doubtful if any parent is ever able to accept completely the 'different' baby" (Moffat, 1951, p. 7). Studies of the impact of the birth of a child with a cleft (Hill, 1956; Clifford, 1969b; Slutsky, 1969) showed that parents reacted less favorably to the child with clefts of both prepalate and palate than to the child with a cleft in only one area. However, until parental feelings can be measured under more controlled conditions, one may be forced to conclude that "it has not been clearly demonstrated that parents of cleft palate children harbor feelings that are more negative than those held by parents of normal children" (Phipps, in Irwin, 1965, p. 107).

Some parents do not realize, at first, the problems they will face in caring for the child born with a cleft. Others give disproportionate emphasis to the difficulties, expenses, and responsibilities they foresee for themselves when they learn that their child has a congenital deformity. Some parents know so little about clefts that they cannot formulate questions and do not understand explanations that may be provided. Some overprotect the child; few will reject him completely. Relationships between husband and wife may be affected by the birth of a child with a cleft, and attention to the child with special problems may interfere with the fair distribution of attention to other children in the family. Conversely, a family may be unified by mutual concern for one of its members.

Although the general characteristics of "cleft palate children" have been described, not all of these characteristics are the results of the clefts. Some are part of each child's inheritance from his parents. Others are concomitant to the cleft, appearing with some frequency in children who are born with multiple anomalies. The child's intelligence, whether or not it is affected by pre- or postnatal environment, is determined in part by parental intelligence. Certain physical characteristics, unrelated to the cleft, are transmitted by the parents to the child. Dental anomalies thought to be the result of the child's congenital malformation may be reflections of the dental structures of the parents, and tendencies toward hearing impairment may be genetic. Strabismus, hypertelorism, or deviations in weight and height may be hereditary, appearing as individual differences in parent and child.

However, certain physical anomalies seem to appear more often in children with clefts than in the noncleft population. Many aborted fetuses have been found to have clefts in addition to other severe physical defects, and some surviving infants present clefts in combination with other malformations. An early treatise (Mason, 1877) spoke of other deformities that sometimes accompanied prepalatal clefts, listing an extra thumb on each hand, internal squint, and a large birthmark as deviations and "a cyanotic condition of the child" as another complication. Concomitants of palatal clefts were congenital fissure of the lobe of the ear, talipes calcaneus, and hypospadias; and, in "one curious instance," a patient with a complete fissure of the palate and bilateral cleft of the prepalate also showed eversion of the lower lip with two openings of buccal glands. Others (Berry and Legg, 1912) pointed out that deformities such as spina bifida and clubfoot were typical of children with clefts, and their observations on the absence or irregularity of an incisor tooth as a concomitant or family trait foreshadowed later investigations (Woolf and others, 1965). Fogh-Andersen (1942) said that "harelip and cleft palate are most likely associated with other severe malformations of any kind in 10 per cent or more of the cases, while the 'normal' frequency of these malformations hardly exceeds 1 per cent" (p. 187). The associated anomalies identified by Fogh-Andersen included clubfoot, polydactyly, syndactyly, inguinal hernia, congenital heart disease, and persistent foramen ovale. Another Danish study of congenital deformities, which investigated deformities of the upper extremities (Birch-Jensen, 1949), stated:

> About the end of the 1930's Stroer called attention to the fact that patients with harelip and cleft palate relatively often have extremital defects as well. Vershuer calculated that 1 out of about 12,000 have the combination of harelip and/or cleft palate and extremital defect, which strikingly often is a defect of the radius. [Pp. 155–156]

More recently, malformations accompanying clefts have been described in even greater detail. In 100 patients with clefts drawn at random from a total of 127, one investigator (McNeil, 1954) found such additional physical malformations as deviant upper lateral incisors, webbed toes, deformed ears, inguinal hernia, heart and eye defects, macrostomia, and deafness. Others (Holdsworth, 1963; Gorlin, 1968) listed, as some of the complications found with clefts, underdevelopment of the maxilla on the side of a unilateral cleft, asymmetry of the skull, anomalies of the brain such as microcephalus, defects of the external ears or the tongue, microstomia, spina bifida, clubfoot, congenital lip pits, premaxillary agenesis, the Pierre Robin syndrome, abnormal digits, congenital hernia, ectopia cordis, and mongolism. A report from a New York hospital (Stark, 1968) included, in the list of the most common associated physical anomalies in 100 children with clefts, clubfeet, micrognathia with Pierre Robin syndrome, and congenital heart disease. The children in this study presented a total of forty-eight associated anomalies, in comparison with seventeen anomalies found in a noncleft control group. In another group of 100 patients with clefts, 31 percent had additional congenital malformations, those of the musculoskeletal system being most common (Pannbacker, 1968). A summary (Greene, 1963) of congenital anomalies associated with clefts listed syndactylism, supernumerary digits and teeth, and congenital heart disease as some of the concomitants; and clefts, clubfoot, polydactylism of the fingers, spina bifida, and hypospadias have been called the "Big Five" in congenital anomalies (Ivy, 1957).

Lis (in Irwin, 1965) divided the associated congenital anomalies of children with clefts into four categories: defects in tissues or organs of branchial origin such as the microtia syndrome and facial deformities, chromosomal abnormalities such as the oro-facial-digital (OFD) syndrome in females, defects involving the central nervous system such as encephalocele, and defects in such distant structures as the heart and genitourinary systems. He also mentioned concomitant physical conditions that may be noted as the child grows: hearing loss; dental caries; the results of accidents and infections; sensory, motor, or perceptual neurological disturbances; and inadequate functioning of such vital organs as the heart, lungs, and kidneys. Summarizing, Lis said, "Although most children with clefts present problems primarily referable to this malformation, a large spectrum of other complications may also be found in this group" (p. 102).

Major defects seem to be associated more with cleft palate than with prepalatal clefts or the combination of the two. In one extensive study, congenital anomalies other than clefts were found in 9 of 124 control children and in 58 of 166 children with clefts (Drillien and others, 1966). Among the associated malformations appearing with greatest frequency in the children with prepalatal clefts were inguinal hernia and strabismus, while hypertelorism appeared with greater frequency than other defects in the children with clefts of both prepalate and palate. In the total of 166 children with clefts, 28 percent of those with cleft lip only and 23 percent of those with clefts of both prepalate and palate had associated anomalies; but 47 percent of those with isolated cleft palate had one or more accompanying defects. An earlier analysis (MacMahon and McKeown, 1953) indicated that the highest percentage of anomalies accompanied combined clefts. Among 276 children with congenital clefts in that study, 9.1 percent with prepalatal clefts, 14.9 percent with palatal clefts, and 21 percent with combined clefts had accompanying physical anomalies.

One may expect, therefore, to find other physical deviations in some of the children with congenital clefts. The different types of clefts may show differing concomitants, but some children will present congenital clefts as their only defects.

Whether the health and growth, the intelligence, and the social adjustment of "the child with a cleft" will be affected differently by the various types of clefts is a matter for careful investigation. Until research can provide more definite answers, descriptions of these characteristics must be general. Some writers emphasize the similarity of children with clefts to their noncleft peers. Others find differences that they consider significant.

In describing the general health and growth of children with clefts, one writer (Olin, 1960) stated, "Except for their lips and palates, children born with clefts are just like other children" (p. 6); and another (Birch, 1952) said, ". . . there is no substantial evidence that a cleft palate or cleft lip will usually prevent a child from becoming a healthy and happy and useful citizen" (p. 6). Some are less optimistic, pointing out that the child born with a cleft "is severely handicapped and presents a serious problem to the parents and the community" (Levin, 1962, p. 761). One text (West and Ansberry, 1968) spoke of "problems so numerous and so varied that they can be solved only by the integrated services of the cleft palate team" (p. 380). These generalizations, each with its own point of view, suggest that the problems and handicaps of the child born with a cleft may be manageable or almost insurmountable, depending on the writer.

Some children with congenital clefts have initial difficulties in nursing, but some can be fed with relative ease. If early nutritional deficiencies cannot be overcome, the child may be smaller in size than others of his age; but he may eventually reach wide normal limits in height and weight. His general health may be impaired by recurring upper respiratory infections, but he may be comparatively free from such disturbances or show no lasting ill effects from those he experiences. He often seems to be more susceptible to colds, otitis media, and other infections; and his general health may be less than satisfactory. In any clinical group, some children with clefts will be healthy; some will not. Some will be average or better-than-average in size; some will be small and thin. Their differences from the average child, in terms of general health, size, and growth, will probably be in degree rather than in kind; and, although the child with a cleft may be less robust than others, he will probably be able to attend school and take part in most of the activities of his peer group.

Measurements of the intellectual capacities of children with clefts are affected by the many variables that characterize all evaluations of intelligence. Additionally, the child with inadequate speech may present difficulties to the examiner who cannot understand him. Perhaps the factor of selection of children from groups that are readily available affects evaluations of intelligence in the same way that it affects the apparent socioeconomic status of their families.

One point of view is that children with clefts show some mental retardation. Such statements as the following are representative: "Mental deficiency is eight times as common as with uncleft people" (Holdsworth, 1963, p. 33); ". . . most agree that cleft-palate people tend to have lower scores on mental tests than their normal peers" (Westlake and Rutherford, 1966, p. 16); and ". . . the performance of cleft palate children on IQ tests which place emphasis on verbal skills shows impairment of from 2 to 11 IQ points" (Phipps, in Irwin, 1965, p. 105). However, others believe that "the most reliable and extensive investigations show their curve of learning potential to be comparable with that for the general school population" (Berry and Eisenson, 1956, p. 324).

Some investigations have provided specific information about the intellectual capacities of children with congenital clefts. One report (Munson and May, 1955) indicated that nearly 63 percent of the children with clefts in the group tested were of normal, above-average, or superior intelligence and that the mean intelligence quotient for 132 cases was 96.2. Another investigator (Lewis, 1961) obtained a mean IQ of 94 for 548 children with clefts, 10 points lower than that obtained by the siblings of these children. In a group of 200 German children with clefts, 20 percent had low intelligence, 67 percent were within the average range, and 13 percent were above average (Schweckendiek and Danzer, 1970). Two other studies (Phipps, in Irwin, 1965; Ruess, 1965) found that children with clefts functioned within the range of normal intelligence.

When different types of clefts were considered in the measurement of intelligence, lower scores were obtained by those with clefts of the palate, according to some investigations (Goodstein, 1961; Drillien and others, 1966); but these findings were not supported by other studies (Means and Irwin, 1954; Lewis, 1961). However, the possibility that children with palatal clefts may be less intelligent, in combination with evidence that such children present more concomitant physical anomalies and that palatal clefts differ morphologically from clefts of the prepalate, suggests the need to determine whether or not the type of cleft has a direct effect on intelligence. A review of research on the intellectual capacities of children with clefts (Goodstein, in Spriestersbach and Sherman, 1968) summarized as follows:

> Despite the differences in methodology and procedure . . . children with cleft palate in general yielded strikingly similar results with the reports of mean IQ ranging only from 94 to 99. The findings of these studies do suggest a generally mild to moderate degree of intellectual impairment, with the distribution of IQ for the group of children with cleft palate displaced to the lower end of the entire distribution. Such intellectual impairment appears to be more pronounced in the verbal area than in the performance area and raises important practical questions in the development of therapeutic and educational plans for children with cleft palate. [P. 212]

Any group of children, with or without clefts, will include some who are well-adjusted and socially adequate, some who relate poorly to those in their environments, and many who are at neither extreme. Children with clefts vary as greatly in social adjustment as the noncleft, and those who are maladjusted might have been so if they had not had the congenital malformation. "The data do not lend support to the assumption that the social adjustment of cleft palate children is markedly inferior to that of other children" (Sidney and Matthews, 1956, p. 10); and no differences in traits measured by the Rodgers Personal Adjustment Inventory were found among boys with palatal clefts, boys with other chronic physical differences, and those with no known physical differences (Watson, 1964).

Conversely, children with clefts have been described as frustrated, shy, timid, and lacking in initiative if they have poor speech (Vaughan, 1940). The "cleft palate patient" has been described (Barber, 1969) as a person who, throughout life, has had many different people "show considerable interest in the status of his oral cavity" (p. 320) and may be fearful and insecure as a result of "the plethora of attention given to him by surgeons, pediatricians, speech therapists, dentists, orthodontists, and his own family" (p. 321). If such feelings exist among children with clefts, they do not seem to be major factors in adjustment. Twenty children with clefts, for example, were asked to evaluate various concepts related to physical disabilities; and they rated "cleft palate" slightly more positively than "cleft lip" and both of these concepts slightly higher than "asthma," "amputation," and "cripple." Conceptually, however, "cleft palate" and "cleft lip" were, to these children, in the range of mild illness and close to the concept of "headache" (Clifford, 1967). A study that investigated the dropout rate of high school students found that 25 percent of those with clefts left high school without completing the senior year but that 42 percent of the siblings of these adolescents were dropouts. The investigators (Demb and Ruess, 1967) suggested that family patterns, rather than the presence of a cleft, were responsible for determining whether or not a child will complete a high school education.

Studies of the social adjustment of children with clefts have not usually considered the type of cleft. One might assume that the child with obvious scars on his lip would be affected by his difference in appearance, but some children with palatal clefts and relatively normal facial appearance may be misjudged if their speech is deviant without any visible reason for the lack of intelligibility or the undue nasality. Children with palatal clefts, according to a study of the impact of anomalies (Clifford, 1969a), felt that their parents were more accepting of them at birth than did children with clefts of the prepalate and palate. However, no significant difference was discerned between these two groups in self-concept; and all the children in the study rated themselves in a self-accepting manner.

In any event, the child with a repaired prepalatal or palatal cleft will probably adjust to his social environment and his appearance in terms of his own potential and the way in which he is treated by family, friends, and those he encounters outside the circle of everyday acquaintances. Leonard Goodstein (in Spriestersbach and Sherman, 1968) summed up the matter of adjustment by saying, ". . . it appears safe to conclude that as a group children with cleft palates are not typically maladjusted or seriously disturbed emotionally, although they may have some problems of social acceptance" (p. 217); and an earlier study using projective techniques (Hackbush, 1951) found "no such entity as a cleft palate personality" (p. 7).

THE CHILD BORN WITH A CLEFT MAY RESEMBLE OTHER CHILDREN MORE THAN HE DIFFERS FROM THEM; BUT HE WILL USUALLY PRESENT DIFFERENCES IN APPEARANCE, DENTAL STRUCTURE, HEARING, SPEECH, OR LANGUAGE AND MAY PRESENT ALL THESE PROBLEMS.

This combination of deviations from the normal affects oral communication particularly, and inadequate speech may be the outstanding characteristic of the child who fails to use structures brought to potential adequacy by various forms of management. One plastic surgeon (Sullivan, 1961) emphasized this point when he said,

> We all have patients with poor speech following closure of palate clefts. We have this, in spite of excellent technical procedures, careful handling of tissues, reduction of trauma to a minimum, and preservation of good blood supply. [P. 31]

The child's appearance will depend on his inheritance, the type of cleft, and the effects of management. Some children are more attractive in facial appearance than others, whether or not they present a congenital anomaly of the face. The child born with a bilateral cleft of the prepalate may be quite deviant in appearance, in spite of the best plastic surgery; and the child whose lip is intact but whose inadequacy in velopharyngeal closure leads him to compensate by facial grimaces may also be noticeably different in appearance. A study of the oral image of children with clefts (Palmer and Adams, 1962) did not support the hypothesis that these children have significantly greater degrees of unresolved feelings regarding their oral structures than do structurally normal children; but attempts to hide labial scars and dental distortions may result in atypical behavior as the child covers his mouth with his hand, hangs his head, or holds his lips in an abnormal position.

Whatever their feelings about their appearance, children whose facial structures remain deviant even with good management probably receive special notice from those they meet. The child may have accepted himself as he is and may not be aware of his own differences in appearance, but comments and unspoken reactions from strangers or friends may have adverse effects that could result in speech that is slurred or rapid or in immobility of the lips and other structures in an attempt at concealment.

Surgeons continue to seek ways of eliminating scars, revising noses, improving the shape of the lips, and bringing about the best possible appearance in terms of the tissue available. The difficulties in improving appearance were recognized by Veau when he wrote, in 1938:

> In the case of cleft lip, even with great effort, one does not always achieve a completely normal structure. I realize that function is a goal that can be reached more easily than form, but who is ever satisfied with the appearance of his own face? [P. vi]

The advisability of postponing cosmetic surgery until growth has occurred complicates the problem, but the young adult whose facial and dental disfigurements have been minimized with surgical and dental management may well be able to take his place in a social or employment setting and be accepted by those with whom he associates.

Dental problems are characteristic of children with clefts of the prepalate and may also appear in those with palatal clefts. These children will probably have dental anomalies and are often described as having severe caries. However, a study of 285 children, with various types of clefts, showed no significantly greater DMF index (number of decayed, missing, or filled teeth) than was found in 300 children without clefts; and the type of cleft did not influence the number of carious lesions (Lauterstein and Mendelsohn, 1964). In another study of dental malformations in a population with clefts, defects of the alveolar ridge were not associated with dental abnormalities more than labial or palatal clefts; and the fact of cleft, rather than the nature of the cleft, was considered the significant factor (Jordan and others, 1966).

Descriptions of the dentition of children with congenital clefts have listed, among the anomalies that may be present, the following: lack of the normal complement of teeth, some degree of hypoplasia of one or more teeth, cross-bite, Class III occlusions (Angle's classification), projection of the premaxilla in bilateral clefts of the prepalate, and supernumerary teeth (Harkins, 1960; Olin, 1960; Lauterstein and Mendelsohn, 1964; Pruzansky and Aduss, 1964; Handelman and Pruzansky, 1968; Ridley, 1968).

The maintenance of good dental health is particularly important for children born with clefts because of the kinds of problems just cited and because of the importance of the teeth in the attachment of prostheses. In addition, orthodontic and prosthetic treatment may make the child's teeth more vulnerable to food entrapment, which is considered a predisposing cause of tooth decay.

The dental anomalies associated with clefts or remaining in spite of changes brought about by revision of structures may distort appearance, interfere with articulation, permit tongue protrusion, or affect the child in other ways. If malocclusion increases as the child grows or if appliances for revision of dental structure impede articulatory activities, the effect of dental anomalies may be increased.

Most writers agree that many children with palatal clefts, repaired or obturated, will have some problems in hearing, although the child with a cleft of the prepalate may hear normally. Impairments of hearing, often fluctuating with physical condition and the presence or absence of infection in the middle ear, are typical. The universality of otitis media, observed clinically, seemed to be confirmed by a study (Paradise and Bluestone, 1968) that led to the conclusion that chronic otitis media, either serous or suppurative, develops in all infants with cleft palate, usually before three months of age. The incidence of hearing loss among those with congenital clefts, however, has been variously reported, with a wide range. Among eight groups of subjects of various ages, with clefts of various types, hearing losses were found in 28.75 percent (Graham, 1964), 38 percent (Nylén, 1961), 39 percent (Skolnik, 1958), 40 percent (Linthicum and others, 1959), 42 percent (Loeb, 1964), 62 percent (Holmes and Reed, 1955), 74 percent (Halfond and Ballenger, 1956), and 90 percent (Sataloff and Fraser, 1952). Variations in procedure, in the age of the subjects, and in the definition of hearing loss were probably responsible for this lack of agreement.

Some of the studies just cited considered the effect of the type of cleft on hearing, but others did not. However, clefts of the palate are probably more often accompanied by hearing losses than clefts of the prepalate. When an otologist and a surgeon (Stool and Randall, 1967) studied the tympanic membranes and middle ears of twenty-five infants with palatal clefts prior to surgery, they were impressed with the high incidence of pathological conditions they found. In forty-seven of the fifty ears they examined, appreciable amounts of mucoid material were present; and ten biopsy specimens showed abnormal tissue in the middle ear. These anomalies were not found with any frequency in the ears of babies with clefts of the prepalate.

Reports from other studies have confirmed the observation that prepalatal clefts have less effect on ear disease and hearing than clefts of the palatal area. Evaluation of the hearing of 190 children who ranged in age from eight to fourteen years revealed no hearing loss at 500, 1,000, and 2,000 cycles per second (Hz) in those born with prepalatal clefts (Graham, 1964); and other studies showed hearing loss to be relatively high in groups with cleft palate (Sweitzer and others, 1968; Pannbacker, 1969).

The type of cleft thus seems to have some relationship to hearing loss, but other factors have been studied for their influence on auditory acuity in the cleft population. The age of the child when the palate is repaired is not related to hearing loss, according to one report (Holmes and Reed, 1955); but another (Masters and others, 1960) indicated that the incidence of hearing loss appears to rise almost by arithmetic progression if palatal reconstruction is delayed beyond eighteen months.

The effect of obturation on hearing also has been debated. On the basis of a study of 134 cases, a group of plastic surgeons (Masters and others, 1960) stated that closure of a cleft by prosthesis is less effective than closure by surgery in preventing hearing loss. A group that included dentists (Graham and others, 1962) found that no infections of the middle ear developed after provision of prostheses for the fifty-four patients they studied. They stated:

> If individuals with cleft palates are followed otologically from infancy, if their ear problems are treated . . . and if obturators are inserted after the age of 4 years, it appears safe to conclude that an obturator may be worn with the knowledge that there will be no adverse effects on the otological condition of the cleft palate patient. [P. 358]

Another group (Spriestersbach and others, 1962), basing their conclusions on thresholds of hearing for 163 children who had various types of management for clefts of the prepalate and palate, did not find a clear relationship between the type of physical management and hearing loss.

Hypertrophy of adenoidal tissue also has been considered a factor in hearing loss, for children with and without clefts. If the adenoidal pad is used to assist in velopharyngeal closure, it may be an important adjunct to speech (Subtelny and Koepp-Baker, 1956); and removal of the adenoids sometimes results in hypernasality in children whose palates, although intact, are short in relationship to the depth of the nasopharynx. Preservation of this pad of tissue may be important to the speech of the child with a repaired or obturated palatal cleft, but growth of adenoidal tissue may block the entrances to the Eustachian tubes and bring about hearing loss as a result of poor ventilation for the middle ear. The surgeon is thus faced with the alternative of preserving the pad as an aid to velopharyngeal valving and increasing the chances of middle ear infection or removing the adenoids and risking a hazard to valving. In some instances, a solution to the problem may be found by removing the parts of the adenoidal mass that impinge on the Eustachian tube area and leaving the central portion to assist in velopharyngeal closure.

A recurrent or chronic hearing loss, even if it is not severe, may interfere with the development of linguistic and articulatory skills; and the child born with a cleft of the palate may develop a pattern of poor attention to the auditory cues that are difficult to hear when his hearing is depressed. If this pattern of poor attention to sound persists to school age, the child may fail to achieve at his best intellectual level even if his hearing reaches wide normal limits. Although the hearing of children with repaired clefts apparently improves with increases in chronological age (Spriestersbach and others, 1962; Graham, 1964), the impairments in hearing that are often found in young children with clefts add a complication to the learning of skills in speech and language.

The middle ear pathology that characterizes the child with a palatal cleft continues to diminish as he grows older, and adults with treated or untreated clefts of the palate do not present serious hearing defects that are direct results of the congenital anomaly. A group with a maximal age of twenty-one years showed that hearing losses accompanying clefts, although such losses were mild to moderate, might reduce the precision of speech production (Halfond and Ballenger, 1956). However, another group, ranging in age from sixteen to seventy-five years, with repaired palatal clefts, had hearing and auditory discrimination within normal limits (Goetzinger and others, 1960). In a group of sixty-nine adults with untreated palatal clefts, evidence of previous ear infection could be seen in almost one-third; but hearing losses were not prevalent (Ortiz-Monasterio and others, 1966).

One might judge, then, that the child born with a palatal defect will be liable to middle ear infections and hearing impairment even though he may have adequate hearing when he becomes an adult. The lack of consistency noted in reports on the incidence and extent of hearing loss in individuals with clefts suggests the need for further investigation to determine, more exactly, the effect of the type of cleft and the type of management on hearing. Variations in the definition of "hearing loss" and lack of differentiation between the types of clefts have limited the value of some of the studies on relationships between clefts and hearing acuity (Hayes, in Irwin, 1965). In addition, the incidence of hearing problems in children with palatal clefts may have been emphasized by the frequency with which their hearing is tested, audiograms being usual parts of any review of the status of a child who is under surgical or dental management. Although the reports of hearing loss in these children are undoubtedly accurate, they may be based on testing that is more frequent than tests of hearing for the general population.

Some differences of opinion are evident in the reports on the effects of clefts on appearance, dentition, and hearing; but most specialists agree that speech is frequently affected. The effects will vary with the individual, with the type and time of management, with the evaluator's opinion, and with many other factors; but the topic "cleft palate speech" has received comment from surgeons and dentists as well as from speech pathologists.

Historically, as indicated in Chapter One, interest in the speech of persons with congenital clefts became widespread during the nineteenth century. One of the advantages of early surgery was said to be that the child would have "the ability to acquire the power of speech or articulation of sounds much more perfectly" (Davis, 1847, p. 37). Those who advised obturators stated that impaired speech was the major problem for speakers with palatal clefts (Kingsley, 1880) and that, among the difficulties that could be remedied by obturation, were "defective articulation and enunciation" (Rhone, 1894, p. 545). Other specialists in the fields of surgery and dentistry, in the early twentieth century, made similar comments. A surgeon (Brophy, 1923) referred to clefts of the prepalate and palate as "one of the most distressing deformities which befalls mankind" because they brought about "inability to speak distinctly enough to be understood" (p. 73). A dentist (Fitzgibbon, 1923) stipulated that a "perfect result" in surgical management meant "perfect speech, delivered without effort or embarrassment on the part of the patient" (p. 718). Another surgeon (Veau, 1931) predicted that an adequate and mobile palate would assure good speech, even without *"éducation phonétique"* (p. 464).

Books and articles appearing after 1950 gave additional evidence of the fact that specialists in professions other than speech pathology were increasingly concerned with the speech of children and adults with congenital oral clefts. Goals of plastic surgeons have included provision of a mechanism requisite to the establishment of normal speech (Slaughter and others, 1956), a palate "long enough to meet the wall of the pharynx and flexible enough to come and go at considerable speed" (Holdsworth, 1963, p. 8), and an adequate speech mechanism that is ready to function when the child first learns to speak (Oldfield, 1959). The importance of speech was stressed in statements that "speech results after operation for cleft palate form the greatest if not the only criterion of success" (Steffensen, 1952, p. 383) and that " . . . the three aims of cleft palate surgery are to make the patient speak well, eat well and look well, in that order of importance" (Kilner, 1958, p. 205).

As the cooperative efforts of several disciplines have been focused on the child with a congenital cleft, references to the effects of the anomaly on speech have been made with greater frequency in dental and surgical journals, at conferences, and in texts. Evidence of this increase in interdisciplinary interest will be presented in Chapter Five; but dentists, surgeons, and speech pathologists now seem to agree, even more than in the past, that speech is a major consideration in the habilitation of the individual with a congenital orofacial cleft.

The person who presents, as one of many individual characteristics, a cleft that was present at birth and has been modified by one or more forms of management, may have many, few, or no difficulties in communicating with those in his environment. He is just as subject to disorders of communication as anyone else, and he may have special problems in some aspects of oral communication. His capacities to use voice, articulation, and language may be impaired by the neurological, physiological, and psychological factors that can affect the communicative skills of any speaker; but he may present deviations that are directly related to the present status of structures that were inadequately formed at birth.

If oral communication, including both speech (articulation, resonance, and phonation) and language (comprehension and expression of auditory symbols), is defective, then the person with a congenital cleft has a communicative disorder, whether or not his physical equipment is within normal limits in structure and function. If he has disordered communication, then the child or adult born with an oral cleft may present problems that are like those of others; and he may also present problems that result from differences that remain after modification of structures.

Most of the investigations of the communicative skills of individuals born with clefts have given major consideration to articulation and resonance; few have been concerned with phonation and language. Some evaluations have been made by those with special interest in the results of surgical or prosthodontic management, and these specialists have attended more to general intelligibility than to specific elements. Detailed study of phonatory and linguistic aspects is relatively recent.

Groups that are representative of the cleft palate population include individuals with wide ranges in age, varying types of clefts, differing forms of management, variations in intelligence, and unequal amounts of speech training. Thus, the judgments of specialists, who hear a limited sample of speech in a structured testing situation, may differ from those of laymen, with whom the child talks most often and perhaps more freely. The complexities of research on the typical communicative disorders of the cleft palate child are evident when one considers the variability that exists in a group of cleft subjects. Comparisons of reports, therefore, are limited by the multiplicity of factors that are involved in studies of the communicative skills of these subjects. However, certain similarities and certain differences become evident when cleft and noncleft groups are compared in terms of articulation, resonance, phonation, and language.

If articulation is considered apart from resonance, certain characteristics of "cleft palate speech" can be discerned. Those with congenital clefts involving only the lip are relatively free from articulatory disorders associated directly with such clefts if repair of the lip is successful. Those whose congenital defects are in the alveolus and the palate have articulatory disorders that, in some ways, resemble those presented by noncleft persons. These similarities are found chiefly in the sounds that are misarticulated and in the changes that occur with increasing age.

Descriptions of articulatory errors usually cite, as the sounds most frequently deviant in the general population, /s/, /z/, /θ/, /ð/, /ʃ/, /ʒ/, /tʃ/, /dʒ/, /f/, /v/, and sometimes /k/, /g/, /l/, and /r/ (Hall, 1938, Roe and Milisen, 1942; Van Riper, 1963; Van Riper and Irwin, 1958). Table 4-1 shows that children and adults with clefts make errors on many of the sounds that are most often defectively produced by noncleft speakers.

Errors on /s/, /z/, and /ʃ/ are characteristic of almost all the groups studied; and, in addition, /θ/, /ð/, /ʒ/, /tʃ/, and /dʒ/ are typically deviant in the speech of children, with or without clefts, as shown in Table 4-2.

The number of deviant sounds decreases as the noncleft child grows older, as Table 4-3 shows; and the effects of maturation are evident also in children with congenital clefts (Van Demark, 1969). Adults with congenitally intact palates probably make more errors on /s/, /z/, /ʃ/, /ʒ/, /tʃ/, and /dʒ/ than on other consonant sounds (Hall, in Travis, 1957); adults born with palatal clefts also present characteristic deviations on these sounds (McWilliams, 1958; Counihan, 1960).

TABLE 4-1 ARTICULATORY ERRORS CHARACTERISTIC OF NONCLEFT AND CLEFT SPEAKERS

	Studies of articulatory errors									
	In noncleft speakers						*In cleft speakers*			
Deviant phoneme	*1*	*2*	*3*	*4*	*5*	*6*	*7*	*8*	*9*	*10*
f		x	x			x				x
v		x	x	x		x				x
s	x	x	x	x	x	x	x	x	x	x
z	x	x	x	x	x	x	x	x	x	x
θ	x	x	x	x		x	x			x
ð		x	x	x		x	x	x		x
ʃ	x	x	x		x	x	x		x	x
ʒ	x		x		x	x	x			x
tʃ	x	x	x	x	x	x	x		x	
dʒ		x	x		x	x	x		x	
k		x	x			x	x	x		
g		x	x			x	x			
l			x			x				
r	x	x	x			x				

1. Hall, 1938
2. Roe and Milisen, 1942
3. Van Riper, 1947
4. Sayler, 1949
5. Fairbanks and Spriestersbach, 1950
6. Van Riper and Irwin, 1958
7. Spriestersbach and others, 1956
8. McWilliams, 1958
9. Counihan, 1960
10. Morley, 1967

In describing cleft palate speech, several writers have referred to groups of sounds rather than to individual phonemes. If the sounds shown in Tables 4-1, 4-2, and 4-3 are classified by manner of production, the similarity between cleft and noncleft groups is maintained. Fricatives and affricates seem to pose the greatest difficulty to children and adults with and without clefts, according to the studies from which thc tables were drawn. Other investigators (Van Demark and Van Demark, 1967; Philips and Harrison, 1969a) have reported similar findings. However, children without clefts

TABLE 4-2 DEVIANT PHONEMES IN THE SPEECH OF NONCLEFT AND CLEFT CHILDREN

	Studies of the articulation of children						
	Without clefts				*With clefts*		
Deviant phoneme	*1*	*2*	*3*	*4*	*5*	*6*	*7*
f		x					x
v		x	x			x	x
s	x	x	x	x	x	x	x
z	x	x	x		x	x	x
θ	x	x	x	x	x		x
ð		x	x		x	x	x
ʃ	x	x			x	x	x
ʒ	x				x		x
tʃ	x	x	x		x	x	
dʒ	x	x			x	x	
k		x			x		
g		x			x		
l				x			
r	x	x		x		x	
t						x	

1. Hall, 1938
2. Roe and Milisen, 1942
3. Sayler, 1949
4. Van Riper, 1963
5. Spriestersbach and others, 1956
6. Byrne and others, 1961
7. Morley, 1967

seem to have more problems with /l/ and /r/; and children with clefts encounter more difficulties with some of the plosive sounds.

The observation that sound substitutions are common types of articulatory errors in the deviant speech of small children (W. Johnson and others, 1967) was made also in studies of the articulation of children born with palatal clefts (Spriestersbach and others, 1956; Bzoch, 1965). The high incidence of sound distortions thought to characterize the deviant articulation of the noncleft adult population was found also in a group of adults with congenital palatal clefts (McWilliams, 1958). The relative incidence of errors of omission in the two populations is obscured by the difficulty in identifying such deviations with accuracy, particularly when judgments are made from recordings. In fact, "some omissions, when closely examined, turn out to be oral or lingual postures without the breath or voice of the correct sound" (Van Riper and Irwin, 1958, p. 78). However, omissions were more frequent than substitutions or distortions in the speech of two groups of children

TABLE 4-3 DEVIANT PHONEMES IN THE SPEECH OF NONCLEFT AND CLEFT ADULTS

	Studies of adult articulation			
	Without clefts		*With clefts*	
Deviant phoneme	*1*	*2*	*3*	*4*
s	x	x	x	x
z	x	x	x	x
ð			x	
ʃ	x	x		x
ʒ	x	x		
tʃ	x	x		x
dʒ	x	x		x
k			x	

1. Hall, 1938
2. Fairbanks and Spriestersbach, 1950
3. McWilliams, 1958
4. Counihan, 1960

with palatal clefts (Rouse, 1956; Spriestersbach and others, 1956) and were more characteristic of a group of children with clefts than of their noncleft controls (Philips and Harrison, 1969a). Difficulties in using consonant sounds in rapid sequence in "consonant blends" or "consonant clusters" have been noted in the speech of noncleft children and also in the speech of individuals born with clefts (Counihan, 1960; Spriestersbach and others, 1961). In the kinds of articulatory errors they make, speakers with and without clefts present more similarities than differences.

Judgments of articulatory defectiveness may be influenced by resonatory factors; and, unless speakers with congenital palatal clefts have achieved adequate velopharyngeal closure, some listeners may be unable to separate articulatory errors, in terms of positioning and movement, from errors that are the result of insufficient breath pressure through the mouth or of undue nasal resonance. When the influence of articulation and nasality on each other is minimized, judgments of accuracy of articulation and degree of nasality appear to be independent; but speakers with superior articulation have been judged as having less nasality, judgment of the degree of nasality tending to vary with judgments of the accuracy of articulation (Van Hattum, 1958). When the resonatory factor is reduced by the presence of adequate velopharyngeal closure in speakers with congenital clefts, listeners are not consistent in identifying speakers as having clefts. Judges who evaluated the speech of two groups of children, one group with functional articulatory disorders and the other with congenital clefts but adequate velopharyngeal closure, categorized the speech of the children with clefts, in two-thirds of the judgments, as representing either normal speech or functional articulatory disorders (Van Demark and Van Demark, 1967). The investigators concluded that, when a child with a cleft palate achieves velopharyngeal closure, it is "difficult to differentiate his speech from that of a child with a functional articulation disorder" (p. 37).

Although some reports have separated the articulatory aspects of speech from the resonatory aspects, others have considered the two processes as integrally related. In considerations of the speech of children born with clefts, this relationship is particularly important; and descriptions of the speech disorders presented by children with repaired or obturated cleft palates are made more complete by combining articulation with resonance.

If a child produces /s/, for example, by directing the stream of air through the nasal cavities as well as through the mouth, the acoustic result will be deviant even if an acceptable articulatory position is achieved. Conversely, /s/ will be deviant if the airstream, coming through the oral cavity without being diverted to the nasal passages, is impeded or directed in such a way that the result is /θ/ or lateralization. If /b/ is articulated in the conventional manner but loses some of its plosion and is resonated in the nasal cavities as well as in the mouth, then /b/ is acoustically deviant. If the valve used to stop the airstream for /k/ is the glottis, then the release of the impounded air will result in a plosive that differs from /k/ and that may, in turn, be emitted both nasally and orally. If, in the production of /ɑ/, the stream of sound is resonated in the nasal cavities as well as in the mouth, then /ɑ/ may retain its identity; but it will not be the same /ɑ/ as that produced without undue nasal resonance by most speakers. Whether the inappropriate coupling of the nasal cavities to the oral cavity is called "nasal emission," "nasality," "hypernasality," or "rhinolalia" and whether this coupling occurs on consonant sounds or on vowel sounds, the result is speech that is difficult to understand or distracting to hear. Hence, although deviations in the speech of individuals with congenital clefts can be described in terms of articulation and in terms of resonance, a combination of the two factors seems more appropriate.

When articulation and resonance are considered together, the similarities between individuals with and without congenital palatal clefts are exceeded by the differences. Groups with congenital clefts make certain kinds of errors that seem typical for them, among these being undue nasal resonance on vowel sounds, nasal emission of consonant sounds, and substitutions resulting from lack of adequate velopharyngeal valving.

Most children with normal structures use vowel sounds acceptably; children with clefts may add undue nasal resonance to mouth resonance in their use of vowel sounds. If vowel sounds are nasalized, the high vowels such as /i/ and /u/ will seem more deviant than the low vowels in the speech of those with clefts (Spriestersbach and Powers, 1959b), although just the opposite has been noted in the nasalized speech of noncleft speakers (Lintz and Sherman, 1961). For vowel sounds with comparable tongue height, cleft palate speakers will seem to have more nasality on front vowels than on back vowels. The nasality that characterizes cleft palate speech is particularly evident on vowel sounds, which appear with such frequency that they give a coloration of nasality to the total speech pattern.

Children with congenital clefts of the palate may make some of their articulatory errors by using substitutions, distortions, or omissions. They may also combine nasal emission with proper positioning to produce errors in articulation-resonance. In addition, they may use unconventional substitutions such as a glottal stop or a pharyngeal fricative in place of a plosive or fricative that requires mouth pressure (Bzoch, 1959; Sherman and others, 1959). These patterns of substitution may develop early as the child seeks a way of impeding or impounding the stream of air or sound (Bzoch, 1959), but the development of velopharyngeal competence may allow the child to eliminate these errors (Van Demark and Van Demark, 1967). Use of the pharyngeal fricative is probably less common than use of the glottal stop, but it is present with some frequency in the speech of children and adults who cannot maintain velopharyngeal closure and use pharyngeal constriction for sounds that require sustained pressure (Bzoch, 1959).

So common were the substitutions of sounds not usually present in American English in the speech of individuals born with palatal clefts that two investigators (Counihan, 1960; Bzoch, 1965) evolved ways of designating these errors. Special symbols were used to designate glottal stops, pharyngeal or velar fricatives, and "nasal snorts." In one group of preschool children with congenital clefts of the palate, use of the glottal stop, the pharyngeal fricative, and the nasal snort accounted for almost two-thirds of the errors that were called substitutions; and distortion from nasal emission was typical of 45 percent of the errors made by these children (Bzoch, 1965). Nasal emission was also a significant factor in the deviant articulation noted in a group of adolescents and young adults (Counihan, 1960).

The deviations in articulation-resonance that differentiate speakers born with clefts from their peers affect the general intelligibility of speech as well as the specific sound units. This factor of intelligibility has been determined in various ways, for various purposes, in studies of the cleft palate population. A review of reports on intelligibility (Nylén, 1961) indicated that, from 1902 to 1931, surgeons noted good or improved speech in as many as 60 percent of their patients. In the surgeons' evaluations, general intelligibility, rather than specific errors, served as the basis for judgment. When intelligibility was assessed by speech pathologists, in the period from 1947 to 1959, normal speech was found in 32 to 83 percent of those evaluated; and "poor" or "bad" speech was noted in no more than 30 percent. Among subjects with palatal clefts in Scotland, 69 percent were considered to be "intelligible," 30 percent "just intelligible," and 11 percent "unintelligible" (Drillien and others, 1966). A review of surgical procedures for 612 Canadian children indicated that, according to the examining surgeon, 69 percent had acceptable speech, with 40 percent having speech that could be considered normal (Lindsay and others, 1962). Among a large group of patients at a cleft palate clinic in Pennsylvania, one-third had adequate speech at the time of evaluation (Takagi and others, 1965).

In spite of the high degree of adequacy reported in some studies, the intelligibility of the speech of children whose palatal clefts have been repaired does not equal that of noncleft children. Evaluations of connected speech showed that fifty-nine children with repaired palatal clefts, ranging in age from three to six years, were less intelligible than the noncleft children with whom they were compared. The subjects born with cleft palates, even at six years of age, did not achieve the speech intelligibility of the three-year-old noncleft group (Philips and Harrison, 1969a).

Most children born with palatal clefts will speak in ways that differ from those of their noncleft peers, whether the differences are in articulation, resonance, articulation-resonance, or general intelligibility. They will vary in their errors, but they will present certain deviations all their own as well as some of the articulatory differences that characterize many noncleft children.

In addition to deviations in the articulatory-resonatory aspect of speech, the child born with a palatal cleft may present vocal disorders. If "voice" includes both phonation and resonance, then the hypernasality characteristic of the vowel sounds in the speech of the child with inadequate velopharyngeal valving could be considered a vocal disorder; and nasal emission of consonant sounds also might be so classified. However, each writer who discusses voice establishes his own categories; and classification of vocal disorders will vary with the author.

One way to resolve some of the problems that have resulted from the varying methods of classifying disorders of voice is to make a division between phonation and resonance. Although this differentiation may be arbitrary, it does help in considering the characteristics of children born with palatal defects by distinguishing vocal defects resulting from laryngeal dysfunctions from those brought about by deviant resonation. In such a division, vocal disorders could be limited to those of phonation; and resonation could be combined with articulation.

The resonatory defects that characterize the speech of those with congenital clefts of the palate have already been described in conjunction with articulatory problems. Phonatory defects will not be frequent in these individuals, but one of the responsibilities of the speech pathologist is to recognize chronic or developing phonatory problems and make appropriate referrals for medical attention.

The child born with a palatal cleft is often susceptible to upper respiratory infections, and he may be liable to the laryngeal pathologies associated with such disease. Repeated use of the glottal stop as a substitution for plosive sounds has not been specifically reported as a cause of phonatory problems in children with congenital clefts, although studies of those who habitually use the glottal plosive might reveal evidence of vocal strain. Additional research could provide useful information about the various types of phonatory disorders associated with clefts, but

> as with vocal pitch and intensity characteristics, there are no systematic studies which indicate that voice quality disorders other than hypernasality are more prevalent among speakers with cleft palates than among those without clefts. [Moll, in Spriestersbach and Sherman, 1968]

Children with congenital clefts may be slow in linguistic development. The physical anomaly, although it provides an explanation for defective articulation-resonance in many instances, does not explain the delay in expressive and receptive language found in the relatively few studies of the psycholinguistic abilities of children with congenital clefts (Philips and Harrison, 1969b). The means of evaluating linguistic skills may have influenced some of the results of these studies, but evidence of linguistic retardation in children born with palatal clefts is apparent in most of the reports available.

Two different groups of children with clefts obtained higher scores on the performance subtests of the Wechsler Intelligence Scale for Children than on the verbal subtests; but, in each group, the mean verbal IQ was within wide normal limits (Goodstein, 1961; Morris, 1962). Another group made better scores on tests of vocabulary recognition than those made by their noncleft controls but did less well in tests of vocabulary definition (Spriestersbach and others, 1958). When 136 children with various types of clefts were given the Illinois Test of Psycholinguistic Abilities, they showed a general depression in language, particularly in vocal expression, gestural output, and visual memory (Smith and McWilliams, 1968); and, in this group, performance became poorer as age increased. Another group of children with clefts, however, lagged behind their noncleft controls until they reached the age of five, at which time the differences between the groups were no longer existent (Shames and others, 1968). Another investigation, however, found that cleft palate children functioned below the noncleft children with whom they were compared and also below their own chronological age levels in both receptive and expressive language skills (Philips and Harrison, 1969b).

The linguistic retardation found in children born with clefts may be a true deficit or may be a reflection of the child's reticence to use language that is not easily understood. Inhibition as a result of past experiences in unrewarding speaking situations may be a factor (Spriestersbach and others, 1958), or the child may "reject his own distorted sound production" (Stryker and others, 1968, p. 18). Sex, race, social maturity, and socioeconomic factors also may affect the linguistic development of children with clefts; but reports that children from upper socioeconomic levels tended to use fewer words may indicate that their parents are more critical and less accepting of their speech than parents at lower socioeconomic levels (Philips and Harrison, 1969b). Additional influences may come from hospitalization, separation from the family, and other psychosocial factors. The development of new measures of psycholinguistic ability, particularly of the linguistic abilities of children beyond the age of six or eight, may enable those who study children with clefts to determine patterns of linguistic development more specifically.

NO DESCRIPTION OF THE "TYPICAL" CHILD WITH A CONGENITAL CLEFT CAN BE COMPLETE OR ENTIRELY ACCURATE, BUT ATTEMPTS AT SUCH DESCRIPTION MAY BE USEFUL AS A REVIEW.

The typical cleft palate child would be one of several children born to a middle-class family in which no previous congenital anomalies were known. He would have clefts of the prepalatal and the palatal areas. He would be somewhat slow in physical development and would have frequent upper respiratory and middle ear infections. He would have some difficulty in nursing at first but would eventually overcome any problems of malnutrition. During his first three months of life, his prepalatal cleft would be surgically repaired; and, before he was three years of age, he would have had some surgical management of his palatal cleft. His linguistic development would be slower than that of his siblings, but he would be using some words meaningfully before his third birthday. As he learned to talk, he would be more difficult to understand than the child without a cleft because, in addition to making the articulatory errors that characterize the speech of many young children, he would misdirect the voiced or unvoiced stream of air for vowel and consonant sounds and thus produce hypernasal vowel sounds and consonant sounds that lacked plosion or friction. In his attempts at articulation, he might use such nonstandard sounds as the glottal stop and the pharyngeal fricative.

By the time he was ready to enter school, he would have been hospitalized for two or more operations, provided with orthodontic appliances to modify dental structures or with a prosthesis to cover a fistula or supplement velopharyngeal closure, examined by a group of specialists on several occasions, and admitted to a program of speech training. Any child who had such experiences prior to school age might understandably be somewhat different from his siblings and playmates; but the cleft palate child would be surprisingly well-adjusted at the time he entered school, would be interested in the kinds of games and activities that caught the attention of his peers, would be willing to communicate with friends and strangers, and would be as eager to begin educational experiences as any other child.

During the years of his elementary education, the typical child born with clefts of the prepalate and palate would encounter some difficulties in learning but would make relatively steady, if slow, progress. Absences from school for medical and dental appointments and additional hospitalization, frequent ear infections with accompanying reductions in auditory acuity, assignment to the school's remedial speech program, and problems in communicating verbally with his teachers and classmates would characterize his elementary school experience. As he entered adolescence, he would become more aware of his differences in appearance and would accept additional surgical and dental management with more understanding of the purposes of the treatment and of the importance of his cooperation in the several kinds of assistance being provided for him. He would complete a high school education and find employment, assume responsibility for financing additional surgical or dental management to improve his appearance, marry, and have a family. In many ways, he would resemble his noncleft peers; in some ways, he would be different from them.

Each of the foregoing assumptions could be challenged, and each could be modified or qualified. "She" could replace "he" because clefts of the facial area are not limited to males. "Palatal cleft" or "prepalatal cleft" might replace "clefts of the prepalate and palate," with "palatal cleft" being more appropriate if the child being described was "she."

Many babies born with clefts are more than somewhat slow in development, but many are average and above average in this factor; and the incidence of infections of the respiratory system and middle ear reported for children born with clefts may be no higher than for noncleft children who, because they present no specific physical anomalies, endure colds and "croup" and "risings in the ears" without the attention that may be given to the congenitally deviant child. Nursing problems, frequently encountered in the past, seem to have been minimized for cleft palate babies by new methods of feeding.

The time for surgery to the congenitally cleft lip, too, has changed; and some babies are provided with appliances to modify and stabilize the alveolar processes before the cleft in the lip is closed. Since no single time schedule for surgery to the palate has been established and accepted, closure of the palatal cleft may be accomplished early or late or in several stages; and the time and success of these surgical procedures may permit the acquisition of skills in the production and use of speech sounds at the rate usually followed by most average, normal children. Linguistic patterns, too, will vary; and the child born with a cleft of the prepalate or palate may use language early or late or may develop linguistically within the time schedule of his peers.

Some children born with clefts may be very successful in school, and they may not need the special services available in many school systems. Others will encounter serious difficulties in learning and will be retarded academically. Some will continue their education beyond high school. Others will not be able to achieve beyond the elementary level. Adults with congenital clefts that have been successfully managed may attain success in business or professional endeavors, but those with inadequate oral communication may be prevented from reaching the potential determined by intelligence and personality.

The differences in causal factors, family attitudes, achievement, opportunity, financial assistance, encouragement, surgical and dental management, speech training, and many other aspects undoubtedly outweigh the similarities; and one might well conclude that no typical cleft palate child exists. Even if one seeks a common denominator in "cleftness," he cannot find it. The varieties in the types of clefts are equaled by the differences in the effects of these anomalies on the individual and his associates and by the variations in the types and results of management provided by members of cleft palate teams.

CHAPTER FIVE

The Cleft Palate Team

THE MANAGEMENT OF CONGENITAL MALFORMATIONS OF THE PREPALATE AND PALATE AND OF THE CHILDREN WHO PRESENT THESE DEFORMITIES REQUIRES THE EFFORTS OF MANY SPECIALISTS.

When representatives of several disciplines work together with a common interest, as a team, their success depends on many factors, among them good communication. Whether the team is a small group or includes many members, each specialist needs to supplement his knowledge of his own field with understanding of the reports made by others.

The emergence of cleft palate teams, from their beginnings shortly after 1940, has been the result of recognition of the fact that no one person is equipped to deal with a child who requires prolonged management and presents a "complex medical, dental, emotional, social, educational, and vocational problem" (Lis, in Curtin, 1962, p. 291). The development of teams concerned with care for children with clefts was facilitated by federal support, by state services for crippled children (Dodds, 1946; Chenoweth, 1964), by intensive programs established in several states (Wells, 1945; Luban, 1955; Keys, 1960; Kobes and Pruzansky, 1960), and by the establishment in 1943 of an interdisciplinary organization now known as the American Cleft Palate Association. Earlier biases and conflicts have been replaced with team efforts, in which the child is the focus of attention.

In 1969, a total of 244 facilities providing services for children with congenital clefts existed in the United States (National Institutes of Health, 1969). Among the 2,224 professional workers affiliated with these facilities, 53 percent were specialists in plastic surgery, prosthodontics, orthodontics, or speech pathology-audiology. Most of the teams included at least one member from each of these four specialties; and 86 percent of the professionals employed at the facilities came from one of five general fields—medicine, dentistry, speech pathology-audiology, social work, or psychology. The majority of the directors of the teams were from medicine, dentistry, or speech pathology. Although the kinds of services varied, the establishment of at least one facility in each of the fifty states and in the District of Columbia, Guam, Puerto Rico, and the Virgin Islands indicated that the needs of many children with congenital clefts were being met through the concerted efforts of several disciplines.

Other evidences of the interdisciplinary approach to clefts can be seen in the publications of the several disciplines, in conferences held throughout the country, and in activities of organizations whose members are affiliated with cleft palate teams. The relationships among team members have been discussed in articles written by representatives of the various disciplines (Kessler, 1954; H. K. Cooper, 1946; Harkins, 1946; Kemper, 1946; Frank, 1955; Lis and others, 1956; Randall, 1957; Vincent, 1960; Curtin, 1962; Gruber and others, 1966; Adisman, 1968; Biron and Felix, 1968; Converse and Horowitz, 1969). Reports concerned with clefts in *Plastic and Reconstructive Surgery* increased from 6.5 percent of the total number of articles in 1947 to 18.7 percent in 1968. In the first six years of publication of the *Cleft Palate Journal,* the senior authors of articles represented the three major disciplines of the sponsoring association almost equally; and articles with multiple authorship were often prepared by members of more than one of the professions. Special conferences attended by representatives of the several disciplines that constitute cleft palate teams, an international congress on cleft palate in 1969, and the annual meetings of the American Cleft

Palate Association have provided additional opportunities for interdisciplinary exchanges of information. Texts written or edited by dentists (Olin, 1960), physicians or surgeons (Drillien and others, 1966; Stark, 1968), and speech pathologists (Westlake and Rutherford, 1966; Morley, 1967; Lencione, 1968; Spriestersbach and Sherman, 1968) have contributed to the understanding of individuals born with prepalatal and palatal clefts and of the role of each of the members of the team. Retrieval systems have facilitated the preparation of information about medical genetic units (Lynch, 1969) and of bibliographies on disorders of communication (Johns Hopkins Medical Institutions, 1968) and on craniofacial anomalies (Georgiade, 1968). These interdisciplinary activities have assisted the several professions represented on cleft palate teams to provide better diagnosis, prognosis, and treatment.

American and Canadian plastic surgeons indicated their confidence in the team approach to cleft palate in their responses to a questionnaire about management of clefts sent to them in 1962. Of 309 responding, 30.4 percent stated that they felt the team was essential; 49.2 percent reported that they considered it helpful; 13.6 percent said that it was complicating; and only 6.8 percent said it was unnecessary (Lewin, 1964). Some have insisted that the team approach is excellent in professional education and research but not practical for efficient treatment. However, if the team becomes "the nucleus of a center for cleft palate research and training" (Chenoweth, 1964, p. 303) while maintaining its efficiency in treatment, the team and the child can profit from the interdisciplinary approach.

No team is without its problems. In their concern for their own positions, some team members can lose sight of the child, for whom the team exists. Leadership may become vested in one individual or one discipline, and representatives of the other professional fields may believe that they and their contributions are not receiving adequate consideration. Teamwork takes a great deal of time, not only for the discussions that lead to decisions about management but in the maintenance of records that permit exchange of information. The team is not a panacea (Koepp-Baker, in Morris, 1965); but, if channels of communication remain open and are freely used, it can be effective. This factor of interdisciplinary communication, although it can lead to "stylized verbal rituals" (Spriestersbach, in Spriestersbach and Sherman, 1968, p. 274), can lead also to improved research and training and to better service to children with clefts.

Those who participate most often on cleft palate teams have special competence in one field but try to understand the functions of the other disciplines. The plastic surgeon, orthodontist, prosthodontist, and speech pathologist can provide information for each other; but they also need information from social workers, psychologists, psychometrists, teachers, parents, and children. They may obtain assistance, also, from others within their own disciplines, such as the otolaryngologist, pediatrician, nurse, psychiatrist, general practitioner in medicine, oral surgeon, pedodontist, general dental practitioner, and audiometrist (Ivy, 1950; H. K. Cooper, 1951; Kessler, 1954; Marcks and others, 1955; Trusler and others, 1955; Keys, 1960; Biron and Felix, 1968; others).

Each of these contributors to the work of the cleft palate team has a special function, some providing information, others providing management. In some localities, a child born with a cleft of the prepalate or palate will be reported to state agencies by means of the birth certificate. This report will call into action a field representative of the state service for crippled children, a nurse or a social worker who will confer or correspond with the parents to give them information about assistance that may be available to them. Shortly after the child is born, an obstetrician, a pediatrician, a plastic surgeon, a social worker, a speech pathologist, or several of these team members will discuss with the parents the kinds of management that will be needed. Arrangements for the first surgical procedures will be made by the plastic surgeon and other members of a hospital staff, and these procedures will be carried out in accordance with the schedule determined by the surgeon in consultation with the parents. Financial arrangements, if the family qualifies for assistance from a state agency, will be made by a social worker, a field nurse, or some other representative of the agency. Instructions to the mother on feeding and caring for the child will be given by a nurse or the surgeon, and the parents will be advised by a psychologist if they need counseling.

Later, the speech pathologist will suggest ways of encouraging speech and language; and regular evaluations of the child's physical, intellectual, and psychosocial status will be made. Each time the team members see the child, at intervals from a few weeks to several months, they will determine his progress and his needs. The pediatrician, audiologist, otologist, psychometrist, and pedodontist may join the orthodontist, prosthodontist, plastic surgeon, and speech pathologist in these evaluations; and referrals may be made to radiologists for films to supplement direct observations. Teachers and school counselors will take part in the collection of additional information and in direct educational assistance to the child; speech clinicians in the school will provide a program designed to improve speech and language.

Additional surgery may be provided, and appropriate modifications of dental structure will be made by members of the team.

> All patients with cleft lip and palate, except perhaps in the initial stage of treatment of the cleft lip, which is primarily surgical, should have the benefit of the consensus of opinion of all specialists concerned after consultation by the group. [Ivy, 1950, p. 537]

Thus, all the members of a team can contribute information that will lead to plans for the habilitative process, although the execution of the plans may be the responsibility of a limited number.

The group that ultimately carries out the decisions about specific forms of management is usually made up of members of those disciplines that are concerned with modifying structures or changing behavior. Hence, the following discussion, while recognizing the importance of all the potential and actual members of a cleft palate team, will emphasize the relationship between the work of surgeons and dentists and that of the speech pathologist.

THE SURGEON, AS A MEMBER OF THE CLEFT PALATE TEAM, MODIFIES STRUCTURES THAT ARE INITIALLY DEVIANT OR THAT HAVE BEEEN PREVIOUSLY TREATED.

He uses "primary" or "secondary" procedures, depending on the point at which he sees the patient. Initial surgical management of a congenital cleft of the prepalate or palate is a "primary procedure"; additional management of these same structures is "secondary."

As the surgeon contemplates the repair of a congenitally cleft prepalate or palate, he considers many factors. He wishes to provide for good deglutition and appearance. He must preserve the innervation and the blood supply to the various parts. He attempts to minimize scarring and tension. He tries to avoid interference with growth. He hopes to provide structures that the patient can use for adequate speech.

The surgeon's task is complicated by many factors: the limited size of the field in which he works, the relative inaccessibility of many of the structures, problems of anesthetization, the anatomic variability of the patients, and others. He must seek new methods, modify those he has found useful in the past, and defend his choice of procedure against the judgment of those who propose other ways of achieving satisfactory results (Kaplan and others, 1969).

When he writes or talks about his work, the plastic surgeon may refer to certain procedures by using the names of those who evolved or modified them. He may also use descriptive terms, speaking of "a push-back," "relaxing incisions," "retropositioning," or "cartilage pharyngoplasty." The speech pathologist should be familiar with both kinds of terms, supplementing his basic knowledge with reference to surgical literature if his communication with the surgeon is to be most effective.

The operative procedures and the time for surgery are determined by the surgeon, in consultation with others who can provide information about the physical status of the child and his ability to tolerate surgery. Repair of labial clefts usually precedes surgical management of clefts of the alveolus and of the palate, if all these areas are affected; but some procedures provide for closing clefts in the lip and the alveolus at the same time.

For many years, closure of the prepalatal cleft has been an early procedure, often taking place before the baby left the hospital in which he was born. Some surgeons believed that nutrition was improved when the baby could nurse more easily, that closure of the labial cleft prevented drying of the nasal mucosa, that the repaired lip would exert a molding influence on the cleft maxilla, and that the improved appearance of the child could minimize the impact of the congenital anomaly on the family (Brown, 1938; Cannon and others, 1951; Stark, 1968). Recent recommendations about modifying the maxilla and retropositioning (moving back) the protruding premaxilla have sometimes led to postponement of surgery to a labial cleft until the child is several months of age (McNeil, 1954; Peet and Patterson, 1963; Burston, 1965; others). However, these recommendations, which will be discussed later in the chapter, have not changed the general time schedule for surgery to labial clefts. Almost all the members of the American Society of Plastic and Reconstructive Surgery who responded to the questionnaire on the management of patients with clefts agreed that a unilateral cleft of the lip should be surgically repaired before the child was six months of age (Lewin, 1964). Although 43 percent of the group stated that repair of the lip should not be undertaken until the child was six weeks old, the usual time reported for surgery to labial clefts was between two and six weeks after birth. The weight of the baby seemed to be one important factor, with 7 to 10 pounds being the minimum required by most surgeons for the primary closure of the labial cleft (Bauer and others, 1953; Lewin, 1964; Wilhelmsen and Musgrave, 1966).

The principal objectives of surgery for clefts of the lip are to obtain a symmetrical lip with a centered Cupid's bow, a vermilion border that is bounded by a white line, a philtral ridge and dimple, a symmetrical nose, and eventual normalcy of appearance (Slaughter and others, 1956;

Maisels, 1967; DeHaan, in Stark, 1968; Crikelair, 1969). In attempting to achieve these objectives, surgeons have used several different procedures, changing them as new methods have been developed. Of the 315 surgeons who responded to the questionnaire sent out in 1962, 211 indicated that they had changed their methods of operating on labial clefts at least once during the decade preceding their reports. In summarizing the responses on this topic, the investigator said,

> The most frequent pattern of change is from the Blair-Mirault-Brown-McDowell procedure to the Hagedorn-LeMesurier to the Tennison-Randall or the Millard procedure. In bilateral cleft lip the trend is evidently away from the Hagedorn procedure. [Lewin, 1964, p. 388]

The names cited in this report are those of surgeons whose procedures for closing labial clefts have been accepted in the period from 1844 to the present.

The "Mirault procedure," described by a French surgeon in 1844, was used also by the twentieth-century American surgeons whose names are connected with it. The procedure involved the use of two flaps, one from each side of a unilateral labial cleft, brought together and interwoven to close the cleft (Brown and McDowell, 1950; LeMesurier, 1955). The "Hagedorn procedure," presented in 1884 in Germany, was improved by A. B. LeMesurier of Canada and widely adopted after 1955. This operation brought a rectangular flap from the cleft side to the normal side of a unilateral labial cleft, with rotation of a portion of the vermilion border on the uncleft side to assist in the formation of a Cupid's bow (LeMesurier, 1962). The procedure used by C. M. Tennison (1952), Peter Randall (1959), and others also transferred a flap from the affected to the unaffected side of a unilateral labial cleft; but, before incisions were made, a bent wire was used as a stencil to define the shape of the flap and its eventual location. The procedure described by D. Ralph Millard (1964b, 1968) involved shifting tissue into a normal position by downward rotation of the Cupid's bow-philtrum-dimple component of the noncleft side and medial advancement of the upper lateral portion of the lip, with its attached alar base. This rotation-advancement principle, recommended for unilateral labial clefts, was also adapted to bilateral clefts of the lip.

Reviews, comparisons, and modifications of these procedures suggested that, for unilateral labial clefts, several methods of closure could be satisfactory (Davis, 1951; Bauer and others, 1953; Brauer, 1953; Wang, 1962;

Musgrave, 1963; Holdsworth, 1963; Davies, 1965; Cronin, 1966; Trauner and Trauner, 1967a; Hoffman and others, 1968; Williams, 1968); and one of these writers echoed a point made by those who cited objectives for surgery to the lip, saying, "A cleft lip repair is only as good as the ultimate appearance of the lip after growth" (Wang, 1962, p. 335).

In several of the procedures just described, and in others, the incision is made in the form of a Z to prevent tension. Some surgeons use the term "Z-plasty" when they speak of any of the several forms of surgical management for labial clefts in which this kind of incision is used. The Z avoids contractures and provides for the outward "pouting" that is typical of the normal upper lip (Davis, 1951; Musgrave, 1963; Stark, 1968). In contrast to the Z is the vertical, linear, or "straight-line" closure, in which the margins of the cleft are trimmed and brought together in a perpendicular line. This procedure has been advised only for repair of a minimal unilateral cleft of the lip without distortion of lip or nose or notching in the alveolus (DeHaan, in Stark, 1968).

When he describes the surgical correction of a bilateral cleft of the lip, the surgeon may remind his reader or listener that this kind of cleft differs from the unilateral in several ways. The physiological landmarks of the upper lip that is bilaterally cleft may be poorly defined, the prolabium may be small, and the sulcus between the lip and alveolus may be absent (Rees and others, 1962; Stark, 1968). The columella, serving as the central prop for the nasal tip (Millard, 1963b), may be unduly short; and the nose may be flattened, with flaring nostrils. The premaxilla, the architectural keystone of the upper dental arch (Barsky and others, 1962), may protrude, with the prolabium also in a forward position. The primary surgical management of the bilateral labial cleft, although it may not solve all these problems, may be accomplished in one operation; or closure of one side may convert the bilateral to a unilateral cleft, with the second side being repaired a few weeks later.

In his text on cleft lip, Victor Veau (1938) cited several of the problems involved in repair of unilateral and bilateral labial clefts, saying that he knew how to construct a lip that was nearly normal but that he had difficulty in getting symmetry of the nostrils in complete unilateral labial clefts. Veau recommended primary surgery to labial clefts when the patient was four weeks of age, with closure of the second side in bilateral clefts three months later. Veau's procedures for closing labial clefts were described in his text, but these procedures were not as widely accepted and used as those that he recommended for closure of palatal clefts.

Some surgeons will close the labial cleft without dealing directly with the protruding premaxilla, judging that the repaired lip may exert pressure that will move the premaxilla into a more suitable position. Some have believed that the establishment of an intact circumoral muscular complex as the result of closure of the labial cleft will provide a molding action that can narrow the palatal cleft, although the growth of the palatal shelves may also contribute to the decrease in the width of the cleft in the palatal area (Rees and others, 1962; Mazaheri, Harding, and Nanda, 1967; Aduss and Pruzansky, 1968).

In closing a bilateral cleft in the lip, surgeons may use a straight-line repair, an adaptation of the Tennison procedure, or the Millard rotation flap (Cronin, in Converse, 1964). In some instances, the premaxilla can be moved into position by light manual pressure; and the repaired lip can hold it in place, or it can be maintained in position by extraoral pressure. In others, the protruding, or "free floating," premaxilla can be repositioned by resectioning of a block of the vomer to provide space into which the premaxilla can be moved (Barsky and others, 1962). The retropositioned premaxilla can be stabilized by use of the vomer as an autogenous graft (Walden and others, 1968); or pins through the cheeks, with traction by rubber bands, can position and hold the markedly protruding premaxilla (Georgiade and others, 1968). If presurgical maxillary orthopedic management is being considered, surgery to the lip may be postponed beyond the usual time. Later discussion will amplify this point.

Other considerations of importance to the surgeon as he closes a bilateral labial cleft are preservation of the orbicularis oris muscle, prevention of flaring nostrils or a fistula from the labial sulcus into the floor of the nose, and provision of a philtrum and a labioalveolar sulcus (Brown, 1938; Glanz, 1959; LeMesurier, 1962; Berson, 1963; Cosman and Crikelair, 1965, 1966; Spina, 1966; Fára and Šmahel, 1967; Trauner and Trauner, 1967a; Climo, 1969; Neuner, 1969; Pennisi and others, 1969). Procedures used to meet these objectives may be primary or secondary.

In the management of bilateral labial clefts, secondary surgical procedures may be needed more often than in the closure of unilateral clefts. Improvement in appearance through provisions for symmetry, establishment of proportionate lengths of the two lips, and minimizing of scars may require surgery, sometimes referred to as "cosmetic," that is undertaken several years after the original repair of the lip.

One of these forms of management, the "switch-flap" or "Abbe flap," has been used as a primary procedure (Antia, 1966); but it is more commonly employed to modify earlier management. Whether the procedure is identified as the switch-flap, Abbe flap, Sabatini-Stein-Estlander-Abbe procedure (Smith, 1961; Harding, in R. T. Millard, 1964; Millard, 1964a), or Estlander-Abbe technique (Estlander, 1872; Abbe, 1898), it is designed to move tissue from the lower lip to the upper to correct flatness of the upper and reduce the redundancy of the lower or even to serve as a simulation of the philtrum.

When the protrusion of the premaxilla is extreme, the surgeon may work with the orthodontist in a procedure known as early, or presurgical, maxillary orthopedics. This approach has been widely discussed by surgeons and dentists; and the speech pathologist, reading or hearing their reports, will find that the topic has been the source of some controversy.

Recommendations in a thesis submitted for the degree of doctor of philosophy at the University of Glasgow by C. Kerr McNeil and appearing in a subsequent text (1954) started the trend toward a combination of efforts by "surgeons, oral surgeons, and dental prosthetists," as they were termed, to provide an intact upper dental arch prior to closure of a labial cleft. The procedure was designed to align the lateral maxillary segments and the premaxilla, with stabilization later by bone grafting in some cases.

In early maxillary orthopedic treatment, an intraoral appliance, usually made of transparent acrylic, is inserted shortly after the child is born. It serves as a temporary anterior palate for feeding, prevents the typical collapse of the lateral segments behind the premaxilla, provides space for moving the premaxilla into position, and can be expanded by an inset jackscrew manipulated by the parents in accordance with a schedule provided for them. The inserted plate is held in position by dental powder or external straps and is removed only for cleaning during a period of several weeks, after which the labial cleft is closed surgically.

Some of the American and Canadian surgeons who answered the 1962 questionnaire (Lewin, 1964) indicated that they had not used early maxillary orthopedics, in spite of their interest in the procedure, because of the lack of necessary cooperation from dentists; but, in several centers, the appliances are being used either before or after surgery to labial clefts, particularly with children who present bilateral complete clefts of the prepalate and palate and who frequently have medial displacement of the maxillary segments of the upper arch (Foster, 1957).

In the period following 1954, particularly in England, some orthodontists used maxillary appliances during the first three months of the child's life, preceding surgical closure of the labial cleft (Burston, 1965; Burston, in

Wallace, 1960; Latham and Burston, 1964); and some surgeons adopted the plan of referring all cleft cases to an orthodontist as soon as they were reported, usually within forty-eight hours after birth, for consideration of maxillary orthopedics (Osborne, in Wallace, 1960; Maisels, 1966). In the United States, several individuals and groups adopted or modified these procedures. One team, for example, used a special feeding plate for three months and an expansion plate when the child was four months of age (Spira and others, 1969). Others suggested fixing a controlled expanding appliance in the newborn at the time of closure of the labial cleft, with bone grafting as a supplementary procedure (Quinn and others, 1967; Mylin and others, 1968). The use of a prosthesis after surgery to the lip and before bone grafting has also been recommended (Georgiade, 1964). Orthodontists proposed placement of an orthopedic appliance following lip closure but prior to closure of the palatal cleft in patients with complete unilateral clefts of the prepalate and palate (Rosenstein and Jacobson, 1967); and a group including an orthodontist and a surgeon, after investigating the value of an orthodontic appliance inserted as early as thirteen days, with tape on the outside of the lip to provide pressure, concluded that such a procedure seemed to facilitate nursing, kept the tongue out of the cleft, decreased the size of the defect in the soft tissues, and provided time for growth (Crikelair and others, 1962).

Arguments for and against the use of early maxillary orthopedics were presented at the Annual Meeting of the American Cleft Palate Association in 1963. Those who defended the procedure stated that, although not all newborn cleft palate patients are suitable subjects for early orthopedic correction, those for whom such management is advisable seemed to benefit. The anticipated objections of parents to the postponement of closure of the labial cleft did not occur, they reported, adding that observations of parent-child relationships revealed "a relaxation of tensions, a feeling of accomplishment, and a better adjustment to this abnormality when compared with the conventional approach" (Shiere and Fisher, 1964). One group reported that the use of a preliminary prosthesis immediately after birth retarded collapse of the maxillary segments and guided occlusion; and this team recommended that bone grafting be undertaken when the child was six months of age, with orthodontic care later (Horton and others, 1964). Two plastic surgeons, describing their work, said that maxillary orthopedics in the newborn and orthodontic procedures in the four-year-old child were becoming part of the routine care of patients with clefts (Brauer and Cronin, 1964).

In dissent to these opinions, Samuel Pruzansky reviewed the arguments in favor of presurgical orthopedics and presented his rebuttal (1964). He asked for evidence to substantiate the claims that orthopedic appliances facilitate lip repair and alar reconstruction, improve sucking and swallowing, facilitate speech development, are of psychological advantage to the parents, and minimize the need for orthodontic treatment. He suggested that collapse of the maxillary segments, said by proponents of maxillary orthopedics to be an undesirable result of closure of the labial cleft, might be desirable in its facilitation of velopharyngeal reconstruction.

Continued study of early maxillary orthopedic management has been recommended by almost all those who use or oppose it; and, in time, enough evidence from children who have undergone such treatment and then have grown to adolescence will be available to provide a basis for evaluation. Until that time, affirmations or modifications of previous points of view will continue to be presented by those on both sides of the question and on both sides of the Atlantic.

Since 1963, proponents and opponents of maxillary orthopedics have provided additional information. One study of the change in size and shape of the predeciduous maxillary arch in children with unilateral clefts provided no evidence that orthopedic appliances stimulated the growth of tissue (Huddart, 1968). Rather, the effect of the appliance was to minimize the increase in the width of the upper dental arch, with growth at the cleft margins serving to narrow the width of the defect in the palate (Neumann, 1967; Huddart, 1968; Monroe and others, 1968). Other changes that seemed to result from early maxillary orthopedic management included restraining of the forward growth of the premaxilla (Robertson and Hilton, 1968), more normal feeding patterns because of the function of the appliance as a feeding plate (Spira and others, 1969), reduction of occlusal anomalies (Ozerovic and Markovic, 1967), and prevention of lateral collapse of the maxillary arch (Latham and Burston, 1964).

Since the use of the maxillary orthopedic appliance was recommended in 1954, changes have taken place in the type of appliance, the time at which it is inserted, and the sequence of events related to this form of management. In Germany, one method of treatment is to insert a plate that covers the vomer immediately after birth and leave it in place until the labial cleft is closed surgically four to six months later (Hotz, 1969). Appliances held in place with extraoral headbands to provide pressure against the protruding premaxilla and move it into place have been used in the United States (Garner, 1964; Jacobson and Rosenstein, 1965). Rapid expansion of the maxillary arch, often accomplished in a three-week period, has been continued in England (Broadway, 1967; Moss, 1968). Appliances have been inserted before surgery to the lip, according to reports from France and the United States (Brauer and others, 1962; Crikelair and others, 1962; Petit and Psaume, 1967); and surgical closure of the lip has preceded insertion of the appliance (Bay, 1967; Jacobson and Rosenstein, 1965; Monroe and others, 1968).

Those who questioned the use of presurgical maxillary orthopedics have presented several additional points in support of their opinions. They have found no appreciable effect of such treatment on the facial growth pattern, for example (Ross and Johnston, 1967). They have contended that the premaxilla will usually come into position without orthodontic aid after closure of the labial cleft (Thilander and Stenström, 1967). They have stated that the collapse of the maxillary arch is not an inevitable sequel to surgical repair of the lip and palate, that children who do not use feeding appliances will gain as much weight as those who do, and that the value of presurgical orthopedic treatment has not been clearly demonstrated (Pruzansky and Aduss, 1967). Thus, the arguments for and against early orthopedic management continue; and the speech pathologist, with special awareness of the importance of the intact and well-aligned upper dental arch to articulatory activities, should be able to participate in discussions of these procedures with other members of the team.

Another approach to the management of prepalatal clefts, that of bone grafting, has been adopted relatively recently. In combination with maxillary orthopedics or as a separate procedure, bone grafting can be used to stabilize the segments of the maxilla if they are in good relationship or after they have been brought into position by other procedures. Alveolar clefts accompanying labial or palatal clefts have usually been repaired during surgery to the lip or palate; and, in some instances, the alveolus seemed intact postoperatively because the mucous membrane covering hid the bony defect. However, in these cases, the premaxilla was not firmly attached to the maxillary segments. In unilateral clefts, the lack of bony contiguity might not be serious; but the separation of the premaxilla from the maxillary segments sometimes resulted in lack of stability of the alveolus. Hence, the use of bone grafts at the point or points of bony discontinuity seemed desirable to provide a stable dental arch, furnish support to teeth adjacent to the graft, fill out the contour of the alveolar ridge, and establish a bony framework for surgical improvement of appearance (Bäckdahl and Nordin, 1961; Brauer and Cronin, 1964; Horton and others, 1964; Schultz, 1964; Muir, 1966; Pickrell and others, 1968).

The materials used for grafts to connect the premaxillary and lateral maxillary segments are frequently autogenous, being taken from one part of the patient's body for insertion elsewhere. Pieces of bone from a rib, the crest of the hip bone, or the leg are used for these grafts; and the wedge of borrowed bone is inserted in the space between the premaxillary and maxillary segments, with bone chips being packed into any remaining space (Johanson and Ohlsson, 1961; Brauer and Cronin, 1964; Converse and others, 1964; Georgiade and others, 1964; Matthews and Grossman, 1964; Schrudde, 1965). Because this procedure has been used for only a short time, its effects cannot be determined until the children with whom it was used reach maturity (Robertson and Jolleys, 1968). The speech pathologist can contribute to the evaluation of this procedure because of the value of his judgments on the articulation of children treated by bone grafting.

Palatal clefts, remaining after closure of defects in the lip and alveolus or existing as isolated anomalies, are usually treated surgically. More than one operation may be needed to complete the closure of the hard and soft palate and provide for adequate velopharyngeal closure, and prostheses may be used to supplement surgical management.

The time for closure of clefts in the palate is determined by such factors as the location and extent of the cleft, the opinion of the surgeon on the effect that surgery may have on growth, and the physical status of the child. For many years, primary surgery to the palate was performed when the child was eighteen months old or in an age range from twelve to twenty-four months (Cannon and others, 1951; Trusler and others, 1955; Bill and others, 1956; Metzger, 1957; Millard, 1962; Peet and Patterson, 1963; Lewin, 1964; Stark, 1968; others). Some variations in this time schedule exist, in the United States and elsewhere; and closure of the palatal cleft is sometimes postponed until the child is three, four, or six years of age or even older (Krogman, 1954; Lewin, 1962; Hoppe, 1965; Fára and Brousilová, 1969).

Whereas closure of the labial cleft is undertaken to improve appearance and facilitate feeding, one of the main objectives in surgical repair of the palate is the provision of structures that can be used effectively for speech. As a result of emphasis on the need for adequate velopharyngeal valving for speech, surgery to the soft palate has often preceded closure of a cleft in the hard palate if two operations are contemplated (Slaughter and Pruzansky, 1954); and recommendations for closure of the velar cleft before the child reaches twenty-four months of age have been based on the time schedule for the acquisition of speech and language.

Although a major goal of surgical repair of the palate is "to construct a competent, functioning, air- and watertight valve at the junction of soft palate and pharynx" (Stark, 1968, p. 153), the surgeon has other purposes in closing palatal clefts. He hopes to provide for normal hearing, to assure development of the central part of the face, to encourage functional dentition and normal contour of the palatal vault, and to give the child an opportunity to have oral structures that are as nearly as possible within normal limits.

In describing the procedures used to meet these objectives, surgeons may classify their work in various ways. Descriptions of early methods have been reported in reviews of cleft palate surgery (Dorrance, 1933; Blair, 1937; Brown, 1938; Aufricht, 1946; Ivy, 1950; Cannon and others, 1951; Steffenson, 1952; Nylén, 1961; Harding, in R. T. Millard, 1964; Letterman and others, 1964; Edgerton and Zovickian, 1965; Saunders, in Stark, 1968; others). Some of these methods, such as the technique of compression (Brophy, 1923), have been abandoned; but others are still being used as they were originally proposed or in modified form, as primary or secondary procedures.

Reports of methods used to close palatal clefts, when they are presented to a cleft palate team, may include the names of the surgeons who introduced the procedures or terms that describe the techniques briefly. In some instances, both the name and the description are used, as in a set of forms proposed for reporting surgical procedures for data processing (Millard and others, 1967). Most of the procedures now employed can be placed in one or more of five categories to indicate the purpose of the operation: to close an anterior cleft, to close a cleft in the velum, to lengthen the palate, to connect the velum and the posterior pharyngeal wall, and to reduce the distance between the pharyngeal wall and the soft palate.

In closing a cleft in the anterior palate, after repair of the velar cleft or at the same time, a surgeon may use sliding mucoperiosteal flaps or bone flaps. If he loosens the mucoperiosteal covering of the palate by making incisions along the inside of the upper alveolar arch, he can free the mucoperiosteum and move it toward the midline to cover the defect in the bony palate. The surgeon may report this kind of repair by saying that he used a modified von Langenbeck procedure or the Veau-Wardill-Kilner modification of the von Langenbeck. If he moves the bone as well as its covering, he has used a bone flap and may call the technique the Dieffenbach-Warren-von Langenbeck procedure. In either of these approaches, he may choose to fracture the hamular processes to permit better movement of the palatal shelves in a median direction, a method that is employed by approximately two-thirds of the surgeons who reported their choices of surgical management in 1962 (Lewin, 1964). The surgeon may close an anterior cleft by creating a flap from the vomer, using the method described by Veau (1931) or the Wardill-Kilner modification. Another technique, in which flaps are created from the mucoperiosteum of the anterior palate and rotated to cover the cleft in the hard palate, is called the Wardill four-flap procedure.

Some of the methods just cited provide for closure of the soft palate as well as for covering or filling the defect in the hard palate. If the velum is cleft but the anterior palate is intact, incisions may be used to relax tension and permit the approximation of the edges of the velar cleft, which are then pared and sutured at the midline. The hamular processes may be divided in this procedure, also. The goal in this type of surgery to the soft palate is to provide a velum that has mobility as well as length.

Because velopharyngeal closure is facilitated if the palate is long enough and mobile enough to participate in valving, the surgeon may wish to move the velum in a backward direction to give it additional length. In such situations, the push-back operation, sometimes called the Dorrance push-back, may be used for retropositioning the palate (Dorrance and Bransfield, 1946). The incisions for the Dorrance push-back are made in a semicircle inside the alveolar arch, and the membrane is lifted from the bony palate and sutured in a position posterior to its original location. This has the effect of loosening and lengthening the soft palate. One modification of this procedure is called the Gillies-Fry technique, in which, after the push-back is accomplished, any defect in the anterior bony palate is covered with a dental plate. Other changes in the push-back procedure are the Ganzer-Veau-Ruppe and the Wardill-Kilner modifications, in which the shape of the incisions resulted in adoption of the descriptive terms "V-Y advancement" and "W-V flap." In both of these forms of management, the palate is moved backward, in spite of the term "advancement." The incisions that free the mucoperiosteal covering go forward along the sides of the alveolar ridge to about the location of the canine teeth and then outline, in general, an area that encompasses the central anterior triangle containing the incisive foramen. Although the incision has been called a V, it is more like W; the name W-V is more suitable, the V being the wedge-shaped outline of the cleft. When closure is completed, the suture lines look like a Y, with the stem at the midline of the palate.

Procedures used to close clefts in the hard and soft palates and to provide additional palatal length often involve flaps of various kinds. Tissue from outside the oral cavity was used by early surgeons who put the patient's little finger or skin from his forehead into the palatal cleft; but modern surgeons who have moved flaps from the neck, thorax, abdomen, or upper arm have not found them entirely satisfactory (Edgerton and Zovickian, 1965). However, tissue from within the oral and nasal cavities can be converted to flaps that will probably not be rejected. In addition to the flaps from the vomer and from the palate itself, already mentioned, the surgeon may report that he has used Esser's nasolabial flap (A. F. Wallace, 1966), nasomucosal flaps (Cronin and others, 1964), flaps from the cheek (Ecker, 1960; Mukherji, 1969), flaps that are turned over so that the raw surface is outermost (Isshiki and Morimoto, 1968), a periosteal flap (Skoog, 1965b), or the Millard island flap that lengthens the palate (Millard, 1963a, 1966; Hage, 1966; Dijkstra, 1969; Georgiade and others, 1969). In making these various modifications of the tissues of the nasal and oral cavities, the surgeon considers the superior, or nasal, surface of the palate as well as the oral surface; and he may line the raw superior surface with mucosa from the vomer or with a skin graft to prevent the stiffening and shortening of the palate that can result from scarring on the nasal side.

The procedure that connects a strip from the posterior wall of the pharynx to the velum, the pharyngeal flap operation or Rosenthal pharyngoplasty, was used and abandoned in the nineteenth century, then revived about 1924 (Broadbent and Swinyard, 1959). The pharyngeal flap was introduced in the United States in 1929 and adopted by many American surgeons after it was described at the Eightieth Annual Session of the American Medical Association (Padgett, 1930). Because the fundamental purpose of the pharyngeal flap seemed to be to provide adequate velopharyngeal valving for speech, many surgeons reserved the procedure for those patients who did not achieve good velopharyngeal control after other forms of surgical management (Webster and others, 1961; Williams and Woolhouse, 1962). Earlier proponents of Rosenthal pharyngoplasty recommended that it be used with children who were at least ten or twelve years old (Récamier, Rosenthal, in Skoog and Ivy, 1957). Others provided a pharyngeal flap for selected children of four to eight years of age (Rubin and others, 1961). More recently, the pharyngeal flap has been combined with other procedures as the first operation on the palate when the child is about one year of age (Stark, 1968, and in Lencione, 1968; Stark and others, 1969).

The decision to use a pharyngeal flap is often based on the child's apparent need, prior to his acquisition of language, for some way of compensating for a short velum or for lack of velopharyngeal closure in the presence of an adequate soft palate (Obregon and Smith, 1959). After language is acquired, if speech training and surgical management have not achieved the desired results, the team may decide that a pharyngeal flap is needed. Evaluation of the efficiency of mesial movements of the lateral pharyngeal walls (Morris and Spriestersbach, 1967; Trauner and Trauner, 1967b) and the use of a temporary prosthesis to determine the effect of additional valving on nasality (Blakeley, 1960; Curtis and Chierici, 1964) have been advised as preliminary measures of the potential for success of pharyngeal flap surgery.

In providing this connective band of tissue, the surgeon takes a vertical section from the center of the posterior pharyngeal wall, leaving it attached at one end, and swings it forward to attach to the velum. This divides the passageway in the oropharynx, with the flap in the center and an opening of 3 to 5 millimeters in width on each side for the passage of air. These lateral openings may increase in size if the flap shrinks, as it sometimes does within the first few months following surgery.

If the surgeon reports that the flap is inferiorly based, he means that the tissue raised from the posterior wall of the pharynx remains attached at the lower end and that the upper end is detached and sutured to the velum. If he speaks of a superiorly based flap, he is indicating that the flap remains attached at the top and swings down to be connected to the soft palate. A flap that is inferiorly based can usually be seen in the oropharyngeal area; one that has its base above may not be visible unless the examiner uses a mirror. Some flaps are attached to the upper side of the soft palate; others are connected to the buccal side. Some are placed in pockets or openings created surgically to receive them. The point of attachment is not necessarily determined by the point of base.

Those who recommend a superior base for the pharyngeal flap have found that elevation of the palate by the upward pull of the flap can result in better velopharyngeal closure (Cox and Silverstein, 1961; Bzoch, 1964b; Skoog, 1965a; Owsley and others, 1966). Those who recommend basing the flap inferiorly have also suggested that speech is improved by this method (Conway and Goulian, 1961) and that the procedure is more easily managed. A summary of studies of pharyngeal flap surgery between 1951 and 1967 (Yules and Chase, 1969) indicated that speech was improved in the majority of the patients, whether the flap was based superiorly or inferiorly, although the methods of measuring improvement varied. Those reporting prior to 1960 used the inferiorly based flap more often; after 1960, the use of the superior base increased. This trend toward preference for a superior base for the pharyngeal flap was shown also in the responses of surgeons to the questionnaire on their management of clefts, 63.4 percent of those using the pharyngeal flap indicating in 1962 that they based the flap superiorly (Lewin, 1964).

Insertion of a pharyngeal flap reduces the total area of the oropharynx, but other forms of pharyngoplasty (Reidy, 1964) may also be reported for diminishing the size of the passageway and permitting the velum to approximate the pharyngeal walls. These surgical procedures bring the posterior walls of the pharynx forward or reduce the side-to-side dimensions of the pharyngeal space.

A procedure used by Gustav Passavant in the nineteenth century created a bar of tissue from the pharyngeal wall in the form of a "caterpillar flap." A more recent technique, which provides a roll of mucous membrane and constrictor muscle that bulges from the pharyngeal wall, is called the "Roll-Y pharyngoplasty" (Hamacher, 1967). Transplantation of the posterior tonsillar pillars with their enclosed palatopharyngeal muscle to make a dynamic muscle sphincter has been described (Orticochea, 1968); and the use of flaps from the lateral pharyngeal walls to form a shelf above the level of Passavant's ridge is called the "Hynes pharyngoplasty" (Hynes, 1950, 1967). In these techniques, the tissue that is used is already present; but its position is modified to reduce the area of the pharynx or to increase the forward thrust of the pharyngeal wall to meet the backward movement of a velum that is mobile but short. In another method, a graft of fascia from the thigh is attached to the temporalis or masseter muscles to provide kinetic energy to a palate that is not mobile and to lift it into a position that permits better function (Kiehn and others, 1965).

Autogenous cartilage may be implanted in the posterior wall of the pharynx (Hill and Hagerty, 1960, 1962; Hagerty and others, 1968; Hess and others, 1968) to reduce the depth of the oropharynx; and other procedures, such as injections of Teflon (Bluestone and others, 1968) and implants of silicone (Blocksma, 1964), have been used for this same general purpose. Of 262 surgeons who responded to a questionnaire on the use of surgery for velopharyngeal incompetence, 50 percent approved the principle of retropharyngeal implantation, 35 percent disapproved, and 15 percent were undecided (Blocksma and Braley, 1969). Implants may be unstable and may move from the position in which they are placed. Injections of Teflon have obtained immediate and demonstrable improvements in velopharyngeal valving, but the long-range results of such management have not yet been determined.

The plastic surgeon may provide other forms of management that may be needed to meet immediately postnatal problems. A child with the Pierre Robin syndrome, with or without a cleft, may have difficulty in breathing and nursing because of the retropositioned tongue and the small jaw (Randall and others, 1965; Takagi and others, 1966; McEvitt, 1968). If conservative management cannot solve the problem, the tongue may be fastened in a forward position by the Beverly Douglas procedure (Douglas, 1946, 1950), some adaptation of that procedure, or the use of a fascial sling (Lewis and others, 1968). Because the Pierre Robin syndrome is frequently associated with a palatal cleft, the child with these multiple problems often comes to the attention of the cleft palate team.

Whatever his choice of procedure for closing clefts of the palate and providing for velopharyngeal valving, the surgeon may consult with other members of the team about the child's status and the probable results of surgery that is contemplated. The speech pathologist should be responsible for evaluating articulatory-resonatory factors when secondary surgery is being planned and for making postoperative evaluations that indicate the effect of surgical procedures on speech. The speech pathologist may also be asked to predict the kind of speech that may be expected if the structures are not modified further or to undertake a trial remedial program that will affect the team's decision to recommend additional surgery. As he reads or hears reports of the procedures used or contemplated by plastic surgeons, the speech pathologist may encounter such statements as the following:

> A palatoplasty (von Langenbeck) with a superiorly based pharyngeal flap was performed.
>
> There is no indication now for an Abbe flap to add tissue to the upper lip. Operation of the Langenbeck type, without pharyngoplasty, was performed. The unilateral cleft lip was repaired with a triangular flap.
>
> Closure of the palate by a Dieffenbach procedure was delayed.
>
> Secondary palatal surgery with a pharyngeal flap and push-back had been performed earlier. An implant of costal cartilage was inserted behind the soft tissues of the posterior pharyngeal wall.
>
> The combination of the lower Z-plasty of Tennison with the upper one according to Trauner or Skoog gives a better nose than the original methods of LeMesurier or Tennison.

If he understands the terms used in such reports, the speech pathologist can participate more effectively in the discussions held by the cleft palate team.

THE ORTHODONTIST'S PARTICIPATION IN TEAM EFFORTS MAY COME EARLY IN THE HABILITATIVE PROCESS OR AT A LATER TIME.

If he takes part in early orthopedic procedures to modify the alveolar arch and align the maxillary processes with the premaxilla, the orthodontist may be involved from the outset (Howard, 1969). Otherwise, orthodontic management of children with congenital clefts is relatively limited in the first six to seven years of life (Olin, in Lencione, 1968).

The orthodontist is interested in the growth and development of the face and jaws (J. A. Cooper, in R. T. Millard, 1964) and in the position, form, number, and caries susceptibility of the teeth (Biron and Felix, 1968). He sees several reasons for orthodontic treatment for children with congenital prepalatal and palatal clefts: the need to align the palatal segments of the maxilla, the importance of freeing impacted palatal shelves that may interfere with normal growth, and the maintenance of gains made in palatodental corrections and in palatal growth (Coccaro, 1969). In more detail, the purposes of orthodontics for children with clefts might be listed under seven general categories: to change the shape of the dental arches, to reposition teeth, to bring the upper and lower dental arches and the teeth they contain into adequate relationship, to provide an oral cavity in which the tongue can move freely for articulation, to furnish support for structures in the oral cavity, to improve appearance, and to maintain modifications that are made in dental structure. In achieving these purposes, the orthodontist correlates his work with that of the other specialists on the team, believing that the "mere construction of a speech appliance with no other consideration is as bad as poorly considered surgery" (H. K. Cooper, 1951, p. 47).

The three phases of treatment related to the orthodontist's objectives are expansion of the maxillary segments when the child is three or four years of age, treatment during the period of mixed dentition, and final correction of the permanent dentition (Conroy, 1951; Pierce and others, 1955; Olin, in Converse, 1964, and in Lencione, 1968; J. Daniel Subtelny, 1966). For children with unilateral clefts, orthodontic treatment before the acquisition of permanent dentition seems to have little effect on facial growth patterns; but early orthodontic management seems beneficial to those with bilateral clefts (Ross and Johnston, 1967).

The orthodontist's reports of his work contain relatively few names, but they do include a number of terms used to describe procedures or identify appliances. The speech pathologist may find such statements as the following in communications from orthodontists:

> Improper treatment of the abutments and poor design of the anterior portion of the prosthetic speech appliance have caused the remaining maxillary teeth to develop severe peridontal involvements.
>
> An extraoral appliance was worn for several weeks.
>
> The mandibular development and the posterior occlusion were normal. However, both of the maxillary cuspids were in lingual occlusion.
>
> The bite plate was removed, and a fixed lingual arch was inserted.
>
> Stainless steel crowns were cemented on the first molars. The maxillary right and left central incisors were banded.
>
> A complete maxillary overlay prosthesis and a full mandibular denture were constructed.

The various forms of malocclusion are known by most speech pathologists, and the names for the various teeth are usually recognized by all members of the cleft palate team. However, understanding of some of the procedures used by the orthodontist and of some of the appliances he uses may enable the speech pathologist to make a better contribution to discussions of orthodontic management.

Although many people say that they wore "braces" on their teeth when they were young, that term does not appear with any frequency in reports of orthodontic management. Rather, references are made to wires, expansion arches, bite plates, expansion screw plates, expanders, intraoral elastics, retainers, and extraoral appliances. Each of these has a purpose, and each may be used at one or more of the stages of orthodontic treatment for children with clefts.

The upper dental arch in the child with a repaired palatal cleft is more often in need of widening than of narrowing if its shape is to be modified. Some orthodontists may report that they used a lingual expansion arch or an expansion plate to achieve a wider upper dental arch. The lingual expansion arch is made of wire that is attached to metal bands placed around the second deciduous molars in most instances. The attachment is made by soldering the wire to a retention lug on the inside of the dental arch, the lingual side, or by running it through buccal tubes that are fastened to the bands. The wire exerts pressure to expand the maxillary arch; and it can be shaped to provide for more expansion at some points, less at others. Additional wires, called finger springs, are sometimes used to obtain greater modification in the arch in certain areas. A similar appliance, the Arnold expander, does not go completely around the inside of the upper dental arch but has a bar that extends from one side to the other, with a small spiral spring to increase the horizontal dimension of the bar as the dental arch moves outward. The expansion plate is not attached to bands on the teeth but is held in place by U-shaped clasps of wire that fit around several of the teeth. The plate is usually made of acrylic and fits into the palatal vault, with its sides against the alveolar ridge to move the dental arch outward. A variation of this appliance is the expansion screw plate, which is split in the middle to allow the two halves to move away from each other as a jackscrew is turned with a "key" made of wire that fits into holes in the center of the screw. As the screw is lengthened, the sides of the plate separate; and the dental arch is enlarged by steady, increasing pressure according to a schedule determined by the orthodontist.

The upper teeth of the child born with a cleft in the alveolus and palate are often out of alignment. Some teeth may be missing; others may erupt in unusual locations, such as the middle of the roof of the mouth or outside the alveolar arch. The orthodontist's task is to bring the teeth into alignment. He attempts, additionally, to correct the deflections of individual teeth from their normal positions, modifying linguoversion, labioversion, and buccoversion. If the teeth are so crowded that removal of some will provide room for the others to be moved into better positions, he may use serial extraction, taking out one tooth at a time and determining the effect of the extraction on alignment before he decides to remove another. He may report to the cleft palate team that he recommends the use of a labial arch wire to reposition teeth that are out of alignment; and he will put bands on the teeth, attach tubes to these bands, run the wire through the tubes, and put the wire into the proper position on the outside of the dental arch, the labial side, to move teeth forward or push them back. If he wishes to correct crossbite, he may recommend an inclined bite plate, placed over the posterior or anterior mandibular teeth to move the maxillary teeth in the proper direction.

Some of the procedures just described will help to bring the upper and lower dental arches into the proper relationship. If additional correction of jaw relationships is needed, the orthodontist may indicate that he has elected to use intraoral elastics to connect bands on the upper and lower teeth and exert a mild directional force provided by the rubber bands to move the lower jaw forward or backward in relationship to the upper.

Provision of an oral cavity in which the tongue can move freely is difficult if appliances must be placed on the lingual side of the alveolar ridge, although the interference from appliances may be justified by the improvement brought about by orthodontic management. If the upper dental arch is widened, if teeth are moved into their proper places or extracted if they are in a position to restrict tongue activity, and if relatively normal dental occlusion is achieved, the oral cavity should be adequate for the various movements of the tongue in articulatory activities as well as in management of food. However, team planning is particularly important in coordinating orthodontic management with speech training during the period for acquiring articulatory skills.

Some appliances that provide support for oral structures may resemble prostheses but can be considered in this discussion of the work of the orthodontist, who may construct devices that do not substitute for missing parts but, instead, give support to the lip or palate. If the upper lip is flat or retruded, the profile is distorted; speech may be affected, also. Even if the upper incisors are present, they may be so far retracted that they do not give support to the upper lip; in such cases, a labial supportive appliance can be used temporarily. This appliance, containing incisor teeth, can improve appearance, facilitate the learning of speech skills, and also serve as a retainer (Adams and Brown, 1965; Rayne, 1966). Other appliances, used with a repaired palate of normal length that is not achieving good function or in cases of velar paralysis, are called palatal lifts, supportive-type speech aids, or palate elevator buttons. They fit against the inferior surface of the soft palate and move it in an upward and backward direction, enabling the patient to achieve the velopharyngeal closure that has been prevented by the lack of velar retraction (Gibbons and Bloomer, 1958; Lang, 1967; Beder and others, 1968; Bloomer and Lang, 1968; Gonzalez and Aronson, 1970).

Orthodontic management can improve the appearance of the child with a congenital cleft, although the process of treatment is long and requires a high level of cooperation from the child and his family. The effect of improved appearance is not only aesthetic (Ricketts, 1968) but brings "psychosocial satisfactions" (Harkins, 1960, p. 3) as well.

Once the dental structures have been brought into relatively normal positions and relationships, fixed or removable retainers may be used to hold the teeth in their places (Curtis, 1968). These may be intraoral plates, small retaining devices called stents, or even extraoral wires that fit around the head and maintain the teeth in the positions to which they have been moved.

These retainers may be worn constantly for a period of time or may be used intermittently. The permanency of results of orthodontic management, in terms of palatal and dental arch form, cannot be evaluated until all of the patient's permanent teeth have erupted and the intradental and interdental relationships can be studied (Coccaro, 1969).

The orthodontist's work depends, to some extent, on the faithfulness with which appointments are kept, on the child's cooperation in wearing and taking care of the appliances, and on the encouragement provided for the family by other members of the team. The speech pathologist can assist by stressing the importance of the orthodontic program to the parents and the child, by explaining methods for cleaning and caring for the appliance in conformance with instructions given by the orthodontist, and by recognizing that necessary orthodontic care sometimes interferes with speech training. Conversely, the orthodontist can consult the speech pathologist about the effect that an appliance may have on acquired or developing articulatory skills. He can modify his program if the speech pathologist indicates that the acquisition of articulatory abilities is more important to the child's eventual habilitation than prosthodontic management at a particular point in time, granting that an orthodontic program that would in any way interfere with speech training "would be contra-indicated until socially acceptable speech is learned" (J. A. Cooper, in R. T. Millard, 1964, not paged). An advantage of the team approach is that the several specialists have an opportunity to exchange opinions as well as information.

PROSTHODONTICS MAY SUPPLEMENT OR REPLACE SURGICAL AND ORTHODONTIC PROCEDURES IN THE HABILITATION OF INDIVIDUALS WITH CONGENITAL ORAL CLEFTS.

By general definition, prosthetics involves the replacement of an absent part with an artificial one. Cleft palate prosthetic management is "the science and art of utilizing artificial materials to provide a separation of the oral cavity from the nasal cavity" (Harkins, 1960, p. 1) or to replace missing or extracted teeth. The prosthodontist attempts to provide structures that will permit the acquisition of socially acceptable speech, restore the masticating apparatus, establish facial and dental harmony, and enable the patient to make a good psychological adjustment. He selects cases for prosthetic management with care, and he does not believe that a prosthetic speech aid should be used just as "a last resort" (Mazaheri, in R. T. Millard, 1964).

If feeding is a problem for the newborn with a prepalatal cleft, the prosthodontist may suggest the use of a feeding obturator that permits the baby to nurse more efficiently before the palate is closed surgically. Specially designed nipples may suffice for adequate nursing, but the construction of temporary obturators for children with clefts or for those with the Pierre Robin syndrome has been described in the past and more recently (Brophy, 1923; Lifton, 1956; Williams and others, 1968; Malson, 1969). Such devices, like the plate used for maxillary orthopedic management, can seal off the nasal cavity and provide a surface against which the nipple can be compressed. The possibility that a prosthesis inserted soon after birth and maintained for about a year could stimulate growth of the maxillary segments was suggested by one group of research workers (McEvitt and others, 1969). Although this appliance was not designed to move the jaw segments into new alignment, it seemed to prevent collapse of the maxillary segments and to cause growth in the tissue adjacent to the anterior part of the cleft. In providing these forms of management, the prosthodontist is involved in the early stages of the child's life; in most instances, his contributions to the habilitative process begin later.

Prostheses to replace teeth are sometimes constructed by the orthodontist; but the prosthodontist also is concerned in determining the need for such replacements and in building them. Some prostheses accomplish more than one task, providing teeth in the anterior section, covering a fistula in the palate, and extending into the pharynx to assist in velopharyngeal closure. Others are designed for one or two needs but not for all three. In some cases, orthodontic appliances are supplemented by prosthodontic additions such as artificial teeth, a palatal plate, or an obturator.

Most team members believe that the form of management should be determined for each patient, although surgery is the first choice in many instances. References to surgical failures are infrequent today; but, in the past, some prosthodontists thought of their services as "the last hope after disaster" (Récamier, in Skoog and Ivy, 1957, p. 184) for patients who could not be adequately treated by the surgeon. The team-oriented prosthodontist of the present is often called on to provide supplements to surgery. If the cleft involves the alveolar ridge, the patient will probably need a fixed or removable prosthesis, sooner or later, to complete the anterior part of the upper dental arch. If the velopharyngeal mechanism is not functioning adequately or if perforations remain in the palate after surgery, a prosthesis can serve as a divider between the oral and nasal cavities, keep food out of the nasal passages, keep nasal secretions out of the mouth, and permit the development of articulation and velopharyngeal valving, with or without speech training (Schalit, 1946; Harkins and Koepp-Baker, 1948; Harkins, 1960; Olin, 1960; Killey, in Holdsworth, 1963).

The team may decide that, for a specific patient, a prosthesis is preferable to surgical management. Some of the factors that affect such a decision include the presence of a wide cleft with insufficient tissue for surgical closure or of a cleft in the hard palate that cannot be closed with tissue from the oral and nasal areas, paralysis or deficiency of the soft palate congenitally or postoperatively, medical contraindications to surgery, and the desirability of postponing surgical management until the effect of the prosthesis as a stimulant to muscular activity can be determined (Mazaheri, 1962). Prostheses can be changed, whereas surgical modifications are more permanent.

Prostheses designed for individuals with congenital clefts may have several parts, palatomaxillary and palatovelar sections serving to hold the prostheses in place and as a base for teeth that may be added and the pharyngeal section functioning in velopharyngeal valving (Aram and Subtelny, 1959). The anterior section may be reduced in size if dentition is adequate and if no fistula exists in the hard palate, but it is still needed to provide attachment to the teeth. In this situation, the speech aid that constitutes the pharyngeal section may be attached to a small anterior section by a central connective strip that follows the line of the palatal vault.

In describing his procedures to the team, the prosthodontist will use some terms that appear in orthodontists' reports and some that apply to his specialty. He may cite the use of bands, clasps, buccal tubes, retention lugs, stents, and finger springs, as the orthodontist does; but, although he may not provide details about the specific materials and tools he uses, the prosthodontist may talk about impressions, models, crowns, thimbles, sections, bulbs, and obturators. His reports may contain statements such as the following:

> Because of the patient's gag reflex, an underextended bulb was put in place for three weeks before the final impression was made.
>
> The stainless steel crowns were cemented on the second deciduous molars, and the palatal portion of the obturator was inserted.
>
> Maxillary and mandibular impressions were made, and a maxillary prosthesis replacing the anterior teeth and an obturator were inserted several weeks later.
>
> Final impressions were made using alginate in an individual acrylic impression tray for the upper dental arch.

In planning a prosthesis, the dental specialist makes preliminary studies and then takes impressions of the mouth of the patient to guide him in constructing the various sections of the prosthetic appliance. Using trays of appropriate sizes and impression materials of various types, he makes a "negative" of the palatal, dental, and oropharyngeal areas from which to build a study model. Teeth that will be used as supports for the prosthesis may be covered with stainless steel or gold crowns to strengthen and protect them. If some teeth are in the palatal vault, where they would interfere with the dental plate that makes up the anterior section of the prosthesis, the prosthodontist may create thimbles, pockets that are the size of the downward-protruding teeth, into which the teeth can fit when the anterior section is in place; or he may fit the thimbles over the teeth and make holes in the plate so that the teeth may come through. He will probably try to avoid removing these misplaced teeth, even though they cause some problems in the construction of the prosthesis, because extracting them might weaken the palatal vault.

Construction of the posterior section of the prosthesis, the obturator or bulb-shaped extension that goes into the pharynx, requires careful attention to size and position. The prosthodontist may report that he formed a ball of soft, pliable material, one brand of which is logically called Adaptol, around a wire loop that extends posteriorly from the velar section of the prosthesis toward the oropharynx. He can then modify the size, shape, and position of the trial bulb before he makes one of more permanent material. In undertaking modifications of the obturator, the prosthodontist may ask the speech pathologist for evaluations of the articulation-resonance achieved by placing the bulb high, low, or in a middle position and by enlarging it or reducing it in size. He may follow recommendations made by investigators who found that articulation scores were better when bulbs were placed below a line drawn from the tubercle of the atlas to the posterior nasal spine (Falter and Shelton, 1964). He may note other studies that showed the best location to be one that takes advantage of posterior and lateral pharyngeal wall movement, regardless of position (Morimitsu, 1958; Mazaheri and Millard, 1965), and that pointed out that obturation was more effective for patients with very short soft palates than for those whose palates were longer and less mobile (Joanne Subtelny and others, 1966). He may also evaluate the "fit" of the speech bulb by x-ray, oral manometer tests, speech tests, or other methods described in Chapter Six. He will undoubtedly check for undue pressure of the muscles of the pharyngeal area against the speech aid and trim the bulb at points of greatest contact to prevent displacement of the soft tissue or irritation from pressure. The speech pathologist, according to one opinion, "has a responsibility to advise the dentist regarding the prognosis for speech improvement with obturation and adequacy of fit for maximum speech effectiveness" (Shelton and Lloyd, 1963, p. 58).

Although some modern prosthodontists have used obturators with sliding or hinged parts (Olinger, 1942; Malson, 1957; Merkeley, 1959), most of the prostheses with speech bulbs to assist in velopharyngeal closure are of the rigid type, sometimes known as Fitzgibbon obturators, that are held in place by various types of clasps around the teeth. The attachment should be firm, and the number of clasps may be greater than for an orthodontic appliance. If the posterior section of the prosthesis moves as a result of activity of the tongue or pharyngeal muscles, the rocking motion can transfer to the teeth to which the anterior section is fastened, with resulting shifts in the positions of the teeth (Rosen and Bzoch, 1958). The weight of the pharyngeal section of the obturator is also a factor in the effect on dentition. The overall dimensions of the bulb can sometimes be reduced after articulatory-resonatory skills have been established with the speech aid (Mazaheri and Millard, 1965; Shelton and others, 1968); and the bulb can be hollow rather than solid to make it lighter (Brown, 1969).

The patient needs time to learn to tolerate the prosthesis and to use it effectively for speech. Trials and changes may continue for months; and the prosthodontist shares the orthodontist's problems of appointments that are not kept, instructions that are not followed, and prostheses that are broken by inept handling. In fact, lack of parental cooperation or mental retardation of the patient may impede prosthodontic management to such an extent that other methods of treatment should be sought (Mazaheri, 1962, and in Lencione, 1968). In most instances, however, if a prosthesis is the indicated form of management, it can be effective, particularly if speech training helps the patient to use it maximally.

AS A MEMBER OF THE CLEFT PALATE TEAM, THE SPEECH PATHOLOGIST HAS SEVERAL FUNCTIONS.

He takes part in the decisions about the most advantageous forms of management. He assesses the communicative abilities of the patient and provides remedial measures to improve speech and language. Additionally, he may serve effectively as a liaison agent between the team and the parents, assist the child to understand procedures that will be carried out by surgeons and dentists, and interpret his terminology and procedures to other professional members of the team (Koepp-Baker, 1946, and in Morris, 1965).

The speech pathologist may be presented with questions about management by the surgeon, the orthodontist, and the prosthodontist. In team discussions, such inquiries as the following may be made: Can this child learn to manage his present structures in such a way that good speech can be anticipated; or should the structures be modified surgically, orthodontically, or prosthodontically? If other treatment is to preface the work of the speech pathologist, should the two forms of management be separate; or can they overlap in time? How well does this child manage the obturator that has been provided? How well could he use it with special training? Are all of the child's deviations in speech the direct result of the palatal cleft, which has been repaired surgically or obturated? How long a period of trial speech therapy should be attempted before a prosthesis is provided? How long should additional surgical management be postponed to permit the speech pathologist to bring about the desired improvements in the child's speech? Will the contemplated orthodontic appliances interfere with the acquisition of articulatory skills or with speech training designed to improve articulation? Is this child capable of acquiring sufficient linguistic skill to justify the long-term surgical and dental management that seems needed? Will postponement of surgery or delay in the provision of a prosthesis create additional problems by giving the child opportunities to practice faulty speech production? Which is the greatest need of the child at the present—more adequate dental structures, better velopharyngeal closure, improved appearance, some combination of these, or some other form of management—in terms of his potential for acquiring speech and language? How can the surgeon or dentist get the child to talk so that he can judge the effects of his management? What should they have him say? How does this child compare with the noncleft child of the same age in speech and language development? These and similar questions are familiar to the speech pathologist who is a member of a cleft palate team.

Assessment of skills in oral communication is not only the responsibility of the speech pathologist but his prerogative. However, as the discussion in Chapter Six indicates, evaluations by others are part of the total process of evaluating communicative abilities. Because one can "interpret the information on the speech learning of cleft palate persons in different ways" (Westlake, in Lencione, 1968, p. 152), the speech pathologist can be the interpreter of findings from various assessments of articulation-resonance. Rather than serving only as a clinician, the specialist in speech has a major function in evaluation.

> It is no mere coincidence that the improvements which have been made in the postmanagement adequacy of the speech mechanisms of persons with cleft palate have resulted in great measure from the change in the role of the speech pathologist from clinician to diagnostician. [Spriestersbach, in Spriestersbach and Sherman, 1968, p. 276]

The next chapter in this text deals with the diagnostic role of the speech pathologist; the final chapter considers his role as a clinician.

In providing remedial assistance for individuals with congenital clefts, the speech pathologist can make still another contribution to the team's efforts. His concern is the modification of behavior, whereas the surgeon and the dental specialists modify structures. Thus, the relationships of the speech pathologist-speech clinician to the patient are possibly more personal and probably longer in total time than those of the surgeon or dentist; and the speech pathologist has more opportunities to inform and influence the child and his parents. If the child is being seen at six-month intervals by the surgeon, at two-month intervals by the prosthodontist, and at two-week intervals by the orthodontist, he may be seen two or three times a week by the speech pathologist. This frequency of contact can make for closer relationships, although the speech clinician may be necessarily more demanding than the surgeon or dentist in terms of the child's behavior. Certainly, the cooperation of the child and his family will be important to the success of any form of treatment; but the speech clinician cannot bring about changes in verbal behavior without the active participation of the child. The discussion of remedial procedures in Chapter Seven stresses this point.

Because he meets frequently with the child and the parents, the speech pathologist is in a position to discuss with them the recommendations made by other team members, to explain some of the procedures used or contemplated, to "keep the child and his family from becoming confused" (Lillywhite, 1956, p. 18), to relay questions from the parents to the team, and to feed back the answers in terms that can be understood by parents whose concern or lack of information may interfere with their best listening in conferences with surgeons or dentists.

The speech pathologist can also help the child to be more cooperative in surgical and dental procedures, which require more than his physical presence in the operating room or dental chair. Following instructions and using information from other specialists, the speech pathologist can prepare the child for maximal participation in treatment procedures and thus save time for the surgeon or dentist.

The importance of communication among members of a cleft palate team has been stressed by those who have discussed the interdisciplinary approach (Lillywhite, 1956; Koepp-Baker, in Morris, 1965; Westlake and Rutherford, 1966; Spriestersbach, in Spriestersbach and Sherman, 1968; Weatherley-White, in Stark, 1968; Westlake, in Lencione, 1968). As a specialist in communication, the speech pathologist carries a particular responsibility. His written and oral reports should be clear, thorough, organized, and well-presented. His questions about the work of the other members of the team can be searching, but they should be tactful. His observations should be in terms of the structural relationships and functions that are adequate or inadequate, not in terms of what other members of the team should have done or should do. His statements to parents should be carefully phrased, to prevent misinterpretation. His approach should be one of considerate interaction, in which he represents a recognized specialty that is an important part of the habilitative process.

If he uses terms that are not familiar, at the outset, to the other members of the team, the speech pathologist may define or illustrate them. He can communicate more effectively if he remembers that plosives, glottal stops, sibilants, pressure consonants, mean sentence lengths, variables, the Templin-Darley, deep testing, the ITPA, and the IPAT may be as unfamiliar to his fellow team members as some of their terms are to him. The purpose of communication, for the team, is the exchange of information. One great advantage of a team is that "it requires a regular and continuing working relationship between specialists who would probably not maintain this contact if it were not formalized" (Westlake and Rutherford, 1966, p. 69); and the relationship that works to the benefit of the patient is strengthened by good communication.

A CLEFT PALATE TEAM MAY SUPPLEMENT ITS SERVICE FUNCTION WITH TRAINING AND RESEARCH.

Each member of the team learns from the others, but each team can also provide opportunities for students in the various professional fields to profit from observation of and participation in the team's activities. Case presentations for students in medicine, dentistry, speech pathology, audiology, otolaryngology, social work, and other training programs can educate the observers without disturbing the child or his family. Data for research can be gathered during a child's visit to the team, and good records can provide information that is useful to the research worker. The introductory statement in the directory of facilities that provide service for individuals with clefts (National Institutes of Health, 1969) stressed the combination of service, training, and research that can result from team action by saying:

> It is hoped that the wide dissemination of this Directory will stimulate increased interest in examining and assessing the existing cleft lip and cleft palate services in the U.S. in relation to the total needs of cleft lip and cleft palate patients. Further, it is hoped that the Directory will (1) stimulate increased collaboration among specialists and among clinics and other service and research facilities and (2) serve to promote the expansion of existing research and service facilities and the development of new facilities devoted to research, treatment, and rehabilitation.

Cleft palate teams have an opportunity to meet these objectives through programs that attempt to achieve the total habilitation of the individual with a congenital prepalatal or palatal cleft through interdisciplinary action.

CHAPTER SIX

Assessment of Speech

EVALUATION OF THE EFFECTS OF A CONGENITAL CLEFT OF THE PREPALATE, THE PALATE, OR BOTH IS THE RESPONSIBILITY OF THE SPECIALISTS WHO WILL RECOMMEND OR PROVIDE REMEDIATION.

Whether their procedures are designed to modify structure or to alter behavior, members of the cleft palate team determine the status of the child as part of the habilitative process. In these assessments, the child is more important than the defect; and, throughout the long sequence of evaluation and management, the team members coordinate their efforts with the child as the focus of attention.

Each specialty has its own methods of assessment; these should be understood, although not necessarily applied, by members of the other specialties. The speech pathologist, drawing from the investigations of the other members of the team, makes his assessment of the child's skills or disabilities as a preface to remediation and determines the child's efficiency or lack of efficiency in using the various oral, pharyngeal, and dental structures modified by other specialists. He also tries to see the factors that, although not directly related to the cleft and its management, may affect the total effectiveness of the child as a speaker.

IN ASSESSING THE CHILD'S ABILITIES AND DISABILITIES IN ORAL COMMUNICATION, THE SPEECH PATHOLOGIST CONSIDERS THE MANY FACTORS, GENERAL AND SPECIFIC, THAT COMBINE AT ANY PARTICULAR TIME TO BRING ABOUT THE CHILD'S LEVEL OF ABILITY TO COMMUNICATE.

In this assessment, certain general principles should govern the various steps that are taken in the process of finding out what the child can do and cannot do. The evaluation of any specific area of ability or disability should be combined with information from investigations of other areas for the broad view of the child and his problems. Evaluation at any one point in time should be correlated with previous observations and plans for future management, to provide a view of the sequential processes that are necessary for this particular child (Litzow and Darley, 1966). The effects of the child's reaction to the specific situation in which the evaluation is made should be a consideration in drawing the conclusions from testing or observation. Evaluations should seek the child's strengths as well as his weaknesses, to provide a foundation for remedial procedures.

All the aspects of the various assessments should be known, if possible, when decisions about speech training are made or as that training proceeds. The child's intellectual and emotional status, the point he has reached in physical growth and development, the results of surgical and dental management, and the child's special needs are important bases for evaluation and for structuring remedial procedures designed to improve oral communication.

If one considers the child and not his cleft, his mental capacities and his emotional state can be determined by those with special training in such evaluations and reported to the speech pathologist. Information about the child's intellectual abilities is perhaps more important than determination of his disabilities if the speech pathologist is to use the child's capacities maximally in therapy, but deficits in intelligence identified by psychometrists will indicate a need for modifications in remedial approaches. Children with congenital clefts may have the same kinds of emotional disturbances that appear in other children; but their needs for social adjustment should be known by the speech pathologist, who can use the information and advice provided by the psychologist or psychiatrist in planning for remediation.

Because retardation in growth and development may typify the child with a congenital cleft, his general health and developmental status should be evaluated by appropriate members of the group responsible for his management. Therapeutic considerations by the speech pathologist will depend on the stage of development the child has reached, as they will for any child with disordered communication.

The results of surgical and dental management have special importance for the speech pathologist. In a concerted approach to habilitation, the child's status as a speaker will depend, to a great extent, on the effectiveness of surgical, prosthodontic, and orthodontic treatment. Modifications in the form and relationships of structures, already completed or contemplated, may affect his communicative abilities.

The speech pathologist needs information about the management provided by other specialists, and he needs to know the recency of these procedures. He may need to recognize, for example, that a prosthesis has been outgrown and is not effective at the time of assessment or that the child's reticence in conversation may be the result of his awareness of facial distortions that will be alleviated by plastic surgery scheduled for a later time.

The needs of the child with an oral cleft may be the same as those of any other child; but he may present certain problems, associated with his congenital anomaly, that must be considered in evaluating his capacities and his disabilities. Most of these special needs differ in degree, rather than in kind, from the needs of noncleft children. Observation of groups of children with clefts suggests that they want favorable attention from those in authority. In this, they do not differ from most children, except that they seem to express their feelings more overtly. The need for being part of a group and for acceptance by peers also seems to be strong in these children. Another need, which may be the result of parental attitudes, is for independence; but, again, advice to parents to avoid oversolicitude is not limited to parents of children with clefts. The need to express ideas, to ask questions, and to indicate wants is strong in these children; but their intelligibility may be so limited that they cannot obtain the responses they seek.

The child born with a cleft may be slow in acquiring skills in language and may have a hearing loss. Because these two disorders affect basic skills in communication, determination of their presence or absence is important to evaluation. Borderline defects in both language and hearing can interfere with the remedial procedures that may be needed for defective articulation-resonance. Attention to serious defects in the use of language and in hearing acuity will probably precede attention to articulation-resonance in habilitation.

Few tests are available commercially for measuring children's expressive linguistic ability, but those that are commonly used can provide estimates that should be helpful to the speech pathologist. Some measures of ability to comprehend language, particularly to understand vocabulary, have been established. Until research produces more testing materials in the area of language, the speech pathologist may request reports from others on linguistic evaluations or make use of some of the available materials cited later in this chapter. Academic achievement may provide some index of linguistic capacity, as well as of intellectual ability; but profiles showing high and low points will be more useful than single scores or grades.

In diagnostic situations that are new and frightening to him, a child may seem linguistically inept because he does not respond readily. In more familiar situations or after he adapts to a new environment, his verbal responses and spontaneous conversation may demonstrate that the apparent linguistic retardation was more situational than real. Trial therapy may reveal that the child with deviant speech, poor language, and a repaired cleft is more proficient linguistically than the testing situation indicated. Reports of adequate use of language from parents and teachers should be accepted with some reservations, although they may be quite accurate. Observation of the child in an unstructured play situation, alone or with parents, siblings, or friends, may lead to the conclusion that language is less affected than the formal testing or structured interview showed. On the other hand, the child with a cleft is not necessarily proficient in language; and his skills in this aspect of oral communication should be carefully evaluated.

The correlation between hearing loss and palatal clefts in children has been well demonstrated. Audiometric measurements appropriate to the child can be made by the audiologist, from whom information about present needs may be obtained. Because the hearing of children with infections of the middle ear, common in those with palatal clefts, is often inconsistent, no single measure of auditory acuity will suffice. Treatment of any hearing loss that may be present in the child with a cleft should be undertaken as soon as the problem has been identified because of the close relationship between adequate auditory acuity and the discrimination necessary for the acquisition of adequate speech and language. Observation can supplement hearing testing, and those in the child's environment can be asked to assist in the identification of loss of hearing acuity. Parents and teachers can assist the speech pathologist and audiologist by describing behavior that might indicate hearing loss, reporting requests for repetition of questions or directions, failures to respond to verbal stimuli when the speaker is not in the child's line of vision, classroom practices of dependence on others for information given orally, responses inappropriate to the inquiries, lack of normal reaction to noise, and other evidences of impaired hearing. The speech pathologist can often detect, in the child's patterns of articulation, specific deviations that suggest the need for thorough investigation of hearing.

Thus, before he makes his own assessment or at any time that the information can be obtained, the speech pathologist should accumulate summary reports from other specialists and should use the information as a supplement to his own detailed investigations. Although he may evaluate phonation, articulation, and resonance within the framework of his own area of specialization, his scrutiny of findings from several disciplines to determine relationships and points of contradiction will facilitate his task.

In spite of all the evaluations that can be made, the ultimate determination of the child's need for training in speech may be based on personal judgments. Speech pathologists have been urged to seek ways of standardizing their tests and the conclusions they draw from their observations, and such standardization is needed (Philips and Bzoch, 1969). One surgeon, for example, stated, "It is difficult to assess accurately the proportion of patients with poor speech results. Evaluation of speech has been a highly subjective process. Even trained speech pathologists, listening to a group of postoperative cleft palate patients, will disagree in a significant number of instances" (Sullivan, 1961, p. 31). Discussions of clinical evaluations of cleft palate patients and their speech have indicated that descriptions of speech are "subjective" and that "normal speech" may be as difficult to recognize as "abnormal" (Vini Coff, 1960). Such terms as "fallibility of personal judgment" and "judgments are precarious" were used to describe the participation of speech clinicians in one study of postoperative patients (Glover, 1961). Even in studies conducted by the speech pathologists themselves, the results of differences in judgment are apparent (Bradford and others, 1964; Philips and Bzoch, 1969).

Instrumentation can supplement the judgments of the speech pathologist; and measurements of air flow, degrees of nasality, tongue positions, velopharyngeal closure, and various aspects of phonation can be obtained with devices described in an earlier chapter and in a later part of the present discussion. Although "none of the mechanical devices for assessing nasality seems satisfactory at this time" (Shelton and others, in Spriestersbach and Sherman, 1968, p. 235), the speech pathologist should make the best possible use of any devices available to him while he attempts to improve his own skill as an evaluator. Surgeons and dentists have some difficulty in evaluating the cosmetic and functional results of their work; and the speech pathologist, while seeking ways of obtaining better assessment in clinical situations, should depend on his training and ingenuity without negating the importance of the opinions of others.

In the final analysis, no one judgment of the adequacy in speech of any child with a repaired cleft palate should suffice. Beauty may be in the eye of the beholder; nasality, and even some articulatory deviations, are frequently in the ear of the listener. Composite judgments from several listeners may be a better indication of the need for speech training than the evaluation made by a single speech pathologist, surgeon, dentist, parent, teacher, or peer; and the speech pathologist should seek such confirmation or refutation of his opinions. However, the determination of the child's present status in speech and his need for remedial assistance is, ultimately, the responsibility of the speech pathologist, whether he works in a setting that provides very adequate consultative and instrumental facilities or in one that does not.

In accumulating information that will facilitate assessment and remediation, the speech pathologist should consider the use of structured forms for reports on the various kinds of management provided or planned for the child with a congenital cleft. These forms, presented in this chapter, have several advantages. They permit the recording of a considerable amount of information on a limited number of pages, they facilitate record keeping and exchange of information, and they enable the speech pathologist to learn more about each child for whom he provides assessment and remediation.

Each speech pathologist will have greater access to some sources of information than to others. He may obtain information from hospital and clinic records, from team conferences, from interviews, or by correspondence; but he may need information, not readily available to him, that can be obtained by requesting information from agencies or individuals and using the reports in planning for evaluation and therapy. The use of a separate page for each kind of report will permit the accumulation of information throughout a period of time, additional reports being put into the collection as they are received. Careful attention to dates for previous management will enable the speech pathologist to see the sequence of procedures used by other specialists prior to his first interview with the child. The evaluation of skills in oral communication is, by itself, a task that should not be impeded by the time required to accumulate information that should be reviewed before the speech assessment.

A standardized report form will save time in record keeping and will permit the addition of information that is obtained during the period of speech therapy. If, for example, the prosthodontist reports that the child is now wearing a new obturator, that information can be noted on the appropriate form. If the child's father, not present at the initial interview, is seen later and is observed to use speech that is deviant in some articulatory aspect, this fact can be noted on the form that includes information about the family. Discovery, during a fifth or sixth remedial session, that the child has developed a hearing loss that was not noted at the time of the original audiometric evaluation can be entered in the daily record and transferred later to the form that contains audiological information.

These forms are useful also in the exchange of information among centers or agencies that provide remedial services for children with clefts. The standardized form, sent from one agency to another, could provide a complete report on the child who moved to a different community and save time for the agency that accepts the child in the new place. However, the standardized form is useful also within a single agency or clinic, to facilitate reevaluation of an individual child, to assure a commonality of information for all members of the staff, and to assist in the accumulation of data for research. Those who are concerned with the communication of the child with a congenital cleft need to strengthen their own lines of communication, and the use of a consistent method of reporting information could be of value to the team as well as to the child.

The speech pathologist who made use of the proposed forms* would not be restricted by them but could find that he knew a great deal about the child when he had accumulated, collated, and recorded the information such a compilation contained. He would see temporal relationships among various surgical, orthodontic, prosthodontic, and educational procedures if the dates of the various types of management were recorded. He would know something about the child's family and about his intellectual and emotional status. He would have information about the child's hearing and language and about his responsiveness to previous speech training, and he

* Copies of these forms, on pages of standard size (8½ by 11), with appropriate spacing for entering information, may be purchased from the author.

could add his impressions to the reports of others as he saw the child initially and observed him in a sequence of remedial sessions.

THE ASSESSMENT OF THE ORAL COMMUNICATION OF CHILDREN BORN WITH PREPALATAL OR PALATAL CLEFTS INVOLVES THE ACCUMULATION AND COORDINATION OF INFORMATION FROM SEVERAL SOURCES.

Whether or not the forms shown in this chapter are used, certain information is important to the speech pathologist's assessment of the oral communication of the child born with a cleft. The following outline cites the information that is needed, and the remainder of the chapter considers ways in which the speech pathologist can gather and use such information.

ASSESSMENT OF SKILLS IN ORAL COMMUNICATION

(Children with Prepalatal or Palatal Clefts)

- General information
  - Malformations present at birth
  - Surgical management
  - Prosthodontic management
  - Orthodontic management
  - General physical management
  - Family history
  - Intellectual and emotional history
  - Auditory acuity and otological management
  - Linguistic abilities
  - Radiological studies
  - Previous speech evaluation and therapy
  - General impressions
- Assessment of skills in oral communication
  - Present status of structures
  - Use of structures for speech
    - Velopharyngeal valving
    - Articulation
    - Intelligibility
    - Visual aspects
  - Summary of assessment

General information should be gathered from all available sources. Such information may be entered on Forms I.A through I.L, although it may not be complete for all forms. The importance of information that identifies and locates the child is apparent; and the first page of the assessment form, serving as a cover sheet, can show any hospital chart number, clinic file number, or other form of coding to supplement the identification and permit easy access to records. Permission from the parents of children not of legal age should be obtained if information is to be sent from one center to another.

ASSESSMENT OF SKILLS IN ORAL COMMUNICATION

(Children with Prepalatal or Palatal Clefts)

____

________________________________ ____________________________
Date of assessment

________________________________ ____________________________
Name and address of center or agency — Speech pathologist

IDENTIFICATION

Name______________________________________ Sex: male____ female____
Last name — First name

Birth date________________ Birthplace__________________________________

Parents: father's name____

mother's name____

Address____
Number and street or route — City — State — Zip code

If either parent is not at the address given above, provide address for:
father____ mother____: ____

School: preschool____ school age but not attending school____

school____
Name of school — Location (city, state)

____
Grade — Academic year — Teacher

Additional information: living in foster home, living with relatives but not parents, changes of address and school within year prior to assessment, other pertinent information to assist in identification____

____

____

____

Hospital chart number__________ ______________________________________
Name and location of hospital

Identification number for center or agency__________

____

____

______________________________ ____________________________

Name and address of center or agency Date

PERMISSION FOR RELEASE OF INFORMATION

I (we) hereby grant permission to

____

Name of agency

to release information about my (our) son____ daughter____

____

Child's name

to____

Witnessed by

____________________________ ____________________________

____________________________ ____________________________

Signature(s) of parent(s)

Classification of the malformations present at birth (I.A) will vary. In some centers, the Veau classification may be used; in others, the congenital clefts may be described generally; in still others, classification may be determined locally. The classifications of the American Cleft Palate Association are recommended, but they may not have been adopted by all centers or hospitals.

INFORMATION FOR: INFORMATION ABOUT:

____________________________ ____________________________

Name of child

____________________________ ____________________________

Name and address of center or agency to which information is to be sent

Names of parents

I. GENERAL INFORMATION

A. Malformations Present at Birth

1. Clefts of prepalate:
   a. Cleft lip: unilateral right____ left____ bilateral____
   Extent: ⅓____ ⅔____ 3/3____
   Describe if above classifications are not used.____________________

   ____

   b. Cleft alveolar process: unilateral right____ left____ bilateral____
   Extent: ⅓____ ⅔____ 3/3____
   Describe if above classifications are not used.____________________

   ____

c. Cleft prepalate (combination of *a* and *b* above): unilateral right____ left____ bilateral____
   Extent: 1/3____ 2/3____ 3/3____
   Prepalate protrusion: none____ slight____ moderate____ marked____
   Prepalate rotation: none____ slight____ moderate____ marked____
   Other____________________
   Describe if above classifications are not used.____________________

2. Clefts of palate (prepalate terminates at incisive foramen):
   a. Cleft soft palate: 1/3____ 2/3____ 3/3____
      Width: narrow____ medium____ wide____
      Palatal shortness: none____ moderate____ marked____
      Submucous cleft: 1/3____ 2/3____ 3/3____
      Describe if above classifications are not used.____________________

   b. Cleft hard palate: 1/3____ 2/3____ 3/3____
      Width: narrow____ medium____ wide____
      Vomer attachment: right____ left____ absent____
      Submucous cleft: 1/3____ 2/3____ 3/3____
      Describe if above classifications are not used.____________________

   c. Cleft soft and hard palate (combination of *a* and *b* above):
      Extent: 1/3____ 2/3____ 3/3____
      Width: narrow____ medium____ wide____
      Description____________________

   d. Facial clefts other than prepalatal and palatal:
      Mandibular process cleft____________________
      Nasoocular cleft____________________
      Oroocular cleft____________________
      (See "Proposed Morphological Classification of Congenital Cleft Lip and Cleft Palate," *Cleft Palate Bulletin*, 10(1):11–16 (January 1960), or "A Classification of Cleft Lip and Cleft Palate," *Plastic and Reconstructive Surgery*, 29(1):31–39 (January 1962). If any other system of classification is used, please indicate the plan for categorizing.)

Additional information about malformations present at birth:
Information about facial clefts____________________
Other congenital anomalies____________________

Information provided by____________________
Name

Address

Date

Reports on surgical management (I.B) need not be detailed. The speech pathologist needs to know when the various operative procedures were carried out, who performed them, where the surgery took place, and the results; but the surgeon's specific procedures or techniques during the operation do not need to be reported to the person who is to evaluate skills in oral communication.

INFORMATION FOR:	INFORMATION ABOUT:
______________________	______________________
	Name of child
______________________	______________________
Name and address of center or agency to which information is to be sent	Names of parents

I. GENERAL INFORMATION

B. Surgical Management

1. Repair of prepalate:
   First operation: date__________ age of child__________
   Place__________ surgeon__________
   Results of surgery__________
   Subsequent operations: date(s)__________ age(s) of child__________
   Place(s)__________ surgeon(s)__________
   Results__________
   ____
   Reasons for additional surgery contemplated__________
   ____
2. Repair of palate:
   First operation: date__________ age of child__________
   Place__________ surgeon__________
   Results__________
   Subsequent operations: date(s)__________ age(s) of child__________
   Place(s)__________ surgeon(s)__________
   Results__________
   Additional surgery contemplated__________
   Alternatives to additional surgery__________

Information provided by__________
Name
____
Address
____
Date

Similarly, the work of the prosthodontist (I.C) and orthodontist (I.D) need not be reported in detail. The speech pathologist should know, generally, the various prosthodontic and orthodontic managements that have been provided in the past, those that are now affecting the child, and those that are contemplated. He does not need to know all the procedures used in such management, but he does need to understand the modifications in structure that have been accomplished and those that will be undertaken during the period of speech training.

INFORMATION FOR: ______________________

____
Name and address of center or agency to which information is to be sent

INFORMATION ABOUT: ______________________
Name of child
____
Names of parents

I. GENERAL INFORMATION

C. Prosthodontic Management

1. Prostheses without "speech aids":
   Age of child when prosthesis provided__________ Date__________
   Type of prosthesis in terms of revision sought__________
   ____
   Is prosthesis still being worn? Yes____ No____ Date of report__________
   State briefly the reasons for modifying or abandoning the prosthesis.__________
   ____
2. Prostheses with "speech aids":
   Age of child when prosthesis provided__________ Date__________
   Describe prosthesis and "speech aid."__________
   ____
   Is prosthesis still being worn? Yes____ No____ Date of report__________
   Is modification or abandonment of the prosthesis with "speech aid" planned?
   Yes____ No____ Reasons for changing or abandoning prosthesis__________
   ____
3. Other information from the prosthodontist pertinent to evaluation of skills in oral communication__________
   ____
   ____

Information provided by______________________
Name
____
Address

____
Date

INFORMATION FOR:	INFORMATION ABOUT:
______________________________	______________________________ Name of child
______________________________ Name and address of center or agency to which information is to be sent	______________________________ Names of parents

I. GENERAL INFORMATION

D. Orthodontic Management

1. Early orthodontic management, prior to eruption of deciduous teeth:

   Age of child when management was begun______ Date______________________

   Duration of orthodontic attention____

   Purposes of early orthodontic management___________________________________

   ____

2. Continuing orthodontic management:

   Age of child when present management procedures were begun__________________

   Duration: from____________________ to_______________________________

   Purposes____

   ____

   ____

   Estimate of duration of orthodontic management from date of this report________

   ____

   Results obtained to date of report____

   ____

   ____

3. Additional orthodontic information pertinent to evaluation of skills in oral communication____

   ____

   ____

   Information provided by____
   Name

   ____
   Address

   ____
   Date

The amount of information about general physical management (I.E) will vary with the programs of speech training being planned. A residential program, for example, would require indications of any chronic physical problems that would restrict activity or of any necessary continuing medication. A child who lives at home and comes to a clinic, school, or center for only part of the day may have special physical problems that should be reported; but, in this instance, the primary responsibility for his general physical care rests with his parents.

INFORMATION FOR:	INFORMATION ABOUT:
____________________	____________________ Name of child
____________________ Name and address of center or agency to which information is to be sent	____________________ Names of parents

I. GENERAL INFORMATION

E. General Physical Management

1. Severe illnesses:

   Type(s) of illness(es): (1)____________ (2)____________

   (3)____________ (4)____________ (5)____________

   Age of child: (1)______ (2)______ (3)______ (4)______ (5)______

   (If additional information is to be provided, place at bottom or on back of page.)

   Medical care needed at present____________________

2. General dental care (not orthodontic or prosthodontic):

   Type of dental care: (1)__________ (2)__________ (3)__________

   Age of child: (1)__________ (2)__________ (3)__________

   Frequency of visits to dentist for checkup____________________

3. Child's general health: excellent____ good____ fair____ poor____

4. Restrictions:

   Dietary____________________

   Activities____________________

5. Other pertinent information about the child's general health____________

   ____

   ____

6. Name(s) and address(es) of family physician(s) and dentist(s)________________

____

____

Information provided by______________________________
Name

____
Address

____
Date

Except for inquiries about the incidence of clefts and other congenital anomalies in the family, the information needed for family history (I.F) is much the same as that needed for any child in any remedial program. Similarly, the summary of the child's intellectual and emotional history (I.G) is the kind of information that is acquired about most children who are to be seen for evaluation and considered for therapy.

INFORMATION FOR:	INFORMATION ABOUT:
____________________	____________________ Name of child
____________________ Name and address of center or agency, to which information is to be sent	____________________ Names of parents

I. GENERAL INFORMATION

F. Family History

1. Incidence of clefts in relatives (describe type of cleft):

Immediate family____________________________________

Grandparents, aunts, uncles (maternal or paternal), cousins (report relationship):

____

____

2. Members of family: mother____ father____ number of siblings____

Names and ages of siblings____________________________________

____

This child was the________in a series of________children.

3. First trimester of pregnancy:

Illnesses of mother (specify)____________________

Drugs taken by mother (specify)____________________

Unusual circumstances (describe)____________________

____

4. Parents:

General health: mother________________ father________________

Physical anomalies other than clefts: mother________________

father________________ siblings________________

Speech: mother________________ father________________

Linguistic abilities: mother____________ father________________

5. Family relationships and socioeconomic status (describe briefly)____________

____

____

____

Information provided by____________________________
Name

____
Address

____
Date

INFORMATION FOR:	INFORMATION ABOUT:
________________	________________ Name of child
________________ Name and address of center or agency to which information is to be sent	________________ Names of parents

I. GENERAL INFORMATION

G. Intellectual and Emotional History

1. Intellectual capacities:

Specific tests given: (1)____________ (2)____________ (3)____________

Dates of tests: (1)____________ (2)____________ (3)____________

Other tests and dates______________________________

Results of testing:

Verbal scores or ratings: (1)______________________________

(2)____________________ (3)____________________

Nonverbal scores or ratings: (1)______________________________

(2)____________________ (3)____________________

Other test scores or levels of achievement______________________________

Recommendations______________________________

____

Information provided by______________________________

2. Emotional status:______________________________

Kinds of testing______________________________

Findings and recommendations______________________________

____

Dates of tests or interviews______________________________

Information provided by______________________________

3. Subjective evaluations:

Intellectual capacities____________________ by_______________

Emotional stability____________________ by_______________

Information provided by______________________________

____

Date

The assessment of auditory acuity (I.H) may be undertaken by the speech pathologist if no audiological services are available. Preferably, an audiologist and an otologist will provide reports on hearing testing and on otological management; and the evaluation of hearing will continue until treatment is no longer needed. The speech clinician needs to be alert to any changes in the child's hearing and to refer for additional evaluations and management that may be deemed necessary by the audiologist or otologist.

INFORMATION FOR:	INFORMATION ABOUT:
______________________	______________________
	Name of child
______________________	______________________
Name and address of center or agency to which information is to be sent	Names of parents

I. GENERAL INFORMATION

H. Auditory Acuity and Otological Management

1. Audiometry:
   Dates of tests: (1)__________ (2)__________ (3)__________
   Types of tests: (1)____________________
   (2)_______________ (3)_______________
   Results (attach audiograms): (1)____________________
   (2)_______________ (3)_______________
   (If additional tests or observations have been made, provide information at bottom or on back of page.)
   Recommendations____________________

   Name and address of audiometrist____________________

2. Otological management:
   Describe briefly otological care provided for the child.____________________

   Additional management contemplated____________________

   Name and address of otologist____________________

____
Date

Evaluation of linguistic ability (I.I) also may come within the province of the speech pathologist. He will undoubtedly wish to supplement the relatively formal testing, whether he or some other qualified individual administers it, with reports on linguistic behavior and linguistic deficits from teachers, parents, and others. The speech clinician will be alert to the child's needs in language and will add to the information gathered prior to or during the initial assessment. He may categorize the linguistic abilities of the child on the basis of such measures of verbal output as the mean length of response, the mean of the five longest responses, and the number of one-word responses (Johnson and others, 1963). He may use an equation proposed for assessing language development or consider the mean length of response as the "best single predictor" (Shriner and Sherman, 1967). He may employ other means of judging linguistic capacity that are available

INFORMATION FOR:	INFORMATION ABOUT:
______________________	______________________
	Name of child
______________________	______________________
Name and address of center or agency to which information is to be sent	Names of parents

I. GENERAL INFORMATION

I. Linguistic Abilities

1. Comprehension of language:
   Methods of determining______________________
   ____
   Dates of evaluations______________________
   Scores, levels of achievement______________________
   ____
   Recommendations______________________
   ____
   Name(s) and address(es) of examiner(s)______________________
   ____
2. Use of language for oral self-expression:______________________
   Methods of determining______________________
   ____
   Dates of evaluations______________________
   ____
   Scores, levels of achievement______________________
   ____
   Recommendations______________________
   ____
   Name(s) and address(es) of examiner(s)______________________
   ____

3. Other information pertinent to the evaluation of skills in oral communication______

____

____

Information provided by____

____
Date

to him at the present time or that result from the increasing amount of research being conducted on this topic (Mecham, 1959; Crabtree, 1963; Anderson and others, 1964; Dunn, 1965; Riley, 1966; Mecham and others, 1967; Kirk and others, 1968; Foster and others, 1969; Lee, 1969).

Information from radiological studies (I.J) of velopharyngeal function should be gathered as part of the total evaluative process or obtained from agencies that have used radiographic procedures with the child. Evidence of closure of the velopharyngeal passageway from single pictures or from films does not necessarily mean that the child's speech will be free from undue nasal resonance or incorrect direction of the airstream, but the cineradiographic films can furnish information about the action of the structures under several circumstances. In addition, cephalometric studies facilitated by radiographic procedures can be used to determine relationship of structures; and reports and interpretations from radiologists can be of value to the speech pathologist.

INFORMATION FOR:	INFORMATION ABOUT:
________________________	________________________ Name of child
________________________ Name and address of center or agency to which information is to be sent	________________________ Names of parents

I. GENERAL INFORMATION

J. Radiological Studies

1. Roentgenograms (single pictures): date____________ place________________

   Area visualized____

   Palatopharyngeal gap: relative amount of closure (by description or in millimeters); if speech aid is used, report (1) without speech aid, (2) with speech aid:

   At rest: (1)________________________ (2)________________________

   In production of______: (1)________________ (2)________________________

   In production of______: (1)________________ (2)________________________

In swallowing: (1)____________________ (2)____________________

Other____

2. Cineradiography (films): date________________ place____________________

Lateral__________ Anteroposterior______________________________

Report (1) without speech aid, (2) with speech aid:____________________

Area visualized____

Palatal movements seen:

In production of__________: (1)____________________ (2)____________________

In production of__________: (1)____________________ (2)____________________

In sound sequences: (1)____________________ (2)____________________

Relative amount of closure: (1)____________________ (2)____________________

Circumstances that provide better approximation of palate to pharyngeal wall________

____

____

3. Cephalometric findings____

____

____

4. Other information pertinent to assessment of skills in oral communication________

____

____

Information provided by____

Name

____

Address

____

Date

Some children referred to a speech pathologist for evaluation will have been seen by other specialists in speech, and reports on previous speech evaluation and therapy (I.K) become important parts of the accumulation of information prior to additional assessment. Repetition of some of the procedures used by other speech pathologists may be desirable, particularly if a long period of time has elapsed since the earlier evaluation or if remedial assistance has been provided. Of particular importance are the estimates, from those who have had experience with the child, of his capacity to profit from additional speech training and reports of his achievements within the limits of the remediation provided.

INFORMATION FOR: ____________________

____
Name and address of center or agency
to which information is to be sent

INFORMATION ABOUT: ____________________
Name of child
____
Names of parents

I. GENERAL INFORMATION

K. Previous Speech Evaluation and Therapy

1. Evaluations:
   Date(s): (1)________ (2)________ (3)________
   Place(s): (1)________ (2)________ (3)________
   Findings (give dates):
   Auditory acuity____________________
   Linguistic abilities____________________
   Velopharyngeal control____________________
   Articulatory abilities____________________
   Other pertinent information from evaluation____________________
   ____
2. Therapy:
   Dates: beginning____________________ ending__________
   Number of clinic sessions______ Length of session__________
   Individual______ Group______ Both______
   Objectives in therapy____________________
   ____
   Achievements____________________
   ____
   Further needs____________________
3. Speech pathologist's estimates:
   Child's capacity for further improvement in oral communication__________
   Child's capacity for cooperation in modification of speech behavior__________
   Parents' interest and cooperation____________________
   Information provided by____________________
   Name
   ____
   Address
   ____
   Date

General impressions (I.L) about the child's appearance, movement, adaptation to various environments, and potential for cooperative response in therapeutic situations that require his active participation should be gathered from several sources. Parents, teachers, acquaintances, siblings, and specialists who conduct various evaluative sessions can provide estimates of the child's behavior; and such reports, once gathered, should be compared. Good interviewing techniques are desirable in conferences with those who can describe what the child does in certain situations and who can report methods of

INFORMATION FOR:	INFORMATION ABOUT:
______________________	______________________
	Name of child
______________________	______________________
Name and address of center or agency o which information is to be sent	Names of parents

I. GENERAL INFORMATION

L. General Impressions

INFORMANT OR OBSERVER

1. Physical status:
   Size (for age): small___ average___ large___ ________
   Posture: good___ average___ poor___ ________
   Coordination: good___ average___ poor___ ________
2. Adaptation to environment:
   To new situations: good___ average___ poor___ ________
   To familiar situations: good___ average___ poor___ ________
   Relationships with others:
   friendly___ average___ withdrawn___
   other descriptive terms________________ ________
   Response to authority figures:
   at ease___ average___ fearful___ ________
3. Characteristic behavior:
   In unstructured situations:
   at ease___ average___ fearful___ hyperactive___ ________
   In structured situations:
   at ease___ average___ fearful___ hyperactive___ ________
   In situations that seem to pose a threat:
   at ease___ average___ fearful___ hyperactive___ ________
4. Estimate of child's capacity to respond in situations that require his cooperative behavior:
   excellent___ good___ average___ poor___
   very poor___ ________

(Use more than one of these sheets, if necessary, or code the responses from several informants.)

management that obtained good or poor responses. Evaluative or remedial sessions in a clinical setting may be new experiences for the child, and information about behavior in informal situations may not be applicable to the more structured environment.

After reviewing and correlating the reports available to him, the speech pathologist undertakes the detailed assessment of the child's skills in oral communication. He needs to see two general aspects of the child's abilities and disabilities in oral communication: the structures that are available for use in speech and the use made of those structures. His description of the child's status at the conclusion of the initial interview will be subject to revision, of course; but he can obtain a series of findings, to be interwoven and given priorities in terms of needs for remediation, through an organized approach to assessment.

In assessing the child's present status in terms of the structures used in speaking, the speech pathologist should evaluate the capacities of the various parts of the "speech mechanism" for function in voluntary and involuntary nonspeech activities as well as in speaking. Scoring or rating is difficult, but the use of a scale can facilitate comparison with findings from reevaluations or with ratings for other children. Consideration of relationships in the activities of the various structures is also important.

Procedures that may be used for determining the status of the labial structures (II.A.1) include asking the child to do what he is instructed to do or to imitate the various activities; recording, or having someone else record, from his own observation or from dictation, the level of competence with which the activities are performed; noting the efficiency with which the child uses his lips in the relatively formal testing situation and in nonstructured situations; modifying the instructions or demonstrations to suit the capacities of the child; using such devices as are available or can be evolved by the speech pathologist to facilitate evaluation. Does the child keep his mouth closed when he is playing, looking at books, chewing, listening? If he cannot bring his lips together on command, can he do so if a piece of paper is placed between them? If he is instructed to blow on the examiner's hand or on his own, does he round his lips for blowing, does he approximate them without rounding, or does he keep them immobile? Are restrictions in labial activity the apparent result of immobilization of the lip by scar tissue, or does the child fail to move his lips because he has apparently not formed the habit of making them active? Are the lips symmetrical or asymmetrical? Is any asymmetry the apparent result of scar tissue?

INFORMATION FROM:	INFORMATION ABOUT:
______________________	______________________
	Name of child
______________________	______________________
	Identification number
______________________	______________________
Name, position, and address of evaluator	Date

II. ASSESSMENT OF SKILLS IN ORAL COMMUNICATION

A. Present Status of Structures

Use a 7-point scale, in which 1 indicates complete adequacy and 7 indicates severe deviation.

	RATING	COMMENT
1. Labial:		
a. Mobility of lips:		
Note the child's ability, following directions or by imitation, to:		
Round his lips, as in /u/	____	____
Protrude his lips, as in /w/	____	____
Retract his lips, as in a wide smile	____	____
Open and close his lips (silent *m-m-m*)	____	____
Note the above activities in nonstructured situations:		
Rounding of lips	____	____
Protrusion of lips	____	____
Retraction of lips	____	____
Opening and closing of lips	____	____
Do inadequacies in the above activities seem to be related to:		
Restriction by scar tissue? Yes____ No____		
Restriction by dental structure? Yes____ No____		
b. Approximation of upper and lower lip:		
Note the child's ability, following directions or by imitation, to:		
Close his mouth completely but easily	____	____
Bring his lips together firmly	____	____
Note the above activities in nonstructured situations:		
Complete, but easy, mouth closure	____	____
Firm mouth closure	____	____
Note the above activities in eating, observing mouth closure in:		
Chewing	____	____
Swallowing	____	____
Note the above activities in blowing, observing whether or not the child:		
Brings his lips together without rounding. Yes____ No____		
Achieves firm approximation of his lips. Yes____ No____		

c. Describe the general appearance of the lips, reporting scars visible, symmetry or lack of symmetry, conditions of nares, presence of nasolabial fistula, other factors.

____

____

____

The speech pathologist does not usurp the functions of the dental specialist when he notes the status of the dental and alveolar structures (II.A.2) in terms of possible effects on speech or in terms of adequate articulation in the presence of dental anomalies. In considering whether or not the dental arches seem appropriate in size to the size of the head and face, the speech pathologist is making a general evaluation of appearance that may lead to recommendation for referral for further dental assessment. The dental occlusion may be an important factor in the child's articulation, or it may have no relationship to it; but the speech pathologist's evaluation

2. Dental and alveolar:
   a. Dental arches:
      Do the arches seem proportionate to the size of the head and face?
      Yes____ No____
      Does the upper arch overlap the lower in the area of the incisors?
      Yes____ No____
      If "yes," is the overlap within the normal limits? Yes____ No____
      If "no," describe the type of relationship between upper and lower dental arches.
      ____
      ____
      Is the upper dental arch relatively smooth and unbroken? Yes____ No____
      If "no," describe the types and locations of the irregularities.____________
      ____
   b. Teeth:
      What teeth are missing?______________________________
      What teeth are deciduous?______________________________
      Is dentition appropriate to age? Yes____ No____
      If "no," what is the status?______________________________
      ____
   c. Occlusion:

	COMMENT
Neutroclusion (Angle's Class I)	____________
Distoclusion (Class II)	____________
Mesioclusion (Class III)	____________

      Additional comments on occlusion______________________________
      ____

should include observation of occlusion and description of it by standard categories.

Lingual motility and control (II.A.3) should be assessed in several ways. The various types of movements are not as important as the demonstration, in several contexts, of the ability to move the tongue. Can the child move his tongue up and down, forward and back, in response to directions or by imitation? Does he show ability in nonverbal activities, such as licking and eating, for tongue movement? Can he move his tongue purposefully and readily from one position to another? In what position does the tongue lie in the mouth when it is quiescent? Does it seem to ride high in the oral cavity? Is the back of the tongue more elevated than the front during rest? Does the position of the tongue, particularly in its relationship to the palate (Falk and Kopp, 1968; Peat, 1968), seem to affect either the articulation of certain sounds or the amount of nasal emission that may accompany them? Does the condition of the lips or teeth seem to contribute to any unusual positioning of the tongue? Have the observations been made several times to eliminate the possibility of chance positioning that is not typical?

3. Lingual:	RATING	COMMENT
a. Motility of tongue:		
Note the child's ability, following directions or by imitation, to:		
Move his tongue upward to the alveolar ridge	______	______
Protrude his tongue	______	______
Move his tongue from side to side	______	______
Repeat the up-and-down movement ten times	______	______
b. Control of tongue:		
Does the child's tongue protrude during nonverbal activities? Yes____ No____		
Note his ability to:		
Lick an imaginary ice-cream cone	______	______
Hold his tongue steady on protrusion	______	______
Hold his tongue steady inside his mouth	______	______
Hold his tongue in a centered position	______	______
Swallow without tongue protrusion	______	______
c. Does inadequacy of tongue movement or control seem related to dental anomalies? Yes____ No____		

If "yes," describe.______________________________

Observations of the present status of the palatal structures (II.A.4) are sometimes difficult and may require time to get the cooperation of the child. Often, scar tissue and restriction in the size of the faucial arch interfere with inspection; but the speech pathologist should do his best to judge the length and control of the palate, particularly in its relationship to the total depth of the oral-oropharyngeal cavity. Both length and mobility are factors in the use of the palate in conjunction with the pharynx to close the passageway to the nasal cavities and permit the flow of air through the mouth. A long but immobile palate cannot participate in such valving; a short but mobile palate cannot reach to or near the pharyngeal walls. Even a long and mobile palate cannot participate efficiently in closure if the depth of the pharynx is so great that approximation of palatal and pharyngeal structures cannot be achieved.

In noting the condition and efficiency of the palatal structures, the speech pathologist is not making an evaluation of the need for additional surgical management or judging the success of previous surgery. He is not attempting to decide how skillful the prosthodontist was when he constructed the speech aid being used by the child. He is trying to determine whether or not

4. Palatal:	RATING	COMMENT
a. Length of palate:		
By general observation	___	___
In relationship to depth of pharynx	___	___
b. Palatal fistula present? Yes___ No___		
If "yes," describe.___		
c. Movement of palate:		
In voluntary activities, does the child:		
Achieve palatal movement on /ɑ/?	___	___
Move his palate without phonation?	___	___
Achieve palatal movement when he inhales through the nose, exhales orally?	___	___
In yawning, does the palate move noticeably?	___	___
In response to tactile stimulation, what degree of movement occurs?	___	___
In response to "threat" of such stimulation, what degree of movement occurs?	___	___
d. Is an appliance or obturator being worn? Yes___ No___		
If "yes," describe effect on speech.___		

the present palatal structures, in conjunction with the pharyngeal walls and with any obturating appliances, can accomplish the valving needed for speech.

In his observation of the pharyngeal structures (II.A.5), the speech pathologist may encounter the same problems that he met in looking for the functions of the palate. He may not be able to see well enough to determine the presence or absence of any bulging of the posterior pharyngeal wall or of movement of the lateral walls. If the child is to enter a program of therapy, observation of structures that are difficult to see may be postponed until such examination can be made without jeopardizing rapport. When the speech pathologist can observe the functioning of the pharyngeal structures or when he views films, he needs to remember that head position may affect the relationships between soft palate and posterior pharyngeal wall during direct observation as well as during cineradiography (Shelton and Bosma, 1962; McWilliams and others, 1968). He should also be concerned with the activities of the lateral pharyngeal walls, as these are seen by direct inspection or by means of anteroposterior films or measured by ultrasound (Minifie and others, 1969; Collins, 1970). If a child has been provided with a pharyngeal flap, the examiner should try to determine

5. Pharyngeal:	RATING	COMMENT
a. Depth of pharynx:		
By observation	________	________
In relationship to palatal length	________	________
b. Lateral wall movement:		
In voluntary attempts to bring walls to midline	________	________
During phonation	________	________
During yawning	________	________
In relationship to radiological reports________		
c. Posterior wall movement or "bulging":		
In phonation	________	________
In response to tactile stimulation	________	________
During yawning	________	________
In relationship to radiological reports________		
d. Is an obturator with "speech aid" being worn? Yes____ No____		
If "yes," describe effect on speech.________		

whether or not the lateral pharyngeal walls are contributing to velopharyngeal closure, even though the presence of the pharyngeal flap may limit inspection of the area.

Direct observation of the laryngeal structures (II.A.6) is not within the province of the speech pathologist, except as he may have an opportunity for such observation during an examination by a laryngologist. In assessment of laryngeal competence, audible cues to possible pathologies or structural deviations can be used to advantage; however, the speech pathologist should recognize that what he hears at any one point in time or the changes he notes in vocal tone give no indication of the exact problem that may exist. Descriptions of faulty phonation are vague, at best; but changes that occur and persist should lead to referral for investigation of the state of the larynx.

6. Laryngeal:
   a. Audible characteristics of sustained vocal tone:
      uneven and interrupted____ "breathy"____ "tense"____ smooth and clear____ free from "breathiness"____ relaxed____
   b. During speech, is any evidence of need for investigation of laryngeal status apparent to the listener? Yes____ No____
      If "yes," describe the audible characteristics that suggest need for laryngological investigation.____
      ____

Respiratory difficulties (II.A.7) will probably be rare in children born with clefts, but the speech pathologist should note those that may be present. Respiratory effort seems to be greater in individuals with velopharyngeal incompetence, probably as a result of higher rates of airflow and prolonged intervals of utterance production (Warren, Wood, and Bradley, 1969). Hence, speech performance may be influenced by respiratory effort. The speech pathologist should also judge vocal volume, which is determined in part by respiratory activities, noting whether volume is insufficient, adequate, or too great in various situations. The adequacy of loudness varies with the speaking situation, the characteristics of the listeners, the surroundings, and the context. It is affected by personality, current emotional status, and the reactions of the listener. It cannot be judged in isolation because it is related to the use of other structures in the larynx and resonating cavities. However, because vocal intensity may be a factor in therapeutic procedures, it should be evaluated at the outset and as it changes in new situations. Audible respiration, wheezing, rattling, and other anomalies noted in nonspeech activities merit investigation by the appropriate specialist.

7. Respiratory:
   a. During sustained conversation, what is the average length of phrases between inhalations?____________________
   b. Can the child sustain a simple vocal tone for 10 seconds? Yes____ No ____
      If "no," how long? ________seconds
      Do repeated trials increase the length of time the tone can be sustained? Yes____ No____
      If "yes," from________seconds to________seconds
   c. Is vocal volume adequate:

	RATING	COMMENT
In responses during testing?	______	______
In play situations, with peers?	______	______
In conversation with those the child knows?	______	______
In emotional situations?	______	______

   d. Are unusual respiratory noises audible:
      During breathing without speech? Yes____ No____
      During breathing for speech? Yes____ No____
      During sleep? Yes____ No____
      Describe.____________________

Additional information obtained on present status of structures for speech__________

Determination of the current status of the oral and pharyngeal structures should be supplemented by evaluation of the child's use of these structures. The speech pathologist, keeping in mind the functions of the central nervous system and the sensory systems in the process of oral communication, should consider specific articulatory-resonatory defects in terms of velopharyngeal valving and articulatory activities, should determine the visual aspects of speech that may interfere with communication, and should determine the intelligibility of the child when articulation and resonance are combined.

Velopharyngeal valving can be assessed in many ways. The types of assessment used will depend on the facilities to which the speech pathologist has access and the importance he attaches to the measures that are available. Instrumentation can provide evidence of the efficiency of valving; judgments based on auditory cues can supplement this evidence.

Although research facilitated by instrumentation has often been directed to measurements of normal velopharyngeal control, as described in Chapter Two, some has been designed to evaluate the velopharyngeal competence of speakers with congenital clefts of the palate. From these studies, the speech pathologist can obtain information to apply in assessing the movement of the soft palate in relationship to the pharyngeal walls, the participation of the tongue in closure, and the flow or pressure of air.

Cinefluorographic films that show the movement of the velum are made in many centers. These films, particularly if they have synchronized sound, can assist the speech pathologist in determining the amount and level of closure and the contribution of Passavant's pad or adenoidal tissue, if either is present, to valving. Even if complete closure is not essential to normal speech, the space between the velum and the posterior pharyngeal wall or the total area of the pharyngeal opening is a factor in undue nasal resonance and inadequate pressure for articulation (Chase, 1960; Blackfield and others, 1962a, 1962b; Weatherley-White and others, 1964; Brandt and Morris, 1965). The amount of palatopharyngeal gap that may be present without interfering with adequate articulation-resonance has been reported as 1, 1.5, and 2 millimeters; and the total area of velopharyngeal opening may apparently reach 19 or 20 square millimeters without producing undue nasality (Hagerty and Hoffmeister, 1954; Joanne Subtelny and others, 1961; Shelton and others, 1965; Warren, 1965; Isshiki and others, 1968). Intelligibility and articulation were not seriously affected by gaps of 0.73 millimeter in children (Shelton and others, 1964) or by gaps of 3 millimeters in adults (Joanne Subtelny and others, 1961).

Films and electromyography have been used to study the influence of tongue position on velopharyngeal valving. In addition to its function as an articulator, the tongue may also participate in the closure of the pharyngeal passageway (Brooks and others, 1965, 1966). Velopharyngeal closure has been found to be less firm if the tongue is relatively low in the oral cavity (Hardy and Arkebauer, 1966); and a high tongue position has been noted in association with a high palatal position (Lubker, 1968). Subjects in one radiographic study who had the greatest perceived nasality also used tongue positions lower and more anterior than those of subjects with less nasality (Dickson, 1969). The functional interconnection between the tongue and the palate, stressed in these studies, points to the importance of considering the position and shape of the tongue as well as the activity of the velum in assessing velopharyngeal competence. The speech pathologist should make careful observations of tongue position as he views cinefluorographic films, although he will probably make little or no use of electromyography in a clinical situation.

Some of the facilities required to obtain visible evidence of valving and tongue position are elaborate and costly, and the assistance of other specialists is needed in making and interpreting the records. Estimates of velopharyngeal efficiency may be made from single pictures or from moving pictures with or without sound, the input may be single speech sounds or contextual utterance, and the information obtained will vary in terms of the techniques and instruments used (Cooper and Hoffman, 1955; Randall and others, 1958; Spriestersbach and Powers, 1959a; Calnan, 1961; Warren and Hofmann, 1961; Kirkpatrick, 1964; McWilliams and Girdany, 1964; Moll, 1964a; Joanne Subtelny, 1964; Fujiki and Wada, 1967; Massengill and Bryson, 1967; Hoopes and Fabrikant, 1968; Lubker and Morris, 1968; Massengill, Pickrell, and Fetterrolf, 1968; Warren and Mackler, 1968; Dickson, 1969).

Other instruments, many of which are in use for research or are being tested for their contributions to the evaluation of velopharyngeal closure, include the sound spectrograph (Bjork and Nylén, 1961; Schwartz, 1968), "nasality meters" (Weatherley-White and others, 1964, 1966), oscilloscopes (Bennett and others, 1966), analog systems (Warren and Devereux, 1966; Warren and Ryon, 1967), devices using ultrasound (Kelsey and others, 1969), and the oral panendoscope (Taub, 1966).

Measurements of the efficiency of velopharyngeal valving may be obtained with instruments that provide other kinds of evidence. The speech pathologist can learn how the child with a repaired or obturated palatal cleft is using his structures by employing devices that record airflow and pressure. The instruments in this category differ in their purposes and in the information they provide. Some show the pressure of the flow of air that is directed into a mask covering the mouth or nose, and these permit the use of speech in testing (Hixon and others, 1967; Machida, 1967). Some indicate the amount of pressure that comes from the nose or the mouth into a tube; these are usually limited to measurements from nonspeech activities (Chase, 1960; Hess and McDonald, 1960; Hanson, 1964; Quigley and others, 1964; Warren and DuBois, 1964; Shelton and others, 1965; Buncke and others, 1966; Hardy and Arkebauer, 1966; Morris, 1966; Pitzner and Morris, 1966; Warren, Duany, and Fischer, 1969). Combined measurements, using oral-nasal airflow and cinefluorography, for example, also have been used in studies of the effectiveness of the velopharyngeal sphincter (Lubker and Moll, 1965; J. Daniel Subtelny and others, 1968; Joanne Subtelny and others, 1969).

Among these devices, the oral manometer is the one that has been used most frequently in clinical assessments of velopharyngeal competence. This instrument permits the computation of scores that indicate whether or not the velopharyngeal valve closes sufficiently to provide mouth pressure with the nostrils open that is equal to mouth pressure with the nostrils occluded. A quotient is found by dividing the amount of pressure, in ounces per square inch or some other unit of measurement, obtained by blowing or sucking with the nostrils open by the amount of pressure with the nostrils closed. A quotient of 1.00 indicates that the velopharyngeal valve is closing the passage to the nasal cavities if a bleed valve, or vent, is provided to circumvent the building up of mouth pressure by tongue positioning that closes off the pharynx (Barnes and Morris, 1967). Quotients less than 1.00 indicate some lack of velopharyngeal valving, and a quotient lower than 0.85 usually indicates inadequate closure. Sounds that require oral breath pressure will usually decrease in consistency of production when the oral manometer quotient decreases (Van Demark, 1969). The oral manometer, with such other devices as the U-tube and various forms of pressure gauges, is limited as a diagnostic tool in several ways (Morris, 1966), chiefly because evidence of valving in a nonspeech activity such as blowing or sucking does not assure valving for contextual speech. In fact, speech may require velopharyngeal behavior that is physiologically different from that required for blowing (McWilliams and Bradley, 1965).

Even if he does not take part in procedures that use these instruments, the speech pathologist can get information from reports he may receive from laboratories that have such equipment. He will probably want to ask, "What is the status of the structures of the velopharyngeal area, and what is their function in speech in this specific individual?" He may request reports on the apparent length and mobility of the soft palate from instrumental measurements. He may ask, "At what level is the contact or near-contact between palate and pharyngeal wall?" He may obtain a description of the way in which the posterior and lateral pharyngeal walls function in relationship to a prosthesis being used as a temporary diagnostic device (Alley, 1965) or as a permanent speech aid. Information about a child who has been provided with a pharyngeal flap can tell the speech pathologist whether or not the lateral pharyngeal walls are participating in attempts at closure. Instrumentation may also furnish answers to questions about the function of the velopharyngeal area in the production of isolated speech sounds, in combinations of sounds, in contextual speech, and in normal and forceful phonation.

If measuring devices are not available, then the speech pathologist will depend on the most common instrument for evaluating velopharyngeal competence, his ear. Listener judgment techniques may provide "the only direct and logically-valid measures of nasal voice quality" (Moll, 1964b, p. 373). Judgments from auditory cues may not always agree with visual or numerical indications of velopharyngeal competence; but the ear of the experienced listener can assess resonance, just as it evaluates articulation.

To supplement his ear, the speech pathologist may use his tactile sense by placing his finger below the nostrils of the child and feeling the escape of air through the nasal cavities. He may also obtain visual evidence of nasal emission of air from movement of a piece of cotton or paper or the clouding of a mirror held under the nostrils. These indications of misdirection of the stream of air or sound, however, are less satisfactory than the evidence obtained from instrumentation and from listening.

Form II.B.1 provides for recording several kinds of evidence of the use of structures for managing resonance. The examiner can indicate whether the airstream is directed through the mouth or through the oral and nasal cavities simultaneously in single sounds, sounds in contexts of varying lengths, and combinations that permit evaluations of assimilative influences. The child can be asked to imitate single sounds produced by the examiner, who can record resonance as primarily oral or oral-nasal. Words can be dictated, or the child can read them. Sentences can be drawn from school texts of appropriate difficulty or from clinical materials used for other kinds of testing. The Iowa Pressure Articulation Test, for example, which was designed to evaluate the adequacy of velopharyngeal closure, includes consonant sounds shown to require the greatest amount of pressure through the mouth. The forty-three words that make up the test include plosives, fricatives, and affricates. In seventeen of the words, single consonant sounds are evaluated. Two-element items, such as /sk/ and /br/, appear in twenty-four words. Two words contain three-element items, /str/ and /mps/. Although no score is obtained, cleft palate speakers with inadequate velopharyngeal closure will make more errors as the number of elements increases (Morris and others, 1961). Determination of the influence of one sound on another (assimilation or coarticulation) can be made with dictated words or phrases or sentences that can be read by the child. In these words, phrases,

B. Use of Structures for Speech

1. Velopharyngeal valving:
   a. In the production of isolated sounds, what is the major direction of the stream of air or sound? (Use *m* for mouth emission, *n* for emission through both oral and nasal cavities.)
      On vowel sounds:
      /i/___ /ɪ/___ /ɛ/___ /æ/___ /ɑ/___ /ɔ/___ /u/___ /ʌ/___
      /ʊ/___ /eɪ/___ /aɪ/___ /aʊ/___ /oʊ/___ /ɝ/___
      On sustained consonant sounds:
      /f/___ /v/___ /θ/___ /ð/___ /s/___ /z/___ /ʃ/___ /ʒ/___
      On plosive consonant sounds:
      /p/___ /b/___ /t/___ /d/___ /k/___ /g/___ /tʃ/___ /dʒ/___
      Note discrepancies between voiced and voiceless members of sound pairs (/p/—/b/, /s/—/z/, for example).____________________

      ____

   b. In the use of sounds in limited sequence, what is the major direction of the stream of air or sound?
      in *up* /ʌ/____ /p/____ (VC combination)
      in *gay* /g/____ /eɪ/____ (CV combination)
      in *easy* /i/____ /z/____ /ɪ/____ (VCV)
      in *cat* /k/____ /æ/____ /t/____ (CVC)
      in *spa* /s/____ /p/____ /ɑ/____ (CCV)
      in *dress* /d/____ /r/____ /ɛ/____ /s/____ (CCVC)
      (The combinations above are examples. Additional words or nonsense syllables should be used to explore capacities in depth.)
      Describe other combinations that produce deviation or improvement.__________

      ____

      ____

   c. In the use of sounds in continuing sequence:
      In contextual speech, the stream of air or sound is misdirected in:
      consonant sounds___ vowel sounds___ both___
      Misdirection of the stream of air or sound is apparent in:
      all speaking situations___ most speaking situations___
      few speaking situations___
      Under what conditions does improvement occur?____________________

      ____

      In contextual speech, the effect of assimilation is toward proper direction of the stream of sound or air when________________ precede(s)____________,
      away from proper direction when________________ precede(s)____________.
      Describe general assimilation noted in contextual speech.________________.

      ____.

and sentences, the effect of nasal consonants on neighboring sounds should be observed. Sentences that do not contain /m/, /n/, or /ŋ/ can be devised or drawn from standard texts. Paired words, such as "bed—men," "pad—pan," "be—me," "cup—come," "hit—him," "suit—soon," may also enable the examiner to hear the effects of nasal and nonsasal consonants on vowel sounds. Determination of sounds that reduce nasal resonance is as important to eventual remedial considerations as locating sounds that increase the amount of air or sound directed through the nasal cavities.

In these listening tasks, the speech pathologist attempts to separate resonance from articulation, to distinguish direction of the stream of air or sound from articulatory positions and movements. Later, he will relate the acoustic evidence of management of the velopharyngeal sphincter to articulatory activities as he considers articulation-resonance as a single entity.

Differentiation between resonatory errors and articulatory errors can be accomplished in several ways. Listening to recorded speech can help the evaluator to focus his attention on the effects of velopharyngeal valving. The use of backward playing (Sherman, 1954) may permit judgment of resonance without the interference of adequate or inadequate articulation. Listening to a child in a play situation without trying to understand what he is saying may help the speech pathologist in the preliminary separation of velopharyngeal competence from articulatory accuracy. Listening from a distance also may help the evaluator to attend to resonance rather than to articulation.

The specific assessment of the articulatory capacities of children with congenital clefts also may be accomplished in several ways. Form II.B.2 indicates that the positioning of sounds should be considered in terms of the sequential use of sounds, as the term "articulation" implies, as well as in the production of isolated vowel and consonant sounds. The purpose of evaluating articulation as a separate factor is fourfold: it enables the examiner to differentiate the articulatory errors that are probably the result of immaturity from those that are brought about by the present status of structures; it can show the relationship of directional errors to positioning errors; it can reveal the consistency and inconsistency of articulatory deviations; and it can aid in determining whether remedial approaches should begin with attention to velopharyngeal valving or to articulation.

The kinds of tests of articulatory proficiency that can be employed in the assessment of positioning skills may be those that are used to obtain a phonetic inventory for any individual, those that evaluate some particular deviation in depth, those that have been designed particularly for evaluations

2. Articulation—articulatory positions and movements as differentiated from direction of the stream of air or sound:
   a. Phonetic inventory:
      Test used________
      Articulatory errors: substitutions________
      distortions________ omissions________
   b. In the production of isolated sounds [indicate (1) with minimal stimulation, (2) with strong stimulation, (3) with directions for "placement"]:
      Labial sounds deviant in position:
      (1)________ (2)________ (3)________
      Labiodental sounds deviant in position:
      (1)________ (2)________ (3)________
      Linguadental sounds deviant in position:
      (1)________ (2)________ (3)________
      Lingua-alveolar sounds deviant in position:
      (1)________ (2)________ (3)________
      Linguavelar sounds deviant in position:
      (1)________ (2)________ (3)________
      Vowel sounds deviant because of errors in shaping mouth cavity________
   c. In the use of sounds in combination—general observation:
      Vowel sounds are deviant.____ Consonant sounds are deviant.____
      Both vowel and consonant sounds are deviant.____ No deviations are noted.____
   d. In the production and use of sounds in combination—specific observations:
      Consonant sounds deviant in position (x) in combination with vowel sounds representing (1) high-front position, (2) low-front position, (3) high-back position:

	(1)	(2)	(3)		(1)	(2)	(3)
/p/	____	____	____	/ʒ/	____	____	____
/b/	____	____	____	/tʃ/	____	____	____
/f/	____	____	____	/dʒ/	____	____	____
/v/	____	____	____	/l/	____	____	____
/θ/	____	____	____	/r/	____	____	____
/ð/	____	____	____	/k/	____	____	____
/t/	____	____	____	/g/	____	____	____
/d/	____	____	____	/h/	____	____	____
/s/	____	____	____	/m/	____	____	____
/z/	____	____	____	/n/	____	____	____
/ʃ/	____	____	____	/ŋ/	____	____	____

   e. Structures that are not well managed in articulatory activities:
      Lips______ Front of tongue______ Back of tongue______
   f. Apparent effect of dental structure on articulation________

   g. In the use of sounds in continuing sequence—in contextual speech, under optimal conditions:
      Vowel sounds distorted________ Substitutions________
      Consonant sounds distorted________ Use of glottal stop for________
      Consonant sounds omitted________ Use of pharyngeal fricative for________

of the speech of children with clefts, and those evolved by speech pathologists on the basis of need for certain kinds of information. No one test can meet all the requirements for complete assessment, and no test can provide results that will correlate completely with observations made by the listener as the child uses speech in situations other than the necessarily artificial environment of the testing room.

Phonetic inventories that provide scores or permit comparison with norms, several of which are available commercially, can be useful in determining the child's efficiency in using structures, can help in the evaluation of remedial procedures, and can reveal improvements that may come from maturation (Barker, 1963; McDonald, 1964; Goldman and Fristoe, 1969; Templin and Darley, 1969; others). These tests were designed for noncleft individuals, but some have been used in studies of the articulation of children with congenital clefts. Some investigators evolved ways of judging the articulatory proficiency of speakers born with clefts to suit the designs of their experiments, using nonsense syllables, counting, passages from texts, sentences containing certain consonant sounds, or other materials devised for specific studies. Children with congenital clefts in the palatal area will present more articulatory errors than those with prepalatal clefts (Spriestersbach and others, 1961); but the speech pathologist, planning methods and materials for assessment, will use, adapt, or design tests of articulation that will reveal both strengths and weaknesses in sound positioning.

Tests intended to provide specific information about the articulatory abilities of speakers born with clefts range from simple to complex. The use of a 1-minute recording of materials using plosive and fricative sounds was recommended by one investigator (Meinhold, 1964). A picture test to evaluate the use of the sixteen consonant sounds most frequently deviant in cleft palate speech was also proposed (Adamson and others, 1966). An articulation test containing forty-three elements to evaluate fricatives and affricates, thirty-four to evaluate plosives, and thirty-two for checking nasals and glides was used in a study of the relationship between velopharyngeal incompetence and articulatory errors (Brandt and Morris, 1965). The preponderance of plosives, fricatives, and affricates in the Iowa Pressure Articulation Test (Morris and others, 1961) suggests that this material might be used for evaluating articulation as well as pressure. Sentences used in a study of listener judgments (Van Demark, 1964) permitted evaluation of fifty-six plosives, thirty-three fricatives, thirty-one nasal semivowels, and twenty-nine glides. Other studies (Shelton and others, 1964; Buncke and others, 1966) concerned with palatopharyngeal closure used sentences containing fricative consonants and words or syllables containing plosives and fricatives. No specific test has been designed and standardized to evaluate the articulation of children with congenital clefts, and the speech pathologist may need to evolve his own materials or adapt those found useful by others. These testing materials should be suitable to the age and reading ability of the subjects; but they should probably contain words that permit evaluation of the accuracy of position and movement for all the sounds of American English, vowel sounds as well as consonant sounds, with particular emphasis on those sounds that influence intelligibility because of their frequent appearance in the language.

Form II.B.2 provides for recording errors in positioning for sounds in various categories, in various combinations, and in context. The efficiency of articulation under varying conditions of stimulus can be shown in terms of the types of sounds that are deviant. The production of isolated sounds requiring the use of various articulators can be judged from imitation of stimuli of differing strengths provided by the examiner. The use of sounds in combination can be observed generally and tested specifically. If consonant sounds are combined with vowels that require varying heights of the tongue, two estimates can be made. The examiner can judge the influence of the height of the vowel on the consonant; and he can also determine whether or not the individual being tested has unusual tongue positioning, thought to be characteristic of some speakers with repaired or obturated palatal clefts, under all circumstances or in certain consonant-vowel combinations.

Standard tests of articulation can be used to obtain information about structures that are managed well or inefficiently for articulatory activities; but, for children, supplementary use of dictated words that are not completely familiar may permit observation of performance that is not influenced by patterns established before modification of structures by surgical or dental management. These words can be chosen from graded vocabulary lists, at a level above the chronological age; or they may be nonsense words that provide for observation of articulatory activities in unpracticed combinations.

Listening to articulation in contextual speech, under conditions that demand the best performance and under those that do not stress careful use of speech sounds, is another way of obtaining information about articulatory abilities and disabilities. In context, glottal stops and pharyngeal fricatives may be used as substitutes for sounds that are difficult to produce and combine in quick sequence; and omissions also may be noted during sequential speech.

The assessment of intelligibility is more general than the evaluation of articulatory abilities. It brings together the factors of resonance and articulation and, if linguistic skills are within normal limits, may be the major determinant of the speaker's capacity to communicate orally (II.B.3).

3. Intelligibility:
   a. Scores or ratings of intelligibility:
      Test(s) used__________
      Score(s) or rating(s)__________
   b. Intelligibility (rate on 7-point scale):
      In controlled situations______ In emotional expression______
      In casual conversation______ In "best performance"______
   c. Intelligibility (rate on 7-point scale):
      When listener watches______ From recorded material______
      When listener does not watch______
   d. Reports on general intelligibility from:
      Those familiar with the child's speech:
      excellent___ good___ fair___ poor___
      Those not familiar with the child's speech:
      excellent___ good___ fair___ poor___

Judgments of proficiency in speech are sometimes complicated by articulatory differences in the presence of adequate velopharyngeal closure (Hanson, 1964), by undue nasal resonance on vowel sounds that are correctly formed, and by nasal emission of air or sound in consonant sounds that are correctly positioned. Hence, a judgment of the total effect of speech may be needed; and a multiple approach that considers both articulation and resonance is useful in summarizing assessment and planning remediation.

Intelligibility may be evaluated in syllables and words as well as in contextual speech, and transcriptions of nonsense syllables and of words can reveal the general degree of intelligibility. In listening to a forty-eight-syllable recording, trained evaluators were unable to transcribe eleven syllables accurately when the speakers were individuals with clefts (Subtelny and Subtelny, 1959). Words from the Fairbanks Rhyme Test (1966), transcribed from recordings, showed that subjects with clefts produced 88 percent of fifty words intelligibly, whereas noncleft subjects produced almost 99 percent of these words intelligibly (Prins and Bloomer, 1968). Relationships found between velopharyngeal competence and articulation (Brandt and Morris, 1965; Pitzner and Morris, 1966) suggested that resonance and articulation combine to produce the total that may be called intelligibility. Judgments made from the reading of a suitable passage or from conversational speech can be made on a 7-point scale at the time of the initial assessment and at intervals during the period of remediation, for comparison of a speaker's general progress in intelligibility. If these judgments are made by several listeners, the intelligibility ratings become more useful; but they do not replace the evaluations that separate resonance from articulation in the total assessment.

Listening may be supplemented with observation that provides visual cues to the effectiveness of articulation or to distracting concomitants related directly or indirectly to articulatory activities. Lack of mobility of lips or jaw may be apparent to the observer without interfering greatly with articulation. Atypical movements of the lips or tongue may also distract the watcher-listener. Tongue thrust behavior and interdentalization, noted as greater in cleft palate subjects than in noncleft controls, may attract undue attention and modify articulation of /t/, /d/, /n/, and /l/ (Marks, 1968). Lingual protrusion in deviant /s/, /z/, /ʃ/, /ʒ/, /tʃ/, and /dʒ/ may also produce an undesirable cosmetic effect. These differences may be found in many children, with or without clefts, who have articulatory disorders; but other observable and distracting behavior is often found in children born with clefts. Constriction of the anterior nares, wrinkling of the nose, and other noticeable facial grimaces often accompany attempts to achieve closure at some point other than the velopharynx (Morley, 1967). Because evaluations based on recordings cannot include the visual aspects (II.B.4), little research

4. Visual aspects:
   Mobility of:
   Lips: good____ fair____ poor____
   Jaw: good____ fair____ poor____
   Unusual movements in facial area: describe.
   ____
   Constriction of nares: absent____ present____
   Note specific activities that elicit this behavior if it is present.____________
   ____

evidence is available on visible concomitants in the speech of individuals with congenital clefts; but clinical evidence of such deviations can be found in many case studies.

A summary of the assessment can be used for reporting and as a guide to planning remedial procedures. In this summary (II.C), the various aspects of oral communication are evaluated from information obtained from other sources or gathered during evaluations. An estimate of the child's ability

C. Summary of Assessment

1. Intellectual capacity: within normal limits____ slightly impaired____ moderately impaired____ severely impaired____
2. Linguistic skills: adequate for age level____ slightly impaired____ moderately impaired____ severely impaired____
   Specific linguistic impairments________________________________
   ____
3. Hearing: within wide normal limits for speech____ slightly impaired____ moderately impaired____ severely impaired____
   Specific auditory impairments________________________________
   ____
4. Status of structures for speech: adequate____ adequate but not used maximally____ adequacy questionable____ adequacy impaired____
   Nature of impairment______________________________________
5. Use of structures for speech: adequate____ adequacy can probably be achieved____ achievement of adequacy questionable____ reason________________________
6. Potential for achievement in speech program: excellent____ very good____ good____ fair____ poor____ very poor____
7. Recommendations____
   ____
   ____
   ____
   ____
   ____

COPY OF REPORT (SPECIFY FORMS) SENT TO:	DATE:
________________________________	________
________________________________	________
________________________________	________
________________________________	________
________________________________	________

to profit from speech training can be made, and recommendations can be presented. This page, with the cover sheet, can constitute a brief report form.

When all the pieces of the evaluation have been assembled, four steps still remain in the total process of assessment. The first of these is the determination of relationships between and among the various items of information that have been obtained (Van Demark, 1966). Confirmations and contradictions should be carefully weighed as a preface to the second step, which is the determination of priority of needs. As earlier discussion indicated, a child whose paucity of language prevents communication that is essential to his progress should be provided with a program of language training rather than with one that emphasizes, at the outset, the other factors in communication. A child with a severe hearing loss may not be able to profit from efforts to develop skills in oral communication until his hearing has been improved by medical intervention or amplification. A child who is wearing an orthodontic appliance designed to correct a dental anomaly may, if the appliance interferes with articulatory activities and if the dental correction can be achieved within a short period of time, be given only minimal speech training, or none at all, until he can use the articulators without interference. A child with an unrepaired palatal cleft or one who is to have additional surgery soon may profit from some general attention to sound discrimination or to control of tongue position and movement, but he may be better able to respond to remedial procedures designed to improve speech when his structures are more nearly within normal limits. A child who cannot accomplish any form of adequate velopharyngeal valving may need to learn this skill before he tries to achieve adequate articulation of sounds that require pressure. A child whose velopharyngeal control is good when he "performs" on command but who does not use his potential skill in contextual speech may need a different point of departure and a different approach from those that might be used with a child who can control the velopharyngeal valve but has formed the habit of using glottal closure to build pressure. Each assessment leads to conclusions that apply to the child being evaluated; and the determination of priority of needs should involve the several specialists from whom the speech pathologist may obtain information in making his decisions.

The third step to be taken after the assessment seems complete is the recommendation of procedures to be followed in remedial sessions, if speech training is to be provided. Although the speech clinician who provides this assistance will determine many of the ways of reaching the goals for the individual child, the judgments of the speech pathologist as a diagnostician also are needed in planning. If assessment is not to be followed by remedial assistance from a qualified speech clinician, then recommendations should be given to parents and teachers, to advise them of what they can do and what they should not do.

Continued evaluation is the fourth step. Progress in therapy can be determined by repetition of evaluative procedures at frequent intervals (Prins and Bloomer, 1965). Additional information from specialists who continue their care of the child can be used in such reevaluations and in modifications of procedures used in speech training. Recommendations for investigation of the advisability of further surgical and dental management can result from evaluations made after a period of trial therapy.

Assessment, then, is a continuing process, begun before the speech pathologist first sees the child and going on throughout any period of speech training that may be provided. It is also a cooperative process in which each specialist relies on the others and contributes his share. It is a process of seeing relationships and of determining needs. It prefaces and supplements remediation. It demands high levels of skill and is facilitated by organized reporting. It must be flexible and not limited, although it is often selective. It is the key to remediation.

CHAPTER SEVEN

Remedial Procedures

EVALUATION AND THERAPY OVERLAP, EACH SUPPLEMENTING THE OTHER, BOTH CONTRIBUTING TO THE HABILITATIVE PROCESS.

Determination of the child's primary needs in speech and language and of his abilities to participate in a remedial program will serve as a preface to therapy. Additional information, gathered as the remedial processes continue, will enable the clinician to determine ways of modifying the original plans or may lead to a decision to terminate or postpone formal therapeutic management.

No one sequence and no single set of procedures will be adequate in every instance (Fletcher, 1966). Just as children differ, so do clinicians and remedial environments. An approach that is useful for one child may not be suitable for another. Occasional therapy differs from intensive speech training. The kinds of procedures used with groups of children differ from those used in individual conferences. The following discussion, therefore, is not intended to be restrictive but suggests remedial approaches to the cleft palate speech problem, with examples of activities that can be used if they are appropriate to the time, place, child, and professional worker.

In planning for therapy, the clinician can adapt the suggestions in this chapter and those in several texts (Berry and Eisenson, 1956; Koepp-Baker, in Travis, 1957; Van Riper and Irwin, 1958; Van Riper, 1963; Westlake and Rutherford, 1966; Morley, 1967; Shelton and others, in Spriestersbach and Sherman, 1968; Westlake, in Lencione, 1968; Zimmerman and Canfield, in Stark, 1968; others). However, he will find few journal articles that provide specific information on procedures for speech training for children with congenital clefts. In a period of thirty-four years, the *Journal of Speech and Hearing Disorders* carried ten articles that dealt with such procedures. Five of these described general and specific methods. Four were concerned with some special approach. One was a discussion of research and clinical implications.

None of the articles dealing with clefts of the prepalate and palate in the first twelve years of publication of the *Journal of Speech and Hearing Research* presented information on remedial procedures. The articles on cleft palate in that journal were concerned primarily with assessment of speech and with characteristics of children with palatal clefts. In the first six volumes of the *Cleft Palate Journal,* less than a dozen articles considered speech training.

Information available to parents of children with clefts through pamphlets prepared by individuals and organizations (Wylie and McWilliams, 1965) can sometimes be useful to clinicians. However, if such informational materials are recommended to parents, the clinician will need to emphasize some of the points, modify some, and negate others.

The similarities between some of the disorders of oral communication presented by children with congenital clefts and those of noncleft children may account, in part, for the lack of detailed discussions of remedial procedures appropriate for cleft palate speech. Ways of encouraging linguistic development and of modifying articulation may not differ greatly for those with clefts and those without, but the combinations of articulatory and resonatory difficulties often present in speakers born with palatal clefts require special kinds of attention in a remedial program.

Information from previous and ongoing assessment will help the clinician decide where to start. One child may have, as his primary need, encouragement to linguistic skills; in this case, speech therapy should be preceded by attention to language. Another may be quite adequate in expressive language but in need of improved velopharyngeal control to make optimal use of his abilities in articulation. Others may need to improve the articulatory aspects of oral self-expression. For some, additional surgical or dental management that is planned or the need for preliminary psychological management will serve as a contraindication to speech therapy (Smith, 1969).

If assessment has been thorough, the clinician can use the measurements of velopharyngeal competence and the information gained from tests of articulation as guidelines for the starting point in therapy. From evidence of the child's ability to accomplish velopharyngeal valving in various nonspeech and speech activities, the clinician can determine whether the first need is for velopharyngeal closure or for improvement of articulation. Questions such as the following may help the clinician in arriving at a decision.

Have surgical and dental procedures reached a point at which the child will have relatively stable structures for a period of time? Do these structures seem adequate for the various activities of velopharyngeal control and articulation, even if they are not now being used efficiently? If so, then speech training should begin, if it is needed. If not, then formal speech training may be postponed until other forms of management have brought the structures to relative stability, with informal environmental stimulation and example being provided during the interim period (Bickel, 1970).

Does the child have sufficient language to use in speech activities that need modification? If language is adequate, even if not completely within normal limits, then speech training can be provided in combination with procedures designed to encourage the development of linguistic skills. If language is so limited that the child cannot express himself, then improvement in articulation-resonance should be secondary to improvement in linguistic skills.

Is auditory acuity adequate for the perception needed for improvement in articulation-resonance? Is auditory discrimination sufficiently mastered to enable the child to use discrimination in monitoring his own speech and that of others? If the first of these factors is deficient, then otological management should precede or accompany speech training; and sufficient amplification should be provided to compensate for depressed hearing. If discriminative abilities are inadequate, special attention to this aspect of the communicative process should accompany other therapy; or, if discrimination is severely deviant, auditory training or ear training may need to be a preface to direct therapy for disorders of articulation-resonance.

Is the child able to achieve velopharyngeal closure? If he can do so in nonspeech activities, can he also accomplish sustained and rapidly changing valving in speech activities at various levels of difficulty? If manometric ratio quotients of 1.00 can be reached, does the apparent facility of the velopharyngeal sphincter extend to single productions of vowel or consonant sounds, to single words, to short phrases, to sentences, to contextual speech? If both nonspeech and speech activities are affected by inadequate valving, the starting point may well be to develop patterns of closure. If valving is adequate for speech activities, then attention may be turned to articulatory deviations, with continued reinforcement of valving.

Is articulation deviant, in terms of positions and movements or acoustic and cosmetic factors, velopharyngeal closure being adequate? If so, then the determination made of the specific articulatory deviations can serve as a guide to the clinician in deciding where to begin. The use of protocols based on the child's ability to use various speech sounds (Van Demark, 1969) can provide information on which remediation for articulatory errors can be built. If, for example, a child uses /k/ correctly 60 percent of the time but uses /g/ correctly only 5 to 10 percent of the time, attention to /k/ may lead to improvement in /g/. If /s/ and /z/ are used correctly in less than 20 percent of the responses in a test situation and other sounds reach levels of correctness well above those for /s/ and /z/, the focus for therapy is relatively clear; improvement in /s/ and /z/ might be the first goal.

Are both velopharyngeal control and articulatory activities deviant? If so, determination of the relationships between valving and the pressure needed for plosive and fricative sounds can be useful in choosing the factor to receive first emphasis. The importance of control of the direction of the stream of air and sound may overshadow, at first, the immediate need for correct articulation. Attempts to eliminate nasal resonance on vowel sounds could well be a first step if velopharyngeal control is inadequate but consonant sounds are well positioned.

The establishment of a starting point will, of course, be related to the long-range goals for the remedial program. These goals, in turn, will be determined by the child's intellectual potential, his needs, the amount of time available for speech training, and the realistic predictions based on assessment.

SPEECH TRAINING FOR CHILDREN BORN WITH CLEFTS OF THE PREPALATE, PALATE, OR BOTH WILL USUALLY HAVE SEVERAL GOALS.

These include:

1. Motivation for improvement
2. Development of awareness of the structures that will be used for new speech patterns
3. Achievement of adequate tonus and movement of the velopharyngeal and articulatory mechanisms
4. Control of the velopharyngeal sphincter
5. Proper direction of the stream of air, with or without voicing, through appropriate resonating, restricting, and impounding channels
6. Adequate production and use of the sound units in syllables, words, and sentences
7. Combination of velopharyngeal valving and articulatory movements in sequences of utterance
8. Ability to monitor performance and compare it with models presented
9. Retention of acquired skills if structures are modified by management or growth
10. Correlation of speech skills with linguistic self-expression in a social environment—the automatization of speech

In attempting to help the child reach the goals he has not yet achieved, the clinician may combine several concepts that facilitate the modification of speech behavior (Fletcher, 1966). He may draw on principles that have been derived from modern learning theory. He may consider speech behavior as a process that is governed by an automatic control system. He may take advantage of teaching machines and devices that permit self-monitoring. He may set out to change speech behavior by other methods. His considerations, however, should be made in the light of what he knows about the child, about the problem, about himself as a clinician, and about the situations in which remediation is to occur.

The use of operant conditioning has not been reported frequently as a means of speech training for children with congenital clefts. However, the tightly sequenced instructional program recommended by some for use in the modification of stuttering or articulation (Gregory, 1968; Sloane and MacAulay, 1968) can be useful to the clinician who is designing a program for the child with cleft palate speech. One report of the use of operant conditioning procedures to eliminate facial grimacing in an adult with a repaired cleft indicated that the approach was not entirely successful (Moller and others, 1969); but the principles of conditioning can be used to advantage in the acquisition of new skills and in the automatization of abilities that have been acquired. Such terms as "discrimination," "successive approximation," "reinforcement," and others are probably familiar to the clinician; and the application of principles of operant conditioning can provide a structure for therapy that, although individually planned, makes optimal use of learning theory.

The consideration of speech as behavior governed by an automatic control system can lead to training that recognizes the existence of receptor, integrator, transmitter, effector, and sensor units (Van Riper and Irwin, 1958; Mysak, 1966) and uses these units to advantage. The clinician can plan remedial procedures that incorporate these concepts as they are applied to the individual and his needs for modification of speech behavior.

Some of the equipment that is used in assessment can be adapted to remediation, but additional devices can be used to establish and automatize adequate velopharyngeal control and acceptable articulation-resonance. Some of these devices, such as palatal lifts, are intended to provide support for the palate or to strengthen it (Blakeley, 1960; Kobes and Kittel, 1966; Lang, 1967; Bloomer and Lang, 1968; Adisman, 1969; Lubit and Larsen, 1969; Gonzalez and Aronson, 1970). Others, such as muscle stimulation units, assist the speaker to gain voluntary control of the circumpharyngeal muscles and then, through operant conditioning, use this control involuntarily in speech (Yules, Welch, and others, 1968). Teaching machines commonly available for clinical procedures can be employed in the modification of the speech behavior of those with palatal clefts, just as they may be used in speech training for disorders of articulation and voice.

The assistance of those in home and school environments can facilitate the work of the clinician, also. With instruction from the clinician and frequent review of the results of adjunctive therapy, changes in speech behavior can be supported and encouraged by parents, siblings, teachers, and peers. Careful patterning of this assistance will make it more useful, and conferences with all those involved in supportive therapy should be held often.

PLANS FOR THE REMEDIAL PROCESS SHOULD CONSIDER THE GOAL SET FOR IMMEDIATE ATTENTION AND THE LONG-RANGE GOALS FOR THE INDIVIDUAL.

If thorough assessment has shown the child's special abilities and his immediate and long-term needs, speech training can be based on his capacities as well as his limitations, the former being used to overcome the latter. The speech pathologist, dealing with behavior, assists the child to modify what he does but is restricted to manipulation of the child himself rather than of his structures. He depends on the child's cooperation, his ability to retain what he has learned, and his ultimate capacity to incorporate his learning into an involuntary pattern that is used in all speaking situations. The speech clinician's procedures require relationships between clinician and child that are personal, continuing, and motivating. Each step in the remedial process depends, to a great extent, on the one before; and, in general, each accomplishment should be well established before the next is attempted, although some goals will be given constant attention throughout the sequence of therapy.

Motivation for modifications of speech behavior, although it may well preface other considerations, is a continuing goal. Research on the motivation for rehabilitation of the individual born with a palatal or prepalatal cleft has not been extensive, but the motivation of those with clefts that have affected their speech may not differ greatly from motivation of others with disorders of oral communication.

Desired behavior can be encouraged by positive reinforcements that provide for consistent attention to improvement. Verbal and attitudinal commendation or token rewards are more suitable than food in a program of conditioning because of the special need for maintenance of dental hygiene in children with clefts. Specific motivational approaches, used before and during a structured program, might include the following:

- The clinician's respect for the child and his consideration of the individual rather than the defect can help to establish the rapport necessary for motivation. The clinician who accepts the child does not necessarily accept all of that child's deviations in communication, but his attitude can promote good relationships.
- The child should know what is expected of him if he is to be motivated to reach any goal that is set. Specific and progressive steps can be made toward an immediate or long-range goal if both the clinician and the child know the destination and the path that is to be followed. Simple explanations of the reasons for asking the child to do the tasks set for him take little time but often motivate effectively.
- The right to make some decisions for himself may serve as a motivating device for the child. If the clinician guides and stimulates but does not assume all the responsibility, the child may consider himself more important in the process of modifying his speech behavior.

- If the child is given a choice, that choice should be respected. The clinician, therefore, should not offer an opportunity for selection if he does not intend to honor the child's decision. To ask "Do you want to tell me about these pictures?" when a negative answer will not be accepted wastes time and does not motivate. The clinician who asks, "What shall we do next?" should be ready to do what the child chooses, having given him the right of selection.
- Commendation is, for many children, a strong motivator. One characteristic that seems unusually prominent in children with clefts is the desire for favorable attention from those in authority. Hence, verbal praise can often serve to encourage continued effort. The clinician may need to guard against constant use of the same phrase or term for commendation. "Very good" or "okay" or "fine" can lose meaning for both clinician and child if the term is overworked or used casually.
- Social acceptance may serve as a motivating device. The opportunity to participate in group activities, to lead the group, to be commended by the group, to make favorable comments about others, to direct the actions of others may encourage the child to use the best speech of which he is capable.
- Recorded evidence of improvement can serve to motivate continued effort. The child who has an opportunity to hear his own speech at various stages of progress may be encouraged to try to exceed his own record and thus to serve as his own pacemaker. The value of the teaching machine is apparent here.
- Penalties, if they are carefully selected and appropriate to the child and the situation, can be useful as motivators. The group or the child may be more effective than the clinician in choosing penalties, but opportunities for reward should not be omitted in emphasis on punishment.
- Motivation, however, is strongest when it results from recognition of the need for better oral communication rather than from a desire to please an adult or receive praise. Any success in controlling his environment by use of better speech can stimulate the child to greater efforts.

The modification of speech behavior for those with residual structural anomalies can be facilitated by awareness of the structures used for articula-

tory-resonatory activities. Learning to manipulate parts of the body and the tools used by those parts, as in scribbling, writing, self-feeding, or playing with toys, is made easier by the relative visibility of the parts. Children learn early that they have hands and fingers; and the visual, tactile, and kinesthetic cues from these parts guide them in their handling of pencils, spoons, and blocks. Most individuals are less aware of the oral and pharyngeal structures they use in producing and combining the elements of speech. Hence, one of the first steps in the habilitative process may well be to help the child to recognize the parts and to understand that they can be controlled and used to advantage in speaking. For the very young child, the procedures can be simple; and the terms can be those he can readily understand. Some older children become quite sophisticated in their use of terminology and find some satisfaction in being able to identify and describe the various articulators, the velopharyngeal valve, and other parts of the facial complex.

Many adults, who may know the names of the structures for articulation and valving, have no real understanding of the functions of those parts. Few people, unless they have some particular reason for the focus, spend much time in investigation of their oral structures. Why, then, one might ask, should the child with a labial or palatal cleft be encouraged to study his mouth, his teeth, his palate? Might not this attention cause undue concern about the facial area? Could the initial emphasis on parts and their movements lead to a purely mechanical approach to speech? Does the child need to know the names of the structures so that he may, in further remediation, be told to put the tip of his tongue on the alveolar ridge or to attempt to move the lateral walls of the pharynx in a mesial direction? Speech is a total process, in which the whole is made up of rapid, sequential, and interwoven activities. No purely mechanical approach can accomplish the totality that is required; and no intent to stress isolated muscular performances should be inferred. However, the child with deviant structures, more than the person who has normal structures but uses them inadequately, needs information about the parts of the mouth, throat, face, and other areas that he must use differently. Such knowledge can provide him with a basis for improving communication; and, although the emphasis should not be so great as to make speech a mechanical process, an understanding of the basic differences with which he was born and of the ways in which he now resembles others and yet differs from them can provide him with a kind of readiness for modifying the use of his structures.

One need have little concern about focusing the attention of the child born with a cleft on his mouth, lips, nose, pharynx, and face. These are areas that have been inspected, subjected to surgical modification, given dental attention, and brought to a high level of awareness in terms of manipulations by others. Now the child must learn to accept them as parts that can be usefully managed for communication, to be aware of what the various structures are doing and can do, and to check the results of changes in behavior with those parts by auditory and visual feedback. Casual and objective reference to the various structures, at first, can establish good attitudes. If the clinician refers to the parts as important elements that most people have in common to help them talk, the similarities between structures that have been repaired or supplemented and those that are intact will be emphasized; and differences can be minimized.

The following kinds of activities can lead to recognition of the parts of the speech mechanism and to awareness of their functions:

- Starting with general considerations, particularly with young children, name body parts that are well known and that can be easily observed. Each member of a group can contribute, or the child and clinician can alternate in such naming. The clinician can then lead the focus to the facial area, if the children have not already done so, and start the naming of lips, teeth, tongue, top of mouth, throat, back of mouth, and so on.
- In another naming procedure, the parts can be identified by pointing to them and naming them. Alternate methods might include having one child name the part and another point to it, either on himself or on another or on a simple chart or diagram. Reversal of the process would call for pointing to a part and having someone give its name.
- Working again from general to specific, the children can tell and demonstrate what they do with various parts of the body—hands, toes, fingers, arms, eyes, ears, mouth, tongue, and others—either in pantomime for others to guess or by verbal description with some demonstration. Again, the clinician can lead the discussion to the structures for speech and begin to focus on the facial area.
- Inspection of the mouth cavity can provide opportunity for further learning about parts and for focus on velopharyngeal activity. Observation of the mouths of others and of his own may help the child to see similarities or to recognize that he is not alone in his differences. Identification by light tactile stimulation may help the child who

has difficulty in recognizing parts that he must learn to manage. Such stimulation, preferably by the child himself after a demonstration by the clinician, can come from a cotton-tipped swab stick or a tongue blade; and the clinician will have further opportunity to note the mobility of the parts as the child shows him where they are and what they can do.

- Names for the various parts may be designated by the clinician; but the children, after they begin to make some investigations, are often ingenious in providing descriptive titles for structures. Participation in so basic a procedure as the identification or titling of parts can often encourage the child to remember what he has named.
- Awareness of the velar and oral structures can be developed directly, but sequencing from other bodily activities to those of the facial area may produce better results. If toes are tapped, hands are clapped, elbows are flapped, and fingers are snapped, the successes in these activities and the identification of the parts as moving structures may facilitate identification of oral structures, provide welcome variations in activity, and serve as a basis for establishing proper tonus and control of the speech musculature. These activities are similar to those cited as the first step in operant conditioning procedures, that of simple nonverbal motor imitation (Sloane and MacAulay, 1968).
- Although no particular minimum level of achievement need be set, attempts to repeat, and to make quick changes in, certain labial, lingual, and palatal activities can be helpful. The child is not left with the impression that isolated movements or positions are sufficient. Rather, he begins to combine and to repeat movements, in nonspeech activities, that remind him that he is using the structures he has identified and that require him to make rapid changes that will be needed for words, phrases, and sentences. Babbling might be encouraged, although another name for it might be preferable. Imitation of nonsense combinations presented by the clinician can be followed by the clinician's imitation of nonsense combinations presented by the child or by group imitation of a child leader. Calling this experience by a special name can identify it for quick referral. Permitting the children to name the activity may be even better; and the name, although it may seem unusual or strange to the adult clinician, may have special meaning for a group or an individual child. This kind of activity is similar to the second step in operant conditioning, the

simple imitation of the placement of the vocal musculature and associated structures (Sloane and MacAulay, 1968).

- Recognition of the dual function of the structures used in speaking as well as in eating permits instruction on the dental care so essential for the maintenance of good oral hygiene. Stress on the importance of the best possible care of the teeth can be an adjunctive value to the development of awareness of structures and their functions.
- Similarly, initial attention to the facial area and the component parts used in speaking can expand to include considerations of caring for dental appliances that are now "parts" of the mouth. Recognition of the value of such appliances to replace, supplement, or modify other parts may facilitate the work of the orthodontist and prosthodontist and contribute to better care of appliances. The speech clinician may, in the environment in which he works, be in a good position to supplement the advice and recommendations of the dental specialist and encourage better management of the appliances provided.

Speech is essentially a muscular activity requiring movement and control during the production of the elements that make up the linguistic whole. If the child's articulatory and valving activities are to be accurate and well-directed, they may need special attention in the early stages of therapy. This step is not an isolated one. It can be combined with other procedures or omitted if it is not needed. However, like awareness, this phase of preparation for the modification of speech behavior, if slighted or overlooked, may result in the building of new skills on a foundation that cannot support them adequately.

The muscular activity of the structures, when they are used for articulation and for control of the direction of the air and sound stream, is different from the activity of those same parts when they are used for chewing, swallowing, yawning, and blowing. Nevertheless, the articulators and velopharyngeal sphincter may be more readily used involuntarily in speech if they have good muscle tone and are under some voluntary control. Separation of the parts of an activity from the whole for the purpose of strengthening the contribution of each portion is defensible if it does not become an end in itself. Reassembly of the component elements of the whole is essential; but, if a chain is only as strong as its weakest link, stronger links can make a better speech chain.

The use of blowing exercises for children with palatal clefts, repaired or obturated, has been the subject of a great deal of discussion and controversy. Those who favor blowing believe that it may strengthen muscles and establish the concept of proper direction of the airstream. Those who oppose blowing believe that the activities involved are not identical with those needed for the rapid control of the velopharyngeal sphincter in speech and that they may result in an excess of air pressure and alar constriction. An early discussion of the rationale of blowing for patients with repaired cleft palates (Kantner, 1947) pointed out that the obvious aim of such activity was to exercise the muscles of the soft palate and adjacent structures having to do with the closure of the opening into the nasopharynx. A second purpose was to establish the idea of mouth direction rather than the physical ability to blow efficiently. The writer suggested that little carry-over value accrued from blowing.

An investigation of the relative effects of blowing, sucking, and swallowing exercises on the size of the velopharyngeal gap in three groups of children with repaired palatal clefts showed that practice in blowing twice a day for almost four weeks produced almost no change in the velopharyngeal opening in the production of two vowel sounds (Massengill, Quinn, and others, 1968b). No evaluations were made of changes in the acoustic end results in speech, the findings being based entirely on measurements of the velopharyngeal gap shown on cinefluorographic film.

A study that combined measurements from films with judgments of speech found that the degree of velopharyngeal closure achieved during blowing with the nostrils open was different from that accomplished during connected speech. The investigators suggested that, because speech demands velopharyngeal behavior that is physiologically different from that required for blowing, blowing exercises could be providing a kind of therapy that is diametrically opposed to the physiologic demands of some speakers (McWilliams and Bradley, 1965).

The evidence suggests that blowing has little value in a speech training program for children with repaired or obturated palatal clefts. If the velopharyngeal gap is not great, other methods of achieving closure may be more useful than blowing. If the gap is wide and the soft palate is inadequate in length or mobility, closure may not be possible for blowing; and attempts to succeed in blowing exercises may result only in further experiences in sending the stream of air through the nose as well as the mouth. Attempts to achieve the valving needed for a nonspeech activity such as blowing can bring about use of the tongue as a stopper and undesirable reinforcement of immobility or poor positioning of the tongue. Additionally, blowing is usually prolonged to provide visual evidence of the oral emission of the airstream; and the rapid alternations of velar closure required for speech receive no reinforcement.

In rare instances, blowing activities might be used to determine the physiologic capacity for velopharyngeal closure; but assessment will already have shown whether or not such closure can be achieved. Indication of the direction of the stream of air can be determined by blowing, but this activity should not be interpreted as having a direct relationship to velopharyngeal closure for speech. Some modifications of blowing are included in the suggested activities in the following pages, but the purpose of these experiences is the establishment of muscular control and not the achievement of blowing as an isolated performance.

Recognizing that the procedures suggested here are preliminaries to the total act of speaking, the clinician may help the child to strengthen the musculature of the velopharyngeal sphincter in the following ways:

- With assurance that the child is not restricted by the surgeon in terms of physical activities, combine general physical movement with speech movements to encourage more vigorous use of the oral and pharyngeal structures.
- Voluntary yawning and stretching with lifted head, inhalation through the mouth, and phonated exhalation provide a combination of movements that stretch the muscles of the soft palate briefly in a nonspeech activity. Attention to kinesthetic cues from the palatal area adds the element of awareness here.
- Introduce the child to the idea of "climbing the ladder" by slapping his ankles, then his knees, then his waist, then his shoulders, then vocalizing briefly and firmly, as in "hah!" Vary this by going "down the ladder."
- Rewards for accurate responses to rapid commands, such as "Touch your knees," "Slap your hip," "Call out your name," or "Whisper a number" will reinforce prompt reactions.
- Imaginative play can be used to encourage imitation of people who have very active mouths or animals that yowl with much lip-rounding or imaginary creatures that swallow large chunks of air and then blow them out to open doors, knock down trees, or crumble walls. Keep the story unstructured, without concern for plot or logic. Let the children have fun with these activities, and they may even extend them beyond the confines of the clinic session.

- With small children, give an imaginary dinner party at which all items of food are chewed vigorously, but without tension, and swallowing requires closed mouth without tongue protrusion. Similar chewing and swallowing activities can be used to illustrate a story told by the clinician, in which animals or unreal creatures or even people eat things that are hard to chew and hard to swallow. Be sure to let the children tell the story occasionally while the clinician follows the directions and participates as a member of the group.
- Combine mouth activity with speech, even at this stage. Although misdirection of the airstream and errors in articulation will be ignored, "big talk" for a short period of time will be noisy but useful. In this situation, everyone, following the example of the clinician, reports some event or idea with highly exaggerated articulatory movements and increased vocal volume. Reverse the situation and use "small talk" for relaxed but purposeful movement of the articulators.
- With a group, present a series of signals or pictures to elicit chewing, yawning, puffing, or swallowing. Show one picture or give one signal at a time for response, then speed up the presentation of the stimuli and indicate one member of the group as respondent. The clinician can serve, later, as scorekeeper or observer and permit the children to present the stimuli and choose the respondents.
- Experience in attempting velopharyngeal closure, although it may not result in complete success at this stage, can be obtained by modified blowing. Sustained exhalation of a narrow stream of air from the rounded lips, with interruption by contraction of the lips, can move a light object jerkily across a smooth surface. The impounding—or attempt at impounding—the airstream at the lips approximates the activities used in the production of bilabial plosives. The object at this time is not to strive for articulation but to encourage such valving action as is present, to identify the kinesthetic sensation of the sphincteric movement that may occur, and to develop muscular control.
- If the interrupted blowing action resulting in an approximation of /p/ can be achieved even partially, variations in activity may be introduced to encourage continued attempts. Even if some of the airstream comes through the nasal cavities, any that comes from the mouth should produce observable results. The child can see a strip of light paper bend if he puffs air against it when he holds it in

front of his mouth. He can feel the emitted puff of air if he puts his finger or the back of his hand in front of his lips. The variations are many, but the objective remains the stimulation of muscular action in the area of the velopharyngeal sphincter and elimination of the immobility that may be the result of hypertension, a low level of awareness, or lack of use of the muscles in that area.

- Alternation of sucking and ejecting movements also can provide stimulation to muscle action. This activity can be performed without equipment by having the child pretend to move liquid from one imaginary container to another by sucking it up from one and ejecting it firmly into the other. Hands or boxes can be the containers, if a focus is desired.

- To supplement awareness and to encourage muscular control of the velopharyngeal sphincter, require deliberate shifts from oral to nasal emission during a sustained tone to help the child sense the movement that occurs.

- For a few minutes let each child use a special language, designed by the clinician for the child's needs. One may use "oo-ee-oo-ee" for his responses, for example; another may say only "wahga-wahga-wahga" when he answers. Within the framework of an imaginary United Nations, converse with the delegates from the various countries and let them reply with their own special kinds of noises. A silent meeting can be a variation on this theme, the responses being given without voice but with increased articulatory vigor.

- Greetings, farewells, and occasional moments of special emphasis provide opportunities for the clinician to stimulate the child or group to use controlled muscle action and to learn social amenities that they can use to facilitate rapport with those they meet. Conditioning to maximum use of muscular skills requires regular attention, and phrases used frequently provide an opportunity for such reinforcement.

- Occlusion of the passageway to the nasal cavities at any point other than the velopharyngeal area should be discouraged. Some children form the habit of closing off the nasal passage toward its anterior end by wrinkling the nose or drawing the nostrils together. Elimination of this incorrectly located valving action is essential, not only to require closure at the proper place but to do away with the distortions in appearance that interfere with the visual aspects of communication. Operant conditioning could be tried to modify this form of undesirable behavior that can be checked visually. Some children find that they can impound the stream of air at the level of the larynx even if they cannot get closure at the level of the oropharynx, and they form the habit of using the glottal stop for many or all plosive sounds.

- Emphasis on the emission of a stream of air or sound through the mouth cavity, with or without interruption, can begin an attack on the habitual use of constriction of the vocal bands to get closure. The free flow of breath or sound from the larynx to the open air can be channeled to the mouth by alternating inhalation through the nose or mouth with exhalation through the mouth. Short practice periods are preferable for this activity, to prevent the transient dizziness that sometimes occurs as a result of sustained inhalation and exhalation.

- When the combination of clinician and group or individual is right, overemphasis can be stimulating to muscular activity. "Wiggle Day" or even "Wiggle Minute" can, under the leadership of the clinician who is willing to serve as example, promote exaggerated articulatory movements, increased vocal volume, wider mouth opening, and release from inhibitions as the children use all the muscles for articulation and valving more firmly and with greater activity. Such overemphasis should not continue indefinitely; but some of it can encourage better use of the parts in the whole of speaking, and alternation with very relaxed speaking will provide contrast in the search for accuracy without tension.

- Articulatory activities, even if they are not used with accuracy in connected speech, should be brought to a level of control. Drills are not particularly helpful, but special attention to certain aspects of articulation may eventually improve general intelligibility and encourage maximum muscular action. Ask the child or the group to "put the tails on the words" spoken by the clinician, who will stop short of the final sound, preferably a plosive, to allow the children to provide it. Accuracy of articulation is not necessarily the goal; rather, firmness of contact, power in expulsion, and general muscular coordination are the aims. "Lee-lay-lie-low-loo" is hard to work into a conversation, but completing words or starting them or making the vowel sounds in them will come closer to the kinds of experiences the child will need to master. Emphasis here should be on strong vocalization, firm contacts of parts, vigorous explosions; increasing rapidity of movement will require control without hypertension.

- Special stimulation can also be used at this point to train the muscles in the oropharyngeal area to operate more effectively as a sphincter. One method of helping the child to gain voluntary control of this musculature uses a muscle stimulation unit that can be applied to the soft palate and lateral pharyngeal walls while the individual relaxes his tongue and focuses on voluntary sphincteric action in the velopharyngeal area (Yules, Welch, and others, 1968). Such training is preliminary to eventual transfer of control to the involuntary level by means of operant conditioning. Other methods that use stimuli from tongue blades or swab sticks encourage the development of voluntary control, with similar transfer to automatization.

Adequate management of the velopharyngeal valve is a goal that, when achieved, can serve as a basis for additional steps in therapy. One of the acoustic results of inadequate management of the velopharyngeal sphincter has been called nasality, hypernasality, or undue nasal resonance. These terms are sometimes used interchangeably, although some writers prefer "hypernasality" to refer to this kind of audible evidence of inadequate control of the velopharyngeal valve, particularly on vowel sounds. The term "nasal emission," as differentiated from "hypernasality," can be used to refer to the audible results of partial direction of breath pressure through the nasal cavities, particularly on consonant sounds. The term "velopharyngeal valving," on the basis of discussion in Chapter Two, can be defined as the closure of the passageway from the oropharynx to the nasal cavities by sphincteric action of the musculature of the soft palate, posterior pharyngeal wall, and lateral pharyngeal walls, with aid in some instances from the adenoidal pad.

The objective of the phase of remediation that stresses adequate management of the velopharyngeal sphincter is to establish the concept of, and skill in, control of the valve for speech activities. Although such management may be established, at first, by direct attention to the activities that bring about velopharyngeal valving, the child who can already achieve closure can go on to the use of this skill in the direction of the stream of air and the modification of the stream by the articulators. If, however, velopharyngeal closure cannot be achieved, the experience of such management serves as a basis for the eventual involuntary control of the valve in speech activities.

Until speech bulbs were provided to supplement inadequate tissue and pharyngeal flaps were reintroduced, much of the training intended to establish valving action in the pharyngeal area was focused on the elevation and retraction of the soft palate. The contribution of the posterior pharyngeal wall was sometimes questioned, and the facilitation of closure by lateral wall action was often neglected. Even for the child with a repaired palate without prosthesis or pharyngeal flap, the upward and backward excursion of the soft palate may not suffice to close off the passageway to the nasal cavities for speech; and such movement in the child who has a prosthetic appliance in the pharyngeal cavity or a pharyngeal flap that divides the cavity into two tracts will not make optimal use of all the sphincteric musculature. The emphasis for training for control of the velopharyngeal passageway may vary with the kind of mechanism that has been provided by surgery or prosthodontics, but the concept of sphincteric closure needs careful consideration in its relationship to oral breath pressure and articulatory activities.

Sphincteric action of the velopharyngeal musculature can be encouraged in several ways if it is not achieved through imitation, discrimination training, or use of key words or sounds that bring about valving and can be used as the desired response for reinforcement. However, one cannot "wait for perfect speech in order to apply reinforcement" (Holland, 1967); and shaping procedures can be used to provide a gradual progression from what the individual can do to the behavior desired of him. Establishment of control of the velopharyngeal sphincter may be one of the first steps in shaping.

One approach is to stress the movements that can be seen and to develop kinesthetic awareness of activities that, although not easily observed, result in greater excursion of the soft palate, the lateral pharyngeal walls, and even the posterior wall of the pharynx. Some of the following procedures can facilitate this phase of speech training:

- Understanding of what a sphincter is may help the child to achieve the kind of all-round closure he needs for adequate valving. Demonstration of the sphincteric action of the lips or the eyes or even of the hand as it is made into a fist may let the child see the kind of movement that he may not be able to observe in the oropharynx. Combinations of activities, one visible and the other in an area that cannot be easily seen, may assist in establishing the concept of sphincteric action. "As the patient masters movement of his lateral walls by thinking 'ugh' (gag or tighten), he usually learns to relax his tongue" (Yules, Welch, and others, 1968, p. 1); and this preliminary step can preface the conditioning of dehypernasality through the method described by Richard Yules and his colleagues or by other means.

- Yawning may bring about closure of the velopharyngeal passageway, and this activity can be used at this stage of training as well as in the development of mobility of the palate. However, the yawns should now be vocalized; and the activity of the palate and pharynx can be observed in a mirror.

- Remembering that, in many instances, any forward movement of the posterior pharyngeal wall may be at a point well above the soft palate and hence not easily seen, stimulate the posterior wall at the highest point that can be reached without gagging the child by touching it lightly with a cotton-tipped swab stick or a tongue blade or a pharyngeal mirror. Use this procedure to stimulate action and provide opportunity for recognition of the movement that may occur, then encourage duplication of the movement without the tactile stimulation.

- Using a simulated speech bulb that can be made of soft wax attached to a tongue blade or a spoon of suitable size, encourage closure around the "obturator." The child can close his lips around the bulb first, then attempt to bring the walls of the pharynx toward it as the simulated bulb is moved to the posterior area. For the child with a pharyngeal flap, this procedure may need modification; the flap itself can serve as the goal for sphincteric closure.

- The use of massage with the finger, although sometimes recommended, seems less desirable than other activities designed to stimulate the action of the soft palate. The child can puff out his cheeks, impound air in his mouth while keeping his tongue low, and push repeatedly and firmly on one cheek. This applies pressure to the palate but prevents the undue pressure that might result from pushing on both cheeks. Holding the air in the mouth against pressure that reduces the size of the mouth cavity requires velopharyngeal valving in a nonspeech activity and may permit recognition of the "feel" of closure.

These preliminary approaches may help to establish the concept of velopharyngeal closure, but they probably will not result in use of the valve in speaking activities. Hence, ways of achieving a transition to actual and involuntary use should be sought. Some of the following procedures may assist in this transfer:

- Combinations of sounds, the first of which facilitates closure (and this may differ from child to child), provide opportunities to experience the use of closure in meaningful sequences. If, for example, the child's use of /g/ seems to help him to achieve better closure, combine /g/ with vowel sounds to make short words. The maintenance of closure through the vowel sound may give the child the experience of speaking even a single word that, recorded and played back for him, helps him to hear the results of better valving and can be used as delayed reinforcement. The first words produced by such combinations should be short, including a single consonant and a single vowel. The words so produced should be meaningful to the child and should get responses from the listener in terms of actions or indications of pictured or printed representations of the words to provide for immediacy of reinforcement.
- Pretending to sneeze, with brief maintenance of the implosive phase and visual evidence of oral emission, may approximate the production of a word.
- The same kind of activity can result in real words—"hot" and "shoe," for example—produced in quick succession and identified as a meaningful utterance. Similar combinations, first as means of establishing closure and then as real words, can result in "catchup," "kitchen," "butcher," "batch," "hatchet," "catch us," and other words and short phrases.
- Any sound that brings about good closure can be used as a key to closure for other sounds. If, for instance, the child is able to achieve adequate closure when he phonates /ɑ/, he can then think /ɑ/ before he attempts to produce other sounds or to combine sounds other than the key sound in simple words or phrases. In this activity, the importance of thorough assessment is obvious. In attempts to find key sounds, do not neglect sounds at the ends of words, where they may be more efficiently produced and directed than when they appear at the beginning of a word and are attacked with a glottal stop. Note differences that may appear between voiced and voiceless

elements of sound pairs, using the member of the pair that produces the more effective closure as a key to the production of the other member.

- Quick inhalation through the mouth can be followed by immediate production of a single sound or short meaningful sound combination. The immediacy of the reversal of the airstream, from intake to output, may permit maintenance of closure established for inhalation, in which the area of opening into the nasal cavities is restricted, the opening into the mouth is increased, and the tongue is kept out of the way of the in- and outgoing stream of air.
- The theme for this particular phase of the remedial process, at whatever point it is used, might be "get it—use it." At first, the clinician may need to provide immediate verbal reinforcement, such as "Good" or "Right." Later, the child himself should learn to discriminate between getting and not getting. The use of such feedback channels as the auditory, visual, and kinesthetic will enable him to assume more and more responsibility for evaluating his own achievements. If he can achieve closure, as it is demonstrated in even a single word or short phrase, the experience can be used for extending control over a period of time.

The child with a repaired or obturated palatal cleft needs control of the direction of the stream of air from the lungs and larynx as a preface to ultimate automatization of the rapid changes in direction needed in contextual speech. If speech required only an open or only a closed passageway between the oropharynx and the nasal cavities, the task of the speaker and the clinician might be much easier. However, control of the direction of the stream of air, voiced or unvoiced, is a matter of rapid adjustments, quick shifts, and constant changes, as the discussion of normal speech in Chapter Two indicated.

In American English speech, most sounds are directed through the oral cavity, the voiced or unvoiced stream of air being impounded, interfered with, released, or modified in a number of ways. Although complete closure of the velopharyngeal passageway may not be necessary for an acoustic result that is acceptable to the listener, the direction of the stream of voiced or unvoiced air is more oral than nasal except for the three nasal consonant sounds. The frequency with which these consonants—/m/, /n/, and /ŋ/—appear in American English complicates the task of shifting from open to closed to open position of the velopharyngeal sphincter in connected speech. Such changes involve alteration of the direction of the stream of air rapidly within phrases and sentences. Most speakers perform these changes involuntarily, and some may even have difficulty in analyzing what they do. However, the simplest conversation usually requires many adjustments of the velopharyngeal valve, as well as of the articulators and other parts of the speech mechanism.

If Joe meets Don on the street in the morning, for example, their social exchange might seem simple; but a review of the velopharyngeal valving needed for adequate speech would show that each speaker, if he is to avoid undue nasal resonance and use sufficient oral breath pressure for consonant sounds, must open and close the passageway to the nasal cavities several times, however brief the conversation may be. If Joe says "Hi, Don," he maintains velopharyngeal closure from the start of the first word to the final sound in his friend's name. At that point, he directs the stream of sound through the nasal passageways at the same time that he goes through the articulatory activities to produce /n/. If Don answers with "Morning, Joe," he begins his contribution to the conversation with a nasal sound, then closes the passageway to the nasal cavities very briefly, opens and closes it again, opens it once more, then closes it for the consonant and vowel sounds in the name of his conversational partner. Even short additional comments require further management of the velopharyngeal musculature. If "How's it going?" is Joe's question, he establishes velopharyngeal closure, maintains it to the end of the phrase, and releases it for the final sound, whether he uses /ŋ/ or /n/. If Don reports that he can't complain, he sets himself a complex task, in terms of velopharyngeal closure. He closes, opens, and recloses the velopharyngeal passageway if he says "can't"; and, for "complain," he retains closure, releases it, reestablishes it, and releases it again.

The difficulties of composing practice sentences that contain no nasal sounds confirm the reports that /n/ occurs with more frequency than any other consonant except /t/ in spoken American English, that /m/ is high in frequency of occurrence in that language, and that /ŋ/ is not the least frequent of English consonant sounds (French and others, 1930; Fletcher, 1929, 1953; Voelker, 1934; Mader, 1954). Analysis of children's rhymes and songs, of their vocabulary, and of their conversations will show that passages containing no nasal sounds, although they could be useful at some stages in therapy, do not approximate actual speech. The shifts from nasal to oral direction of the airstream, then, become important aspects of the process of oral communication. The child who uses /m/, /n/, /ŋ/, and perhaps the glottal stop for many consonant sounds because he cannot achieve closure is difficult to understand. Strong nasal resonance on vowel sounds is distracting to the listener, even if the vowel sounds are intelligible. Lack of pressure for the plosive and fricative elements of consonant sounds, with accompanying nasal emission, also interferes with intelligibility.

The child needs every encouragement to send the stream of air to a point outside the mouth, by way of the mouth cavity. If control of the velopharyngeal sphincter has been achieved, that control should combine with proper direction of the stream of air. External targets can be established to focus attention on oral rather than nasal emission; and visual and tactile sensations can be used to judge the direction of the voiced or voiceless sounds carried by the stream of air, with sufficient breath pressure to permit the articulatory impedances that can result in speech sounds.

Some of the following procedures, adapted to the child and the situation, can be useful in establishing the "orality" of direction that is basic to intelligibility. These approaches may be combined with those designed to establish or stabilize velopharyngeal valving.

- By aiming at targets, real or imaginary, that are external to the mouth cavity, the child may develop the concept of direction of the stream of air through the mouth. A real bull's-eye target can be constructed, a circle of light on the wall can serve, a mark on a paper can be used, or the clinician's hand can be the target.
- Sounds, words, phrases, and sentences can be put into a basket made of the cupped hands held just below the mouth or a real basket or box or other container. Random verbal activities—noises that can be changed rapidly in any sequence or combination—can be used at the outset, with the shift to real sounds and words as soon as the idea of direction has been established.
- Cupping the hands around the mouth, below the nose, as a supplement to the mouth cavity may help to establish the concept of oral emission. Attempts to direct the stream through the mouth cavity may be facilitated by assistance from an imaginary rope or string that is pulled by the hands to bring the air or sound through the mouth cavity to the open air.
- During the time in which facility in establishment of oral breath pressure is being acquired, other means can be used to demonstrate differences between oral and nasal emission. A small piece of card-

board can be placed under the nostrils to keep nasally emitted air from affecting the object to be moved, and sounds or words can be used to push balls of paper or cotton held on the back of the hand in front of the mouth. Many similar devices can be used to provide visual evidence of oral emission of air. Once established, this skill can be stabilized and brought to involuntary management through conditioning procedures.

- With a group, training in discrimination can be combined with practice on proper direction by having the performance of one child monitored and evaluated by others. Recordings of practice can be used in such discrimination training, particularly if the speakers are unidentified and each child judges what he hears without knowing whose speech he is evaluating. Self-evaluation thus becomes more objective, and the child who is highly critical of a certain recorded sequence may find that he is identifying his own errors and successes.
- Maintenance of closure over a period of time, as in phrases and sentences containing no nasal sounds, provides the opportunity for the child to experience closure and direction. Because conversational speech rarely includes sentences with no nasal sounds, the eventual skill to be developed from this experience is in rapid shifts from nasality to orality. However, use of some material without nasal sounds may be useful; and phrases and sentences that can be used frequently in social situations can be evolved. Greetings, for example, could consist of "Hi," "I feel good today," "It's good to see you," and others.
- Description of a picture or naming of objects without using nasal sounds can set a goal for the child and give him some experience in distinguishing between /m/, /n/, and /ŋ/ and sounds that require velopharyngeal closure and the use of oral breath pressure. Although one investigation (Buck, 1953) found no evidence to support the belief that insufficient mouth opening is related to nasality in speakers with congenital palatal clefts, a later report (Spriestersbach and Powers, 1959b) that high vowels are more nasal than low vowels in cleft palate speakers supports the suggestion that wider mouth opening can assist in the establishment of oral breath pressure, at least for some vowel sounds. In combination with what might be called an "open mouth policy," increased vocal volume may lead

to oral emission as the child gives commands to those at a distance, aims at a faraway target, or even whispers so that he can be heard across a room.

- Attention should be given to the possible interference to oral breath pressure by elevation of the back of the tongue. Two postural positions of the tongue have been described for normal speakers: the habitual, in which the tip of the tongue is in contact with the incisor teeth and the dorsum is in contact with the hard or soft palate, and the relaxed, in which the dorsum of the tongue shows more convex curvature and does not maintain contact with the incisors or hard palate (Peat, 1968). However, even in those with normal structures, the dorsum of the tongue was found to be in contact with the soft palate during the relaxed position in 72.8 percent of 103 individuals evaluated. One description of tongue position for speakers with repaired palatal clefts indicated that the tongue was farther from the palate than in speakers with normal structures, with the suggestion that the position of the tongue in those with repaired palates may have been the result of a habit pattern developed during periods of palatal repair, when the child attempted to avoid contact with a healing palate (Buck, 1953). Other investigators hypothesized that both nasal emission and poor articulation resulted from talking with the jaw elevated and the dorsum of the tongue high in the back of the mouth (McDonald and Koepp-Baker, 1951). Although children with repaired or obturated palatal clefts apparently do not have inferior tongue flexibility (Matthews and Byrne, 1953), the use of the back of the tongue to facilitate valving or the habits of retraction and elevation of the tongue developed by some children may require specific attention. Conditioning procedures can assist in maintaining desirable tongue position once it is established.

The production and combination of the sounds used in speech should be brought to a level of acceptability and intelligibility that will facilitate oral communication. Whatever the cause of the articulatory errors that may characterize the speech of the child with a congenital prepalatal or palatal cleft, velopharyngeal closure and modifications of the direction of the airstream, together with improved articulatory positions and movements (McWilliams, 1954), should result in acceptable units that will form syllables, words, phrases, sentences, and connected oral discourse.

The articulatory patterns of the child with repaired structures can result from many factors. The discussion in Chapter Four cited some of these factors, and the speech pathologist and speech clinician who work with the child with a congenital cleft will recognize a number of the following possible causes for defective articulation: The child with a cleft may use speech sounds incorrectly in combination but produce them accurately in isolation. He may make articulatory errors that have only slight relationships to his residual structural anomalies. He may present deviations in articulation—the production and use of speech sounds—because of immaturity or in imitation of models in his environment. Hearing loss or dental irregularities may account for his articulatory differences. In seeking to approximate what he hears but cannot produce, he may invent unusual plosive and fricative sounds that he can make with structures he can control. Provision of dental prostheses or use of appliances to modify dental structure may bring about differences in articulation. Immobility of some of the parts may contribute to articulatory errors. He may achieve or approximate the articulatory positions and movements that would, in the presence of adequate velopharyngeal closure and oral breath pressure, produce acceptable sounds; but, because of lack of orality, the resulting acoustic effect fails to come within normal limits.

In his assessment, the speech pathologist will have determined which of the articulatory errors made by the child with a prepalatal or palatal cleft are the direct result of the physical anomaly and which have resulted from other factors. His evaluation of the articulatory aspects of the total speech process will provide the basis for determining the point at which to start in modifying articulatory behavior, in deciding how to combine attention to articulation with improvement in control of the velopharyngeal sphincter and oral breath pressure, or in choosing to focus on one or the other of these aspects at the outset.

Procedures for improving general skills in articulation and for modifying the production and use of specific sound elements, suggested in the following discussion, are based on the structural deviations characteristic of many children born with clefts; but remedial approaches recommended for articulatory defects resulting from factors other than clefts also can be used and adapted.

The production and use of labial sounds—/p/, /b/, /m/, /w/, and vowel sounds requiring lip movement, for example—may be inadequate because of immobility or restricted activity of the lips as a result of scar tissue, an inadequate labial sulcus, dental anomalies, or a prosthesis or appliance that is designed to move the upper lip in a forward direction. Additional surgical management to improve appearance may modify the upper lip and its relationship to the lower, but the child's acquisition of skill in using his lips and monitoring his speech prior to such revision can help him to adapt more readily to the changes brought about by later surgery. The visibility of labial sounds, while facilitating attempts to bring them within normal limits in use, also requires that they be adequately produced because they are so readily observed by the listener.

- If no additional revision of the lip is contemplated, or if such revision must be postponed for several years, the surgeon may recommend that the speech clinician encourage mobility of the upper lip by finger massage, tongue pressure against the inside of the lip, retraction of the lip in a gliding movement against the upper teeth, and attempts to curl the lips against the teeth while the mouth is held slightly open.
- Observation of the lip area in a mirror, with other areas of the face unseen, will help the child to attend to the parts that, at the time, he is attempting to control. Focusing on his lips, he can move them in as many ways as possible, making them flexible and duplicating, without sound, some of the positions usually used for the production of bilabial sounds.
- Tactile and kinesthetic stimulation, in combination, can be provided by presenting a piece of paper, a straw, a tongue blade, or some other object of appropriate thickness for the child to grasp with his lips, hold momentarily, and return by ejecting it forcefully. If approximation of the lips is difficult, closure around the head of a clean old-fashioned clothespin may be possible, with continued attempts at closure around smaller and smaller objects as mobility of the lips is acquired.
- Cold cream or vaseline for boys and lipstick for girls can be applied to the upper and lower lips to provide stimulus for bringing the lips together and moving them against each other to spread the substance over the entire area of the upper and lower lip. This activity can be practiced with and without visual cues.
- Double stick tape, which has adhesive on both sides, can be grasped by the lips to provide tactile evidence of lip approximation. Pulling the lips apart will require some muscular activity to release the contact, and movement of the lip to which the tape remains adhered will be required to loosen the tape.

- Attempts to hold a piece of paper placed between the lips will require some lip pressure as the clinician pulls on the paper and the child tries to retain it in position. The paper can be varied in width or in position if certain areas of the lip seem to need more stimulation to action.
- The use of "touch points" may facilitate lip closure and contact between the upper and lower lip needed for the production and use of bilabial sounds. With a swab stick or tongue blade or spoon, touch the upper and lower lips firmly and ask the child to put the two touched points together. The tactile sensation provided by touching is momentary, but it can be brought into awareness by practice.
- Words without sound—"silent words"—containing bilabial sounds can be used to check and encourage the use of adequate positioning and movement. Provide a word list or set of pictures for the child to use. If the clinician can speechread the word, he reinforces the behavior in any of a number of ways. Reverse the process to develop the child's ability to recognize adequate lip action for bilabial sounds.
- If, by combining proper direction of the airstream with adequate lip action, the child can produce /p/, he then needs to recognize it as a unit that can be used with other sounds to make words that have meaning and that obtain responses from listeners.
- Although voiced sounds may be less frequently deviant than voiceless in the speech of the child with a cleft palate and might be introduced first, the problem of nasal resonance in voiced sounds if valving is not adequate may make these sounds seem more deviant. Misdirection of the airstream in /p/ can generate some noise, but /p/ may seem less deviant than /b/ because the nasal resonance is minimized by unvoicing.
- Although /m/ is rarely deviant in speech, the child whose lips are immobile or who has a notched upper lip may tend to make this sound labiodentally. Acoustically, labiodental /m/ is acceptable; in terms of visual cues to the listener, it is deviant. Hence, some children with labial clefts may need assistance in achieving the proper visual aspects of /m/.
- Skills in lip-rounding can be used to facilitate the production and use of /w/ and some vowel sounds that require sphincteric closure of the lips. The relationship between /w/ and /u/ can be used to help the child correct the one that may be deviant. Attention

to the "wh" sound can be minimal, because distinctions between "wear" and "where," "wine" and "whine," "weather" and "whether" are relatively unimportant. The context gives the cue to the word that is meant; and, in some areas of the country, the two sounds are not differentiated.

- Any kinds of lip activities that can be evolved by the clinician or child can be helpful in establishing awareness and control of lip movement and positions. In play, many children imitate the noises made by animals and machines. The clinician may find that, in using the sounds he hears in his environment, the child can demonstrate capacities for lip movement that can then be used for acquisition and eventual automatization. Duplication of the clinician's nonspeech-sound movements of the lips—smacking, popping, vibrating, protruding, rounding, and other actions—can provide the child with the experience of lip action that can then be modified for the production and use of the bilabial sounds in context.

Many children whose missing deciduous upper central incisors have not yet been replaced by permanent teeth continue to approximate the labiodental sounds /f/ and /v/, at least acoustically. The child with a prepalatal cleft whose premaxilla is malpositioned or distorted and whose upper central incisors are missing or poorly erupted, may need to give special attention to sounds that usually require upper front teeth. Provision of artificial teeth also may necessitate some modification of speech behavior. One of the best means available to the child for adapting to different or changing structures is his ability to compare his articulation with that of the best models in his environment. Instruction about placement, therefore, should be minimal; and discrimination should be stressed.

- Comparisons between bilabial and labiodental sounds in their effects on word meanings may assist in developing discrimination. Word pairs may be used for this discrimination, with occasional silent presentation of words in which /p/ contrasts with /f/ to encourage use of visual cues.

- The activity that, in combination with pressure through the oral cavity, will produce /f/ and /v/ can be originally established by simple description—"Bite your lip and blow," "Bite your lip and buzz"—or by imitation. If the back of the tongue, held high, interferes with the stream of air or sound that must be impeded by the lips or teeth, preliminary attention to control of the tongue may be needed.

- Any ability to move the lower lip that has been developed previously or can be established will facilitate the production and use of /f/ and /v/. The actual movement is by the lip, the teeth being used for near-contact if they are present.

- Presentation of /f/ before /v/ can be defended on the basis of the acoustic result as a means of judging articulatory accuracy. If valving is inadequate, /v/, like /b/, may seem more deviant because of the nasal resonance of the voicing. Pressure for friction is, of course, important for /f/ as well as for /v/; but the visual aspects of correctly positioned /f/ may compensate for minimal friction. No single position is essential for /f/ and /v/. Some speakers establish the contact that results in friction by bringing the inside of the lower lip to the teeth. Others establish contact between the vermilion border and the teeth. If the combination of acoustic and cosmetic effects is adequate, the specific point of contact is not essential.

- Just as important as the approximation of parts is the capacity to move to and from the contact with facility. Hence, /f/ and /v/ and other sounds that require maintenance of position must be sufficient in length to establish their identities but not so prolonged that they interfere with the rapid transitions needed in contextual speech. If /f/ and /v/ are too brief in duration, they resemble plosives; if they are prolonged unduly, they prevent the sequencing required. Indications of length of maintenance of the /f/ or /v/ can be given visually by a line drawn on a paper or chalkboard, presented tactually by the clinician's finger on the child's hand or arm, or demonstrated for the auditory sense by presentation of the sounds directly to the child's ear through a tube or the headphones of an amplifier. Combinations of such sensory stimuli may be even more effective than presentation through a single avenue. Without firm direction of the air or sound stream through the mouth cavity, /f/ and /v/ will lack the friction that is needed to establish part of their identity. Hence, attention to valving and to the combination of velopharyngeal closure and articulatory activity should be constant.

Absence or distortion of the upper central incisors may have some effect on labiodental sounds; but such anomalies may, more significantly, permit protrusion of the tongue and distortion of linguadental and lingua-alveolar sounds. If lingual protrusion has become habitual and if no modifications in the anterior dental structure are contemplated, the child may need special encouragement to retain the tongue within the mouth cavity and to use his lips as barriers to forward tongue movement. This approach, however, may not be as helpful as the establishment of good management of the tongue for speech and for other functions in which it may be inadequate. If tongue thrust complicates the problem of retention of the tongue in the mouth cavity, recommendations from the dentist may be needed; or the speech clinician may incorporate attention to the problems of "tongue thrust" in the general plan of remediation (Marks, 1968).

The linguadental and lingua-alveolar sounds used in speech are less visible than those for which labial movement is required. Forward motion of the tongue may be desirable for /θ/ and /ð/, but many speakers produce these sounds without actual protrusion of the tongue. Upward movement is needed for other front-tongue sounds, some of which are facilitated by adequate cutting edges of the upper incisor teeth. Some of the sounds that involve use of the front of the tongue are difficult to hear; and lack of visibility, in combination with low acoustic power, can contribute to the problems that any child may encounter in forming and using them.

A child whose congenital structural anomalies have resulted in distortions of the dental arch and poor dental occlusion may, in spite of his differences, be able to achieve some approximation of the customary positions for sounds involving the tip of the tongue. More commonly, however, he will find that the combination of inadequate dental structure, lack of oral breath pressure, and possible reduction in hearing acuity will make the use of these sounds difficult. Furthermore, the requirement of pressure through the mouth for the plosion of /t/ and /d/, the friction for /s/, /z/, /θ/, /ð/, /ʃ/, and /ʒ/, and the combination of plosion and friction for /tʃ/ and /dʒ/ tends to bring about frequent errors in the sounds that usually require agility of the front of the tongue.

Errors on /t/ and /d/ result, in many instances, from the lack of pressure for plosion rather than from poor tongue management. Forward tongue positioning may result in some dentalization of these sounds; but, in general, the problem is one of air pressure through the mouth cavity with sufficient force to produce the characteristic explosion when the stream has been impounded and then released. Emphasis on firmness of contact may get better results than stress on an exact point of contact. Nasal emission of /d/ results in a sound resembling /n/; and, in some instances, /t/ also shows this resemblance. The frequency of /t/ and /d/ in American English increases the need for adequate use of them.

- If /t/ and /d/ lack plosion, seek facilitating sounds that can precede or follow the "t" or "d" sounds to establish the best possible closure to accompany /t/ and /d/.
- Light contact and less pressure may bring about acceptable /t/ and /d/. However, the plosion should be produced by release of impounded sound or air, not just by tongue action, which can accomplish an approximation of plosion.
- If the child uses the glottal stop for /t/ and /d/ in his attempts to build up pressure wherever closure can be achieved, simple exhalation or /h/ can be used to begin the production of /t/; and tongue action can interrupt the stream of air in practice that will permit the child to experience the movements used by most speakers for /t/.
- Minimal tension may help to eliminate the use of the glottal plosive, and shifts from a vowel sound to a consonant /t/ can permit phonation that can then terminate without the glottal attack as the /t/ is produced.
- Alternations of "hard attack" and "soft attack," as in [ˀoʊ]—[d^{h}oʊ] or [ˀaɪ]—[t^{h}aɪ], may call attention to the difference between the glottal plosive and initial /t/ or /d/.
- If some modification in the point of contact seems essential, diagrams or observation of the articulatory actions of others may help the child to see that most people touch the gum ridge with the tongue tip in the production of /t/ and /d/. However, dentalization of these sounds may be a less serious defect than lack of breath pressure which should have attention before changes in positioning for /t/ and /d/ are stressed.
- Isolated sounds, no matter how well they are produced, have little value for oral self-expression. Hence, the syllabic combinations of /t/ and /d/ with vowel sounds and the search for other consonant sounds that may facilitate /t/ and /d/ should be introduced early. In devising combinations of sounds that may improve /t/ and /d/, do not overlook the possibility of combining words rather than putting sounds together to make single words. If, for instance, vowel sounds that usually require a high position of the front of the tongue

enable the child to produce /t/ more efficiently, use phrases such as "point east" or "he told" as well as such words as "tea" or "eat" or "team" or "meat."

- Nasal resonance for /n/, which resembles /t/ and /d/ in some ways, should not be difficult to achieve. However, skill in shifting from velopharyngeal patency to closure when /n/ is used in conjunction with other sounds may require specific practice. The /t/ or /d/ can be impounded but not exploded, followed by rapid opening of the velar passageway for /n/, then by closure for /t/ or /d/ to provide experience in alternation of nasal and oral direction.
- The influence of /n/ on vowel sounds may suggest minimal attention to /n/, which will probably have had considerable use as a substitute for other sounds. Discrimination between /n/ and the sounds for which it may be used could be more important than emphasis on /n/ as a separate sound, and the frequency with which /n/ appears in American English makes such differentiation all the more essential.
- Establishing oral direction for vowel sounds that precede /n/ in words and phrases may lead to more success in controlling the direction of breath pressure than experience with /n/ followed by a vowel sound. Phrases and sentences in which /n/ occurs infrequently may give better practice than "loaded" material in which /n/ appears often.

The pressure required for plosives, such as /t/ and /d/, is brief. That needed for such continuant consonant sounds as /ʃ/, /ʒ/, /s/, and /z/ must be of slightly longer duration. Except for /ʒ/, which appears rarely except in combination with /d/, these sounds are frequently produced and used incorrectly by many children. The child who cannot achieve competent velopharyngeal valving and who has deviant dental structure will be liable to special difficulties with the continuant sibilant sounds. In his attempts to produce the sustained pressure needed for these sounds, the child may wrinkle his nose, constrict his nostrils, or go through other compensatory motions that distract the listener. Establishment and maintenance of velopharyngeal closure is important; but attention to the special articulatory characteristics of /s/, /z/, and /ʃ/ is also needed.

- The clinician who asks the child to imitate a specific position, rather than the total acoustic end result, for /s/ or /z/ may retard the acquisition of skill in the production and use of these sounds. In almost any group of speakers, half will produce /s/ and /z/ with the tongue tip behind the upper teeth; half will place the tongue tip behind the lower teeth. The exact position for /s/ and /z/ is not important, particularly for the child whose dental structures require individual adjustments. The sounds should come within the wide range of acceptability, but no two individuals make these sounds in exactly the same way.

- Attempts to produce the kind of whistle in which the lips are retracted rather than rounded may help the child to approximate /s/. Demonstration of the "two-fingers-in-the-mouth whistle" can be helpful, the child trying to duplicate the sound without the use of the fingers.

- Facilitating sounds should be investigated. If /t/ helps /s/, use combinations of syllables or words that include these two sounds in sequence. Such word groups as "hot soup," "hit song," and "ate some" illustrate this kind of combination. Pluralization of words ending in /t/ also provides experience in following /t/ with /s/ if /t/ is a facilitator, as in "hat"—"hats," "bite"—"bites." Movement from /θ/ to /s/ or /ð/ to /z/ also may provide the experience of /s/ or /z/, but insistence on a certain kind of "tongue placement" is unwise.

- Cues to the point of emission of the airstream for /s/ can be obtained by using a length of syringe tubing to lead the sound from the point at which it is emitted—and this will vary from person to person—to the ear. The clinician should be able to demonstrate this to the child; and so investigation of the point at which the tube should be placed, often below the lips, not directly in front of them, should precede such illustrations.

- Closure for pressure, established by preparation for /p/ or /b/, may continue through /s/ and /z/ as a shift is made from the plosive to the fricative, because the tongue can get ready for /s/ while the lips are occupied with /p/. Pluralization of words ending in /p/ or /b/ or combinations such as "knapsack" or "observe" or "keep some" can be used to provide this experience.

- A swab stick placed on the midline of the tongue and drawn out of the mouth may encourage the stream of air to follow the pathway stimulated by contact of the stick with the tongue and provide the groove down which the airstream can move with rapidity.

- Alternation of /ʃ/ with /s/ or of /ʒ/ with /z/ may, if one of these sounds is more easily achieved than the other, strengthen both.

- Acquired skills in the production of /s/ or /z/ can be incorporated into sequential use in several ways. Responding with plurals to the clinician's dictation of singular nouns ending in /t/ or /d/ may assist in the transfer to use if /s/ and /z/ are made in the "tongue-up" position. Completion of words that end in /s/ or /z/, with a high-front vowel preceding the final sound, may accomplish the transfer if the child makes /s/ and /z/ with his tongue tip low in his mouth. Word sequences also can be devised to require combination of /s/ and /z/ with other sounds; and the clinician's statements such as "The boat is big" or "The road is long" or "My hand looks dirty" can call for responses such as "The boats are big," "The roads are long," "My hands look dirty."

- Lingual protrusion on /s/ and /z/, which is typical in children whose upper front teeth do not present a barrier to the tongue to retain it in the mouth, may be modified by visual and kinesthetic cues. Touching the tip of the tongue and sweeping the upper or lower alveolar ridge with a tongue blade can indicate points that should be in near-contact, not only for some sounds but when the articulatory mechanism is at rest. Sudden introduction of a mirror in which the child can observe the protrusion of his tongue can serve to condition control of tongue protrusion. If the upper dental arch is distorted and the upper central incisors are missing or in poor position, approximation of /θ/ and /ð/ for /s/ and /z/ can be expected.

- Interference with acquisition of skill in using /s/ and /z/ may be posed by dental appliances designed to expand or retain the dental arch, to correct crossbite, or to replace teeth that are missing. In such instances, compensatory activities will be required; and changes in ways of producing and using /s/ and /z/ will be needed as the dental structure is modified or the appliances are revised. Attempts to imitate /s/ and /z/ as they are produced by others cannot be based on duplication of position, but a scatter-gun approach in which all possible positions are explored may help the child to determine ways of producing "s" and "z" sounds that are within acceptable limits if the successful response found by experimentation is reinforced.

- Auditory monitoring of /s/ and /z/ is of particular importance because movements for the production of these sounds are not easily observed. Amplification of sufficiently high quality to permit the child to hear the sounds as he uses them and as they are used by others may be necessary for the child with a hearing loss and desirable for others.

- Modification of the resonating cavities for /ʃ/ and /ʒ/, the first of which is used by itself with some frequency, the second being limited in American English but needed for combination with /d/ in the production of /dʒ/, may be accomplished by giving attention to the additional cavity created by the slight protrusion of the lips for these sounds. Visual cues will show whether or not lip activity is being used.

- The acoustic power of /ʃ/ is greater than that for /s/, and the passageway through which the stream of air comes differs in size and shape. Analogy with the sound frequently used to request silence may help the child to identify /ʃ/ and to move toward accurate production and use of the sound. Alternation of /s/ and /ʃ/ can serve to strengthen both sounds and to distinguish between them.

In spite of their relative lack of acoustic power, /θ/ and /ð/ are less frequently deviant than /s/ and /z/, which they often replace. The characteristic that usually needs some stress if /θ/ and /ð/ are to be produced and used accurately is the duration of the sounds, rather than the way in which they are made. The use of dentalized "t" and "d" sounds as replacements for /θ/ and /ð/ is often noted in those for whom English is a second language or in those whose speech environment includes people who use this substitution. More important than the positioning of /θ/ and /ð/ is the pressure that is needed to make them audible. Hence, oral breath pressure should have more emphasis than position if /θ/ and /ð/ are inadequate.

- Preceding /θ/ with /h/ may establish strong oral direction of the stream of air, which can then be modified by the action of the tongue.

- Protrusion of the tongue between the teeth is not essential for /θ/ and /ð/, and undue forward movement of the tongue can result in a distracting distortion.

- Alternation of /θ/ and /ð/ with other fricatives, such as /f/ and /v/, may promote discrimination of the several sounds and result in differentiation of them.
- The "preparatory set" of velar closure may serve as a useful preface to attempts to produce and use /θ/ and /ð/.

Success in using the elements that make up /tʃ/ and /dʒ/ does not necessarily assure adequate use of the affricatives, which combine plosion and friction in rapid succession. The child who can use /t/, /ʃ/, /d/, and /ʒ/ may not be able to produce and use /tʃ/ and /dʒ/ easily.

- Analogies with sneezes may present the concept of /tʃ/, and "chew" can result from imitations of the noise usually heard from a sneezer. Although /t/ and /ʃ/, separated in time, do not make /tʃ/, /t/ with /ʃ/ and /d/ with /ʒ/ in nonsense words may tend to bring the two elements into rapid approximation. "Tat" followed by "show" makes a nonsense word, but "kit" followed by "shen" and "bad" followed by "zher" make real words. A pause between the two units permits good production of each; the pause can be shortened in successive trials, with visual or tactile cues to indicate the time to be allowed between one unit and another.
- Word pairs that contrast /d/ with /dʒ/ and /t/ with /tʃ/ at the ends of the words may assist in the acquisition of skill in using the affricatives. Such pairs as "hat—hatch," "bad—badge," "Ed—edge," and "eat—each" can demonstrate the need for both /t/ and /ʃ/ in "each" and "hatch" and for both /d/ and /ʒ/ in "edge" and "badge."

Other sounds that involve activity of the front of the tongue—/l/ and /r/—resemble vowel sounds and need adequate valving for oral emission. They also require special kinds of lingual adjustments, complex in nature and difficult to see. The lateral emission of /l/ and the retroflexion for /r/ may be facilitated by descriptions of the movements that result in these sounds; but duplication of the models presented by good speakers should be achieved, if possible, without special attention to placement.

Both /l/ and /r/, even as consonant sounds, have some of the quality of vowels; and both are used as vowel sounds, as in "battle," "candle," "girl," and "mother." If syllabic "l" or vocalic "r" can be produced, they can be used to help the acquisition of consonant /l/ and /r/.

- Inadequacies in dental structure, which may interfere with the lateralization of /l/, may require some modification of the conventional method of producing the sound. Unilateral emission of the stream of sound can sometimes produce an acoustically acceptable /l/. Strong stimulation for the imitation of /l/ may result in adequate production. Direction of the stream of air over the sides of the tongue, as in voiceless "l," may assist in establishing the concept of the sound without the interference of habit patterns of lip-rounding or elevation of the dorsum of the tongue.
- Some vowel sounds, in combination with /l/ may be found to facilitate the production of the consonant. High-front and low-back vowels can be tried as facilitators. Sequences in which syllabic "l" is followed by consonant /l/ may assist in the acquisition of the more deviant of the two sounds. Phrases such as "Call Larry," "a tall lady," "feel luck," and "real lemon" permit, in the prolongation of the final syllabic "l" to the consonant /l/, attempts to bring the sound toward acoustic accuracy.
- Interpolations of /l/ into a sustained /ɑ/ can, if /ɑ/ improves velopharyngeal closure, provide for observation of the upward movement of the tongue in the production of the consonant.
- Combining /l/ with a bilabial plosive provides an opportunity for the tongue to be ready for /l/ as the lips open for the explosion in such words and phrases as "play," "please," "plant," "apply," "supplement," "rope length," "hipline," "blow," "blank," "cub lion," "grab Lucy," and so on.
- Attempts at duplicating /r/ may sometimes result in approximation of the sound, but demonstration of tongue movement and retroflexion is not helpful even in combination with /ɑ/.
- Phrases in which vowel "r" and consonant /r/ can facilitate each other may be tried. "A car ride," "overrun," "all-weather road," "fur wrap," "far-reaching," and similar combinations give the child time, during the prolongation, to attempt modifications and to obtain some kinesthetic cues to combine with auditory cues in judging his accuracy of use of /r/.
- Vowel "r" varies in different geographical regions, but consonant /r/ must come within certain limits to be recognized and accepted by the listener. Attention to the consonantal form might well precede attempts to modify the vowel "r" if both are deviant.

- Interpolations of /r/ into sustained /u/ may make production of /r/ easier because the rounded /u/ focuses attention at the front of the mouth and reduces the size of the cavity in which the tongue must move.

Although linguavelar /k/ and /g/ do not require complex activity of the tongue, several characteristics of those sounds combine to make them difficult for the child with a palatal cleft to produce and use. They require firm velopharyngeal valving. They are difficult to see. They cannot be demonstrated without some distortion. Although they vary in place of production in assimilation with various vowel sounds, they usually require use of the back part of the mouth cavity near the velopharyngeal passageway, thus increasing the possibility of nasal direction. Their backward position makes the glottal stop or a pharyngeal fricative a logical substitute for them, and they appear frequently enough in American English speech to affect intelligibility if they are deviant.

- Because valving must be relatively firm for the adequate production of these plosive sounds, attention to closure should precede, or be combined with, attempts to produce and use /k/ and /g/.
- If elevation of the posterior part of the tongue is habitually used in an attempt at closure, the problem is compounded; but the use of vowel or consonant sounds that bring the back of the tongue down as prefaces to /k/ and /g/ may help to eliminate this problem.
- Contrasting activities, as in /tʌkətʌkə/ or /dʌgədʌgə/ can help to establish the concept of back-of-the tongue movement and might assist in modifying the substitutions of /t/ for /k/ and /d/ for /g/ that are typical of the errors of many small children with or without clefts.
- Immobilization of the front of the tongue with a tongue blade, spoon, or finger can be tried as a means of stimulating movement of the back of the tongue. Such practice should be brief, being used only to establish the kinesthetic sensation of desirable movement.
- Imitation of the sounds of imaginary creatures that use /g/ and /k/ for "communication" may assist the child to experience the activities needed for the sounds. The Google-Gub and the Keekee-Kap can be anything the child wants them to be and can bring along such relatives and friends as the child may invent, just as long as their speech includes /k/ and /g/.

- Transfer to use, once the /k/ and /g/ can be achieved, might be speeded by single-word exchanges in which the clinician presents a real monosyllabic word that, when /k/ or /g/ is used in place of the consonant sound, becomes another real word. "Bait" can get "gate" as a response, and "peep" can get "keep." Identification of the child's responses as real words will assist in conditioning procedures. Short phrases can be evolved to obtain the same kind of response, "I am told" being stimulus for "I am cold," for example.
- The relative lack of visibility of /k/ and /g/ requires the use of sensory channels other than the visual. If the ear is to be used to identify the sounds, /g/ might be used first because it is easier to hear; or amplification may be needed. Tactile stimuli are not particularly useful because the points for contact are not specific, changing with the vowel sounds that accompany /k/ and /g/.
- In the combination of vowel sounds with /k/ and /g/, careful attention should be given to oral direction of the vowel as well as the consonant sound, particularly when back vowels are involved.
- The nasal sound produced at the back of the mouth, /ŋ/, may be well used. If occasional lapses to /n/ for /ŋ/, in "ing" endings are noted, they may be ignored until more important distinctions are established. However, /ŋ/ can be tried as a facilitator for /g/ or /k/ in combinations such as "think," "bank," "thank," or "finger."

Vowel sounds, which pose little interference to the outgoing stream of breath, are not often deviant. Dialectal and imitative differences may be noted in the speech of some children, but the normal mouth usually performs as an adequate resonator in the production of vowel sounds. The major difference in vowel sounds used by children with velopharyngeal incompetence is in the hypernasality that results from the resonation of vocal tone in the nasal cavities as well as in the mouth. This nasalization of vowel sounds is a characteristic of the speech of children with palatal clefts, repaired or obturated, although such nasality may be heard also in the speech of individuals whose palatopharyngeal sphincters are normal in structure but inadequately used.

A report on velopharyngeal closure on vowels suggested that proximity to /n/ causes vowel sounds to exhibit incomplete closure and that isolated vowel sounds tend to show less closure than those in nonnasal consonant contexts (Moll, 1962). Another stressed the relationship between the size of the velopharyngeal opening and the degree of closure of the mouth cavity in the nasalization of vowel sounds, differentiating between openly resonant quality and the kind of resonance that results from an open velopharyngeal area and anterior blockage of the nasal passages. The former, according to the investigator (Moore, in Travis, 1957), is more typical with cleft palate, paralysis of the velum or the velopharyngeal constrictors, congenitally short palate, or perforated palate. Nasalization can be said to occur in vowel sounds when the coupling between the pharyngeal-oral and nasal portions of the vocal tract system is increased sufficiently to produce a perceptually significant change in the speech signal (Curtis, in Spriestersbach and Sherman, 1968). The word "perceptually" becomes particularly significant when one considers that judgments of hypernasality on vowel sounds vary with the listener, that some listeners may accept degrees of hypernasality that others would consider distracting, and that the ear of the listener is probably as reliable as any other measures for the assessment of nasal voice quality (Moll, 1964b).

The goal of therapy designed to improve the production and use of vowel sounds by those with velopharyngeal incompetence, then, is to reduce the nasal components of resonance and increase the oral components. Progress toward this goal may be judged instrumentally or by the ears of several listeners—both sophisticated and naïve—as procedures selected from the following are used:

- Modification of the relationship in size of the velopharyngeal opening and the mouth cavity and opening may increase the oral resonance of vowel sounds and minimize their nasality. Hence, experience in valving may be accompanied by wider mouth opening and, at the outset, with attention to vowel sounds that bring the tongue to a low position. Nasalization of vowel sounds may result in decreased vocal volume, the vowel sounds providing the "carrying wave" for the transmission of speech to the ear of the listener. Increased volume without laryngeal tension may improve the acoustic end result of vowel sounds, particularly if such increase in pressure is accompanied by velopharyngeal activity.
- Some consonant sounds may facilitate the oral direction of vowel sounds. Combinations of vowel sounds with consonant sounds that bring about good closure to produce syllables or words can provide the child with the experience of producing and monitoring better vowel resonance.

- Maintenance of velopharyngeal closure that can be achieved for any vowel sound can be used to improve others. If, for example, /ɑ/ has more oral resonance than /i/, the child can start with /ɑ/ and move to /i/ and other vowel sounds without interrupting the stream of sound.
- Some of the vowellike consonant sounds—/w/, for example—may give the child an opportunity to establish valving and to focus on the front of the mouth as he prepares to produce various vowel sounds in combination with /w/. Perhaps, for some children, another of the semivowels—/l/, for instance—will be more facilitating.
- Alternations between nasally directed consonant sounds and vowel sounds, requiring a wide differentiation in direction of the airstream, may provide opportunities for noting acoustic differences as well as changes in velopharyngeal and oral activities as the child shifts from /m/, /n/, or /ŋ/ to vowel sounds.

The correlation of velopharyngeal control with articulatory activities adds to the complexity of the speaking task but is essential for adequate sequential utterance. Throughout the various phases of therapy that may be presented separately to establish certain skills, attention should be given to the combination of factors that are inseparable in the coordinated act of speaking. Production of isolated sounds may be achieved, and combinations of these sounds in single words or short phrases may be accomplished; but sequential conversational speech requires rapid, controlled activity of many structures while ideas are being expressed in adequate linguistic form. Experience in the transfer of isolated skills into use for self-expression should not be postponed until the skills are brought to total adequacy. Rather, the correlations among the many activities—respiration, phonation, resonation, articulation, mentation, and social interaction—should be established as soon as possible, even if some of the activities are not entirely adequate.

- Asking the child to choose words or phrases suitable for some particular aspect of practice will encourage analysis, even if it must be limited, of the sound units that make up words and, perhaps more importantly, of the words made up of the sound units. The child's choice of words that illustrate a certain motor skill will bring the activity patterns for velopharyngeal control and articulatory activity into his own linguistic areas.

- Separation of the several aspects of speaking may preface their combination. Respiration can be considered as an activity that has more than one purpose. Simple phonation, recommended as the starting point in therapy by one group of investigators (Luse and others, 1964), may assist in reducing undue tension in laryngeal and hypopharyngeal areas. Velopharyngeal valving action, established and practiced in isolation, can develop awareness of this factor. Articulatory activities in the production of isolated sounds can be studied. However, the ultimate goal is the correlation of these aspects; and sequential combinations of respiration with phonation, then of respiration with phonation and alternations of valving, and finally of respiration with phonatory, resonatory, and articulatory activities may bring the whole together and avoid overemphasis of any one of the parts. Establishment of correlated activity for brief periods of time, as in syllables or single words, may serve as a basis for extension of the time period in which control can be maintained. For some children, maintenance of control may be difficult; for others, the extension of time for control may be rapid. However, correlation of the several skills needed for sequential speech may be achieved in stages if it cannot be acquired in one quick transition from parts to whole.
- Deliberate separation of words into single units can demonstrate the difference between sounds and the whole word. Recognition of the fact that /k/ plus /æ/ plus /t/ does not really name the animal or that /s/ plus /p/ plus /i/ plus /k/ does not really name the activity may help the child in his motivation for correlation of activities.
- Preliminary focus on closure of the velopharyngeal passageway before a word or phrase is attempted may be necessary. Single-word responses to questions can be used to provide opportunity for practice in preparatory valving before words are spoken. The questions can be constructed to require, at first, response words in which no nasal sounds occur and that start with various plosive and fricative consonants. "What number comes after 'one'?" "How many fingers do you have on each hand?" and "What direction is opposite east?" are examples of questions that demand, as responses, words in which preparatory valving can be maintained and reinforced.
- Special times or places can provide opportunity for practice in coordination of activities. Short periods of control can be expanded as the child gains skill in using all his newly established abilities at

once. Record keeping may furnish some stimulation for extending the time period in which coordinated speaking is used, and the structured control of operant conditioning can be effective here. Rewards and punishments for combinations of skill in valving and articulation can be simple. The clinician may report that he is unable to hear sequential utterances in which such combinations are not present, once the child has demonstrated some ability to achieve the complex coordinations required for speech. Desired objects can be withheld until coordinated speech activities are used by the child; or collections of awards (beans, stars, poker chips, or cards, for example), received for sequential use of correlated activities, can be traded for something the child wants.

- In groups, each child can serve as a monitor for the others, gaining experience in judging whether or not velopharyngeal valving has been combined with adequate articulation in the sequential speech of his peers, with the possibility that such practice may help him to evaluate his own performance.

Because speech is a learned activity, the models from which it is learned must be readily heard and seen. The child needs to monitor his own performance, also, through several sensory channels. The importance of what has been called ear training, auditory training, auditory stimulation, sound-discrimination training, and integral stimulation has been discussed in several publications (Milisen and others, 1954; Van Riper and Irwin, 1958; Berry and Eisenson, 1956; Van Riper, 1963; West and Ansberry, 1968; others). The child with a repaired or obturated palatal cleft may need auditory training or ear training for the same reasons as those that apply to noncleft children with vocal and articulatory disorders; but the combination of inadequate valving, misdirection of the airstream, and articulatory differences makes the task of identifying his own errors and differentiating them from acceptable resonance and articulation more complex for the child with a congenital cleft. The two major channels for feedback, the auditory and the kinesthetic, may be disrupted in the child born with a cleft. Ability to respond to ear training may be diminished by a hearing loss, or the inconsistent disturbances in hearing that are typical of infections of the middle ear may lead the child to mistrust his auditory sense as a monitor. Although disruption of lingual and palatal taction did not seem to affect the articulation of a group of children with normal structures (Weiss, 1968), children wearing prostheses that cover the anterior section of the palate may need to use sensory feedback from avenues other than the tactile to monitor their articulation (McCroskey, n.d.; Martone and Black, 1962; Hochberg and Kabcenell, 1967). The auditory and visual cues that seem essential to the acquisition of sounds may become less important than the kinesthetic and tactile cues once the sound has been mastered (Van Riper and Irwin, 1958), but the child with a prepalatal or palatal cleft will probably need to use all sensory avenues in his acquisition and automatization of articulatory skills.

- Differentiation between oral and nasal emission can be demonstrated through visual cues if auditory stimuli are not effective. Electronic devices such as flowmeters present visual evidence of orality or nasality. A contact microphone placed on the nose can be used in conjunction with an amplifier that has a volume indicator to show the presence or absence of nasal resonance. Indications of the presence or absence of oral breath pressure for plosion and friction can be obtained with a standard microphone and a meter. A microphone that is hooded to limit pickup to the nose or the mouth will enable the child to see, on the meter dial, general evidence of changes in the amount of oral or nasal resonance or shifts from nasal to oral emission, even if the readings on the instrument do not correlate specifically with the perceptual variations.
- Simpler ways of showing the difference between oral and nasal direction of the airstream also can be employed. Movement of a piece of paper or cotton from the lower of two small shelves, one below the nostrils, the other in front of the mouth, can demonstrate whether or not the stream of air from the mouth exceeds that from the nose. Tactile evidence of oral direction can be obtained by placing the finger or the back of the hand at the point for plosion. Comparison of nasal and oral emission can be made by using two fingers, one under the nostrils and one in front of the mouth. Demonstration of the desired direction of the stream of air by the clinician can be checked tactually by the child, who can then attempt to duplicate the tactile sensation through his own sound production.
- Preliminary attention to general kinesthetic cues can be provided by the child's verbal report of what his hand does when he picks up a pencil or crayon, what position his foot or leg is in when he is suddenly asked to describe it without looking and without moving,

what he feels when he focuses his attention on some one part of the body, what is "tight" and what is "loose" when he points or beckons or claps. Transfer of attention to the pharyngeal and oral areas may be easier if some preliminary training has established the concept of "kinesthesia," whether or not the word is used.

- The auditory feedback mechanism will continue to be important for the child whose kinesthetic sense may be limited by scar tissue or a prosthesis. Self-monitoring will be necessary if he is to maintain good orality, once he has achieved it; and analysis of his own speech in comparison with that of others should become habitual. Devices commercially available or constructed by the child or clinician can serve to send speech from mouth to ear directly; or, in the absence of such devices, the cupped hands held in front of the mouth will help to direct the words to the ear to facilitate judgments of speech efficiency.
- Tape recordings made with and without the child's knowledge help him to hear the speech he uses in unstructured situations. Children who have learned to operate a tape recorder can often prepare demonstrations of their various levels of performance for the clinician. Comparisons of child judgment with clinician judgment provide additional opportunities for evaluation of progress.
- The use of visual cues can assist in monitoring, and adapted approaches to speechreading may encourage the child to watch those who talk to him and to imitate his models more accurately. For those whose hearing losses make some training in speechreading desirable, different methods may be needed; but even those who hear adequately may profit from discriminating between unvoiced words, following simple directions given without voice, or attempting to speechread from silent films. The child can readily learn to differentiate between two words, phrases, or directions that have little resemblance but include visible sounds. "Give me the fish" in contrast with "Give me the book" or "Show me the boy" as differentiated from "Show me the light" or "Wave your hand" in comparison with "Jump up and down" will provide better practice for this phase of training than comparisons and contrasts of homophenous words or phrases.
- Discrimination between nasal and oral direction of the stream of air and sound will need constant reinforcement. The child's recorded

demonstrations of speech "out of the mouth" versus speech "out of the nose and mouth" can provide opportunity for strong immediate approval of the adequate direction. His own evaluations of the differences can strengthen the child's capacity for self-monitoring during sequential speech.

- Auditory trainers with amplification suited to the child's adequate or inadequate hearing can strengthen the signal that is to be evaluated. A tape recorder used as a public address system can let the child hear his own speech through the usual channels of air and ear to supplement listening through headphones.
- The child may assign simple penalties to the clinician, who duplicates the improper breath pressure or inadequate articulation of the child. In turn, the clinician may penalize the child; or the child may penalize himself. The goal of self-monitoring is important in the establishment of independence in modifying speech behavior.

Structures brought to one level of adequacy by surgical and dental management may be further modified, and the child should learn to adapt to changes that occur because of growth or management. The child without a cleft experiences some changes, which are sometimes sudden, as in the loss of deciduous teeth or removal of tonsils and adenoids, sometimes slow, as in the general growth of oral and laryngeal structures. Many children with normal structures require a day or two to adjust to the loss of a deciduous tooth, just as the adult experiences some temporary problems in speaking when he is provided with full dentures. These adaptations, however, are usually unconscious processes, guided by the ear or the kinesthetic sense of the speaker.

Children whose palates are intact but are at a marginal level of adequacy in length or whose pharyngeal space is deep may, after the removal of the adenoidal pad, exhibit some of the speech characteristics of the child born with a palatal cleft. Some adapt rapidly to the new pharyngeal size; others fail to do so. Most of these children, however, after a period of time, return to the speech patterns they demonstrated prior to adenoidectomy.

Children with repaired or supplemented palates may be able to compensate for changes that occur gradually, but they may have some difficulty in adjusting to sudden alterations in structure. The decision to remove the tonsils and adenoids of a child with a repaired cleft palate should be made only by those who are well aware of the possibly devastating effects of such disturbance to already-modified structures (Subtelny and Koepp-Baker, 1956;

J. Daniel Subtelny, 1962); and such a decision requires careful consideration by pediatrician, plastic surgeon, family physician, and others. An appliance to modify dental structures may bring about a temporary or long-term change in articulatory patterns, and a bulb that almost fills the pharyngeal space may change resonance patterns from hypernasal to hyponasal. The structures of a child born with a palatal cleft will probably be changed in several ways during a period of years, and the child may need to compensate for these changes without the assistance of a speech clinician. Hence, some preparation for coping with changes should be provided as part of a sequence of remediation in speech.

Perhaps the best ways to prepare the child to manage modified structures are to improve his discrimination, to explain to him the possible effects of a new appliance or a pharyngeal flap or a prosthesis to help in closing the pharyngeal passageway, to help him to develop a flexible and controlled speech mechanism, to avoid suggesting to him that a speech sound can be produced in only one way, and to develop his skills in monitoring. Explanations to parents can help them to help their children; and information from surgeons and dentists also can prepare the child for necessary changes, gradual or sudden, in his oral, pharyngeal, and dental structures.

Communication involves many factors, which are used habitually and automatically in a social environment. Language that cannot be used effectively because speech is unintelligible or distractingly unpleasant to the listener interferes with adaptation to the environment. Language that is used effectively through the medium of intelligible speech provides a means for social control and interaction that can facilitate learning, promote the development of an acceptable personality, and permit preparation for vocational competence. Language and speech, at an adequate and automatic level, are essential for the child's school progress and his eventual assumption of a position that will make him a contributing member of society. Whether he has good or poor potential for earning a living, he will live in a world that will react to him in terms of the way he talks. The girl who becomes a homemaker and mother will need to communicate with those in her neighborhood and will influence the speech of her children. The boy or girl who is capable of a professional career will have a special need for good speech and language. The child who will need a sheltered environment still needs to communicate with those who care for him. Vocational opportunities will depend, to a great extent, on the adequacy with which the young man or woman can express ideas and talk with others. Remedial procedures for children born with clefts, therefore, are not limited to modification of motor behavior.

They include consideration of linguistic skills and of relationships to a social and occupational environment.

In his concern for improving resonance and articulation, the clinician should not lose sight of the fact that his ultimate goal is to prepare the child to take whatever place he can assume in society to earn a living, to relate to others, to be a total person who reaches his highest level of achievement. Skill in the use of speech sounds and in the proper direction of the stream of air or sound to achieve acceptable control of resonance is certainly desirable; but /t/ and /s/, no matter how well they are produced, do not constitute language. The correlation of linguistic training with the development of motor skills may be more important for children born with clefts than for some other children, if linguistic and intellectual retardation are typical of children born with these anomalies, as some authorities believe.

The ultimate goal of the speech training program for the child with a prepalatal or palatal cleft, therefore, is the automatization of skills that have been acquired. Once established, linguistic, articulatory, and resonatory capabilities should combine in purposeful oral communication that is reinforced by the responses it obtains. At this stage, the use of operant conditioning procedures may be particularly helpful (Chisum and others, 1969). Such procedures require careful planning and strict adherence to the schedule that is set, together with understanding of behavioral principles.

- Behaviorism holds as yet unexplored advantages for the practice of speech correction. In some instances, careful and systematic incorporation of the findings of the behavioral laboratory has a high probability of evolving new methods of clinical management. In others it can help us do our jobs more efficiently. In many others, it can help us to understand why what we are doing produces the results it does (Holland, 1967, p. 16).
- Socially facilitating oral expression can provide rewards that will stimulate continued efforts to improve communication. Greetings, requests, responses to inquiries, and social phrases and sentences that can be used as means of stabilizing motor skills can also facilitate social communication. The child who responds effectively to his social environment and to whom others respond favorably will be encouraged to use his best speech outside the structured clinical situation.
- Self-identification may also provide practice material at any or several stages of therapy. The child's name, age, address, parents' names, school, siblings' names, and other words and phrases with personal

significance can be used to combine motor skills with social facilitation.

- Naming parts of the body, even if the child has known them previously, provides experience in modifying motor behavior patterns and in additional self-identification.
- Certain individuals in the child's environment may provide special stimulation to best performance at any level of achievement. Conversely, meeting and talking with strangers may, if preparation has been good, elicit the child's maximum effort.
- Linguistic skills can be encouraged in all remedial activities. Vocabulary can be increased; and, in some instances, new words may be more effectively used than old words. The pattern of response in which complete sentences are used combines emphasis on transfer of motor skills with experience in linguistic combination.
- The child who is being encouraged to use language effectively should have something to talk about. Whatever his level of intellectual capacity, he needs experiences from which language can result. If he has been culturally deprived, he will need special opportunities to have experiences that he can talk about.
- Grammatical construction can receive emphasis in the total training program, perhaps by example and perhaps by direct attention. Post-stimulation can often help both language and articulation if the clinician, the parent, or the teacher will feed back, in acceptable form, the child's inadequate verbalizations. Parents and teachers may need to be reminded that "Your bike is in the garage" is more helpful than "It's in the garage" if the child's use of "bike" is inadequate. Similarly, responding "Yes, the books are on the shelf" when the child says "The books is on the shelf" permits the child to hear the correct construction without being made to feel that he is being corrected.
- With due consideration for the child's opportunities to take part in the conversation, parents and teachers can provide stimulation by good example through talking to the child. Just as the child with a hearing loss needs the language from others in his environment to instill in him the concept of talking, so the child whose speech and language are inadequate, regardless of the status of his oral and pharyngeal structures, can profit from hearing linguistic and speech models that he can imitate.

- Training in speech and language must extend beyond the clinical setting to the home and school, and the speech pathologist's suggestions to parents and teachers should stress encouragement to the child to use his best speech, good example for the child to follow, wise use of reminders, and insistence on maximum performance. Each home and each schoolroom will provide different kinds of opportunities for reinforcement of the work of the speech clinician, and each should be used maximally for the child who can be influenced by these environments.
- In his concern for the child's language, the clinician will not forget his own. The child must be able to understand the directions given by the clinician, who may need to modify vocabulary, sentence length, and linguistic complexity to suit the capacities of the child at any point in the remedial sequence.
- The child born with a cleft, more than many other children with disordered communication, will need continued attention from the many professional workers who are concerned with his habilitation. The speech pathologist, although he is only one of these specialists, is often in a position to encourage parents to keep appointments with orthodontists and prosthodontists, to stress the importance of maintaining the child's best level of health with aid of the pediatrician or family physician, to explain projected surgical or dental management in ways that can lead to acceptance of recommendations for additional treatment, and to serve as a liaison agent for all those interested in helping the child to attain and retain improvement.

Few clinicians spend all their time on the communicative problems of children born with clefts. In the public schools, the incidence of speech problems associated with clefts will be low. In hospital settings, the duration of stay and the recency of surgery may limit the time the clinician has for providing assistance. In rehabilitation centers or community clinics, the number of children or adults with repaired obturated clefts will not be great. Occasionally, special programs will provide the clinician with an opportunity to work intensively with these children or with young adults with clefts. The complexity of the cleft palate problem, however, justifies extensive attention to it. Speech training provided in any setting should be frequent; it should be correlated with home and school activities; and it should relate to other services needed to improve appearance, assure competent deglutition, restore or maintain normal hearing, promote good educational progress, establish emotional adjustment, and prepare for eventual vocational achievement. One might wish that such a variety of services could be provided for any child with disordered communication; for the child with congenital physical malformations and communicative problems, the multiplicity of services is essential.

IN THE SECOND HALF OF THE TWENTIETH CENTURY, THE CHILD BORN WITH A CLEFT OF THE PREPALATE, THE PALATE, OR BOTH CAN BE THE RECIPIENT OF BENEFITS THAT HAVE ACCRUED TO HIM THROUGH LONG PERIODS OF TIME AND FROM THE EFFORTS OF MANY DEDICATED WORKERS.

The effect of congenital anomalies of the facial area on child and family alike is great; but the efforts of scientists who have contributed to knowledge in such fields as surgery, dentistry, speech pathology, audiology, anatomy, physiology, neurology, embryology, epidemiology, and teratology have reduced the impact of the presence of clefts. Earlier conflicts resulting from claims of priority in evolving certain surgical procedures or forms of prostheses and from interests centered on the remediator rather than on the child have given way to cooperative attempts to prevent and manage congenital clefts of the prepalate and palate and to habilitate children born with these anomalies.

As knowledge continues to increase and as those specialists who are most deeply concerned with children born with clefts continue their joint attack on the problem, the child whose prepalatal and palatal structures were defective at birth can become an adult who is a contributing member of society. The attention of the many specialists whose work has been discussed in this book can assist him in many ways, not the least of which is the acquisition of skill in the most important and frequently used form of communication, the means of exercising control over his environment and those in it, the universal medium of social exchange—adequate oral communication.

Bibliography

Abbe, Robert (1898): "A New Plastic Operation for the Relief of Deformity Due to Double Harelip," *Medical Record,* 53:477–478. Also in *Plastic and Reconstructive Surgery,* 42:481–482[1]

Adams, Richard M., and Laurel E. Brown (1965): "Labial Supportive Appliance," *Cleft Palate Journal,* 2:389–393[2]

Adamson, Jerome E., Charles E. Horton, Hugh H. Crawford, and Mildred Wertz (1966): "A Practical Method of Judging Cleft Palate Speech," *PRS,* 38:544–551.

[1] Hereafter *Plastic and Reconstructive Surgery* will be shown as *PRS.*

[2] Hereafter *Cleft Palate Journal* will be shown as *CPJ.*

Adisman, I. Kenneth (1968): "The Role of Prosthodontists in Hospitals," *Journal of Prosthetic Dentistry,* 20:269–275.

——— (1969): "Prosthetic Stimulation of the Incompetent Soft Palate," paper presented at 1969 International Congress on Cleft Palate.

Aduss, Howard, and Samuel Pruzansky (1968): "Width of Cleft at Level of the Tuberosities in Complete Unilateral Cleft Lip and Palate," *PRS,* 41:113–123.

Alley, Norman R. A. (1965): "The Use of Speech Aid Prosthesis as a Diagnostic Tool," *CPJ,* 2:291–292.

Altemus, Leonard A. (1966): "The Incidence of Cleft Lip and Palate among North American Negroes," *CPJ,* 3:357–361.

Anderson, Ruth M., Madeline Miles, and Patricia A. Matheny (1964): *Communicative Evaluation Chart from Infancy to Five Years,* rev. ed., Educators Publishing Service, Inc., Cambridge, Mass.

Angelici, Dino R. (1968): "Reopening of Fused Palatal Shelves," *CPJ,* 5:205–210.

Antia, N. H. (1966): "Primary Abbe Flap in Bilateral Cleft Palate," *British Journal of Plastic Surgery,* 19:215–219.

Aram, Ali, and J. Daniel Subtelny (1959): "Velopharyngeal Function and Cleft Palate Prostheses," *Journal of Prosthetic Dentistry,* 9:149–158.

Arey, Leslie Brainerd (1946, 1965): *Developmental Anatomy,* 5th ed., 7th ed., W. B. Saunders Company, Philadelphia.

Aufricht, Gustave (1946): "The Development of Plastic Surgery in the United States," *PRS,* 1:3–25.

Azaz, B., and Edith Koyoumdjisky-Kaye (1967): "Incidence of Clefts in Israel," *CPJ,* 4:227–233.

Bäckdahl, M., and K. E. Nordin (1961): "Replacement of the Maxillary Bone Defect in Cleft Palate—A New Procedure," *Acta Chirurgica Scandinavica,* 122:131–137.

Baden, Ernest (1955): "Prosthetic Therapy of Congenital and Acquired Clefts of the Palate," *Journal of the History of Medicine,* 10:290–301.

Baibak, George, and Bertram E. Bromberg (1966): "Congenital Midline Defects of the Midface," *CPJ,* 3:392–401.

Baker, Henry A. (1881): "An Appliance for Congenital Cleft Palate," *Dental Cosmos,* 23:178–186.

Bankoff, George Alexis (1952): *The Story of Plastic Surgery,* Faber & Faber, Ltd., London.

Barber, Thomas K. (1969): "The Handicapped Adolescent," *Dental Clinics of North America,* 13:313–327.

Bardanouve, Venus Tretsven (1969): "Cleft Palate in Montana: A 10-Year Report," *CPJ,* 6:213–220.

Barker, Janet O'Neill (1963): *Arizona Articulation Proficiency Scale,* Western Psychological Services, Beverly Hills, Calif.

Barnes, Ida Jones, and Hughlett L. Morris (1967): "Interrelationships among Oral Breath Pressure Ratios and Articulation Skills for Individuals with Cleft Palate," *Journal of Speech and Hearing Research,* 10:506–514.

Barsky, Arthur J. (1964): "Pierre Franco, Father of Cleft Lip Surgery: His Life and Times," *British Journal of Plastic Surgery,* 17:335–350.

———, Sidney Kahn, and Bernard E. Simon (1962): "Early and Late Management of the Protruding Premaxilla," *PRS,* 29:58–70.

Bauer, Thomas, Harold Trusler, and Sanford Glanz (1953): "Repair of Unilateral Cleft Lip—Advantages of LeMesurier's Technique—Use of Mucous Membrane Flaps in Maxillary Clefts," *PRS,* 11:56–68.

Bay, R. (1967): "Nos Expériences avec la Méthode de McNeil," *Report of the Forty-Third Congress, European Orthodontic Society,* 337–339.

Beder, Oscar E., James A. Carrell, and Jeanne Tomlinson (1968): "The Palatal Elevator Button," *Journal of Prosthetic Dentistry,* 20:182–188.

———, Herbert E. Coe, Richard P. Braafladt, and James D. Houle (1956): "Factors Associated with Cleft Lip and Cleft Palate in the Pacific Northwest," *Oral Surgery, Oral Medicine, and Oral Pathology,* 9:1267–1273.

Bell, Alexander Melville (1897): *The Science of Speech,* The Volta Bureau, Washington, D.C.

Bennett, C. G., M. D. Largent, and L. E. Edwards (1966): "Study of the Oral Conditions with an Oscillographic Analysis of Isolated Vowel Sounds of Repaired Cleft Palate Children," *Folia Phoniatrica,* 18:261–268.

Berry, James, and T. Percy Legg (1912): *Harelip and Cleft Palate,* J. & A. Churchill, London.

Berry, Mildred, and Jon Eisenson (1956): *Speech Disorders,* Appleton-Century-Crofts, Inc., New York.

Berson, Morton I. (1963): *Atlas of Plastic Surgery,* 2nd ed., Grune & Stratton, Inc., New York.

Bethmann, Wolfgang (1969): "Birth Order and Cheilo-Gnatho-Palato-Schisis," *CPJ,* 6:205–209.

Bickel, Jacqueline (1970): "First Results of Early Speech Readiness Program in Cleft Palate Children," *CPJ,* 7:156–160.

Biggerstaff, Robert H. (1969): "Classification and Frequency of Cleft Lip and/or Palate," *CPJ,* 6:40–44.

Bill, Alexander H., Jr., Alton W. Moore, and Herbert E. Coe (1956): "The Time of Choice for Repair of Cleft Palate in Relation to the Type of Surgical Repair and Its Effect on Bony Growth of the Face," *PRS,* 18:469–473.

Birch, Jack (1952): "Personality Characteristics of Individuals with Cleft Palate: Research Needs," *American Association for Cleft Palate Rehabilitation Newsletter,* 2(2):5–6.

Birch-Jensen, Arne (1949): *Congenital Deformities of the Upper Extremities,* Andelsbogtrykkeriet, Odense, Denmark.

Birkenfeld, Werner (1926): "Über die Erblichkeit der Lippenspalte und Gaumenspalte," *Archiv für Klinische Chirurgie,* 141:729–753.

Biron, George E., and Miles Jon Felix (1968): "The Cleft Palate Patient: Theory and Dental Responsibility," *Pennsylvania Dental Journal,* 71:20–22, 29.

Björk, Lars (1961): "Velopharyngeal Function in Connected Speech," *Acta Radiologica,* Supplementum 202.

——— and Bengt O. Nylén (1961): "Cineradiography with Synchronized Sound Spectrum Analysis," *PRS,* 27:397–412.

Blackfield, Harry M., Earl R. Miller, John Q. Owsley, and Lucie I. Lawson (1962a): "Cinefluorographic Evaluation of Patients with Velopharyngeal Dysfunction in the Absence of Overt Cleft Palate," *PRS,* 30:441–451.

———, ———, ———, and ——— (1962b): "Comparative Evaluation of Diagnostic Techniques in Patients with Cleft-Palate Speech," *PRS,* 29:153–158.

Blair, Vilray P. (1937): "Cleft Palate—Its Surgery," *Journal of Speech Disorders,* 2:195–198.

Blakeley, R. W. (1960): "Temporary Speech Prosthesis as an Aid in Speech Training," *Cleft Palate Bulletin,* 10:63–65.

Blechschmidt, E. (1961): *The Stages of Human Development before Birth,* W. B. Saunders Company, Philadelphia.

Blocksma, Ralph (1964): "Silicone Implants for Velopharyngeal Incompetence: A Progress Report," *CPJ,* 1:72–81.

——— and Silas Braley (1969): "Present Status of Retropharyngeal Implantation for Velopharyngeal Insufficiency," *PRS,* 44: 242–247.

Bloomer, H. Harlan (1953): "Observations on Palatopharyngeal Movements in Speech and Deglutition," *Journal of Speech and Hearing Disorders,* 18:230–246.

——— (1968): "Informational Gaps in the Area of Clinical Services," *Asha,* 10:371–374.

——— and Brien R. Lang (1968): "Principles and Procedures in Construction of the Palatal Lift Appliance for Patients with Velopharyngeal Insufficiency or Incompetency," paper presented at 26th Annual Meeting, American Cleft Palate Association.

Bluestone, Charles, Ross H. Musgrave, Betty Jane McWilliams, and Phyllis A. Crozier (1968): "Teflon Injection Pharyngoplasty," *CPJ,* 5:19–22.

Boo-Chai, Khoo (1966): "An Ancient Chinese Text on a Cleft Lip," *PRS,* 38:89–91.

——— (1969): "The Transverse Facial Cleft: Its Repair," *British Journal of Plastic Surgery,* 22:119–124.

——— and Ichiro Tange (1968): "The Isolated Cleft-Lip Nose: Report of Five Cases in Adults," *PRS,* 41:28–34.

Böök, J. A. (1951): "The Incidence of Congenital Diseases and Defects in a South Swedish Population," *Acta Genetica,* 2:289–311.

Borçbakan, Cihat (1969): "An Analysis of 1000 Cases of Cleft Lip and Palate in Turkey," *CPJ,* 6:210–212.

Bosma, James F., and Samuel G. Fletcher (1961–1962): "The Upper Pharynx. A Review," *Annals of Otology, Rhinology, and Laryngology,* 70:953–973, 71:134–157.

Bradford, Lawrence J., Alta R. Brooks, and Ralph L. Shelton, Jr. (1964): "Clinical Judgment of Hypernasality in Cleft Palate Children," *CPJ,* 1:329–335.

Brandt, Sara Dale, and Hughlett L. Morris (1965): "The Linearity of the Relationship between Articulation Errors and Velopharyngeal Incompetence," *CPJ,* 2:176–183.

Brauer, Raymond (1953): "A Consideration of the LeMesurier Technic of Single Harelip Repair with a New Concept as to Its Use in Incomplete and Secondary Harelip Repairs," *PRS,* 11:275–289.

——— and Thomas D. Cronin (1964): "Symposium: Expansion Prosthesis and Bone Grafting—Maxillary Orthopedics and Anterior Palate Repair with Bone Grafting," *CPJ,* 1:31–42.

———, ———, and Edith L. Reaves (1962): "Early Maxillary Orthopedics, Orthodontia, and Alveolar Bone Grafting in Complete Clefts of the Palate," *PRS,* 29:625–641.

Broadbent, Thomas Ray, and Chester A. Swinyard (1959): "The Dynamic Pharyngeal Flap: Its Selective Use and Electromyographic Evaluation," *PRS,* 23:301–312.

Broadway, E. S. (1967): "An Appliance for the Rapid Expansion of the Maxilla," *Report of the Forty-Third Congress, European Orthodontic Society,* 441–443.

Brooks, Alta R., Ralph L. Shelton, Jr., and Karl A. Youngstrom (1965): "Compensatory Tongue–Palate–Posterior Pharyngeal Wall Relationships in Cleft Palate," *Journal of Speech and Hearing Disorders,* 30:166–173.

———, ———, and ——— (1966): "Tongue-Palate Contact in Persons with Palate Defects," *Journal of Speech and Hearing Disorders,* 31:14–25.

Brophy, Truman W. (1923): *Cleft Lip and Palate,* P. Blakiston's Son and Company, Philadelphia.

Brown, George Van Ingen (1938): *The Surgery of Oral and Facial Diseases and Malformations,* 4th ed., Lea & Febiger, Philadelphia.

Brown, James Barrett, and Frank McDowell (1950): "Small Triangular Flap Operation for the Primary Repair of Single Cleft Lips," *PRS,* 5:392–402.

Brown, Janet (1939): "Hypothyroidism as an Etiology of Cleft Palate," *Journal of Speech Disorders,* 4:247–253.

Brown, Kenneth E. (1969): "Fabrication of a Hollow-Bulb Obturator," *Journal of Prosthetic Dentistry,* 21:97–103.

Buck, McKenzie (1953): "Facial Skeletal Measurements and Tongue Carriage in Subjects with Repaired Cleft Palates," *Journal of Speech and Hearing Disorders,* 18:121–132.

Buncke, Harry J., Patricia Page, Barbara Price, Carol Blazine, and Freda Fraser (1966): "The Evaluation and Management of Velopharyngeal Insufficiency," *CPJ,* 3:171–180.

Burdi, Alphonse R., and Kathleen Faist (1967): "Morphogenesis of the Palate in Normal Human Embryos with Special Emphasis on the Mechanisms Involved," *American Journal of Anatomy,* 120:149–160.

——— and Ralph G. Silvey (1969): "Sexual Differences in Closure of the Human Palatal Shelves," *CPJ,* 6:1–7.

Burston, W. R. (1965): "The Early Orthodontic Treatment of Alveolar Clefts," *Proceedings of the Royal Society of Medicine,* 58:767–771.

Byrne, Margaret C., Ralph L. Shelton, Jr., and William M. Diedrich (1961): "Articulatory Skill, Physical Management, and Classification of Children with Cleft Palates," *Journal of Speech and Hearing Disorders,* 26:326–333.

Bzoch, Kenneth (1959): "A Study of the Speech of a Group of Pre-school Cleft Palate Children," *Cleft Palate Bulletin,* 9:2–3.

——— (1960): "Clinical Appraisal of Cleft Palate Rehabilitation Problems," *Journal of the American Dental Association,* 60:696–698.

——— (1964): "The Effects of a Specific Pharyngeal Flap Operation upon the Speech of Forty Cleft-Palate Persons," *Journal of Speech and Hearing Disorders,* 29:111–120.

——— (1965): "Articulation Proficiency and Error Patterns of Preschool Cleft Palate and Normal Children," *CPJ,* 2:340–349.

——— (1968): "Variations in Velopharyngeal Valving: The Factor of Vowel Changes," *CPJ,* 5:211–218.

———, T. M. Graber, and T. Aoba (1959): "A Study of Normal Velo-Pharyngeal Valving for Speech," *Cleft Palate Bulletin,* 9:3–4.

Calnan, James (1953): "Movements of the Soft Palate," *British Journal of Plastic Surgery,* 5:286–296.

——— (1954a): "The Error of Gustav Passavant," *PRS,* 13:275–289.

——— (1954b): "Submucous Cleft Palate," *British Journal of Plastic Surgery,* 6:264–282.

——— (1956): "Diagnosis, Prognosis, and Treatment of 'Palato-Pharyngeal Incompetence' with Special Reference to Radiographic Investigation," *British Journal of Plastic Surgery,* 8:265–282.

——— (1961): "The Mobility of the Soft Palate," *British Journal of Plastic Surgery,* 14:33–38.

Canick, M. Leon (1954): "Cleft Lip and Cleft Palate: A Review of Embryology, Pathologic Anatomy, and Etiology," *PRS,* 14: 30–46.

Cannon, Bradford, David Fisher, and Henry C. Britton (1951): "Plastic Surgery: Harelip and Cleft Palate," *New England Journal of Medicine,* 245:179–185, 215–219.

Carpenter, Mary A., and Hughlett L. Morris (1968): "A Preliminary Study of Passavant's Pad," *CPJ,* 5:61–72.

Carter, Cedric (1963): "Racial Variations in Cleft Lip and Palate (An Annotation)," *Developmental Medicine and Child Neurology,* 5:182–183.

Case, Calvin S. (1903): "New Artificial Palate," *Dental Digest,* 9:48–56.

Červenka, Jaroslav, Robert J. Gorlin, and V. Elving Anderson (1967): abstract of paper, *Oral Surgery, Oral Medicine, and Oral Pathology,* 24:379.

———, Ladislav Růžička, and Olga Klásková (1969): "Seasonal Incidence of Cleft Lip and Palate in Czech Regions," *CPJ,* 6:35–39.

Chase, Robert A. (1960): "An Objective Evaluation of Palatopharyngeal Competence," *PRS,* 26:23–39.

Chase, Samuel W. (1942): "The Early Development of the Human Premaxilla," *Journal of the American Dental Association,* 29:1991–2001.

Chenoweth, Alice D. (1964): "Services for Children with Cleft Palates by State Crippled Children's Agencies," *CPJ,* 1:299–303.

Chierici, George (1967): "Some Observations on the Pharyngeal Airspace," *CPJ,* 4:129–136.

Clifford, Edward (1967): "Connotative Meaning of Concepts Related to Cleft Lip and Palate," *CPJ,* 4:165–173.

——— (1969a): "The Impact of Symptom: A Preliminary Comparison of Cleft Lip-Palate and Asthmatic Children," *CPJ,* 6:221–227.

——— (1969b): "Parental Ratings of Cleft Palate Infants," *CPJ,* 6:235–244.

Climo, Merrill S. (1969): "Diastasis of the Orbicularis Oris Muscle in Repaired Unilateral Clefts of the Lip," *CPJ,* 6:316–322.

Coccaro, Peter J. (1969): "Orthodontics in Cleft Palate Children: A Continuing Process," *CPJ,* 6:495–505.

Coccia, Chester T., and David Bixler (1967): "Cleft Lip, Cleft Palate, and Congenital Fistulas of the Lower Lip," *Oral Surgery, Oral Medicine, and Oral Pathology,* 24:246–249.

———, ———, and P. M. Conneally (1969): "Cleft Lip and Cleft Palate: A Genetic Study," *CPJ,* 6:323–336.

Cocke, William, Jr. (1966): "Experimental Production of Micrognathia and Glossoptosis Associated with Cleft Palate (Pierre Robin Syndrome)," *PRS,* 38:395–403.

Collins, Bill M. (1970): "A Descriptive Study of Lateral Pharyngeal Wall Activity," unpublished doctor's dissertation, University of Missouri-Columbia.

Conroy, Cecil R. (1951): "Three Age Phases of Orthodontic Treatment of the Cleft Palate Child," *PRS,* 7:100–117.

Converse, John Marquis (1962): "Victor Veau (1871–1949): The Contributions of a Pioneer," *PRS,* 30:225–235.

———, ed. (1964): *Reconstructive Plastic Surgery,* W. B. Saunders Company, Philadelphia.

——— and Sidney L. Horowitz (1969): "The Surgical-Orthodontic Approach to the Treatment of Dentofacial Deformities," *American Journal of Orthodontics,* 55:217–243.

———, ———, Cary L. Guy, and Donald Wood-Smith (1964): "Surgical-Orthodontic Correction in the Bilateral Cleft Lip," *CPJ,* 1:153–163.

Conway, Herbert (1958): "Effect of Supplemental Vitamin Therapy on the Limitation of Incidence of Cleft Lip and Cleft Palate in Humans," *PRS,* 22:450–453.

——— and Dicran Goulian (1961): "Experiences with the Pharyngeal Flap in Cleft Palate Surgery," *Cleft Palate Bulletin,* 11:2.

———, P. McKinney, M. Climo, N. Hugo, R. Cole, and D. Goulian (1968): "A Cleft Palate Registry in Action: Analysis of 850 Consecutive Cases," *PRS,* 41:38–49.

——— and Kurt J. Wagner (1966): "Incidence of Clefts in New York City," *CPJ,* 3:284–290.

Cooper, H(erbert) K. (1946): "The Responsibility of the Orthodontist in the Cleft Palate Problem," *American Journal of Orthodontics and Oral Surgery,* 32:675–683.

——— (1951): "Cleft Palate: Dentistry's Opportunity," *Journal of the American Dental Association,* 42:37–47.

——— and F. A. Hoffman (1955): "The Application of Cinefluorography with Image Intensification in the Field of Plastic Surgery, Dentistry, and Speech," *PRS,* 16:135–137.

Cosman, Bard, and George F. Crikelair (1965): "The Reconstruction of the Unilateral Cleft Lip Nasal Deformity," *CPJ,* 2:95–111.

——— and ——— (1966): "Release of the Prolabium in the Bilateral Cleft Lip," *CPJ,* 3:122–129.

Counihan, Donald T. (1960): "Articulation Skills of Adolescents and Adults with Cleft Palates," *Journal of Speech and Hearing Disorders,* 25:181–187.

Cox, James B., and Bernard Silverstein (1961): "Experiences with the Posterior Pharyngeal Flap for Correction of Velopharyngeal Insufficiency," *PRS,* 27:40–48.

Crabtree, Margaret (1963): *The Houston Test for Language Development,* The Houston Test Company, Houston, Texas.

Crikelair, George F. (1969): "Why Repair a Cleft Lip?" *CPJ,* 6:93–107.

———, Adrian F. Bom, Joseph Luban, and Melvin Moss (1962): "Early Orthodontic Movement of Cleft Maxillary Segments Prior to Cleft Lip Repair," *PRS,* 30:426–440.

Cronin, Thomas D. (1966): "A Modification of the Tennison-Type Lip Repair," *CPJ,* 3:376–382.

———, Raymond O. Brauer, John T. Alexander, and William G. Taylor (1964): "Push-Back Repair Using Nasal Mucosal Flaps: Results," *CPJ,* 1:269–274.

Curtin, John W. (1962): "A Surgeon's Evaluation of the Cleft Palate Team," *PRS,* 29:289–292.

Curtis, James F. (1970): "The Acoustics of Nasalized Speech," *CPJ,* 7:380–396.

Curtis, Thomas A. (1968): "Fixed Retention Following Cleft Palate Orthodontics," *Angle Orthodontist,* 38:211–215.

——— and George Chierici (1964): "Prosthetics as a Diagnostic Aid in Pharyngeal Flap Surgery," *CPJ,* 1:95–98.

Davies, David (1965): "The Repair of the Unilateral Cleft Lip," *British Journal of Plastic Surgery,* 18:254–264.

Davies, Jack (1963): *Human Developmental Anatomy,* The Ronald Press Company, New York.

Davis, Albert D. (1951): "Management of the Wide Unilateral Cleft Lip with Nostril Deformity," *PRS,* 8:249–257.

Davis, John Staige (1924): "The Incidence of Congenital Clefts of the Lip and Palate," *Annals of Surgery,* 80:363–374.

——— and Harry P. Ritchie (1922): "Classification of Congenital Clefts of the Lip and Palate," *Journal of the American Medical Association,* 79:1323–1327.

Davis, N. S. (1841): "Case of Congenital Hare-Lip, Double, with Both Fissures Extending through the Roof of the Mouth and the Palate," *American Journal of the Medical Sciences,* 4:371–373.

——— (1847): "Case of Double Hare-Lip," *New York Journal of Medicine and the Collateral Sciences,* 9:36–38.

Demb, Norman, and Aubrey L. Ruess (1967): "High School Drop-Out Rate for Cleft Palate Patients," *CPJ,* 4:327–333.

Denton, George B. (1935): "The Most Famous Dental Book," *Bulletin of the Medical Library Association,* 24:113–123.

DeVoss, Henry (1952): "A Study of the Factors Relative to the Incidence of Cleft Palate Births from 1945 to 1949 in San Bernardino County," *Speech Monographs,* 19:301–308.

Dickson, David Ross (1962): "An Acoustic Study of Nasality," *Journal of Speech and Hearing Research,* 5:103–111.

——— (1969): "A Radiographic Study of Nasality," *CPJ,* 6:160–165.

Dijkstra, R. (1969): "Secondary Lengthening of the Soft Palate Using Millard's Island Flap Technique," *British Journal of Plastic Surgery,* 22:113–118.

Dodds, Paul (1946): "The Responsibility of Public Health Agencies to Cleft Palate Patients," *American Journal of Orthodontics and Oral Surgery,* 32:665–666.

Doig, R. K., and O. McK. Coltman (1956): "Cleft Palate Following Cortisone Therapy in Early Pregnancy," *Lancet,* 271(6945): 730.

Donahue, Richard F. (1965): "Birth Variables and the Incidence of Cleft Palate: Part I," *CPJ,* 2:282–290.

——— (1967): "Birth Variables and the Incidence of Cleft Palate: Part II," *CPJ,* 4:234–239.

Dorrance, George Morris (1933): *The Operative Story of Cleft Palate,* W. B. Saunders Company, Philadelphia.

——— and J. W. Bransfield (1946): "The Push-Back Operation for Repair of Cleft Palate," *PRS,* 1:145–169.

Douglas, Beverly (1946): "The Treatment of Micrognathia Associated with Obstruction by a Plastic Procedure," *PRS,* 1:300–308.

——— (1950): "A Further Report on the Treatment of Micrognathia with Obstruction by a Plastic Procedure: Results Based on Reports from 21 Cities," *PRS,* 5:113–122.

Drillien, Cecil M., T. T. S. Ingram, and Elsie M. Wilkinson (1966): *The Causes and Natural History of Cleft Lip and Palate,* The Williams & Wilkins Company, Baltimore.

Dunn, Lloyd M. (1965): *Peabody Picture Vocabulary Test,* Western Psychological Services, Beverly Hills, Calif.

Ecker, Herbert A. (1958): "Medial Clefts of the Lips," *American Journal of Surgery,* 96:815–819.

——— (1960): "The Use of the Buccal Flap in Cleft Palate Repair," *PRS,* 25:235–239.

Edgerton, Milton T., and Anthony Zovickian (1965): "Reconstruction of Major Defects of the Palate," *PRS,* 17:105–128.

Eichenwald, Heinz F. (1965): "The Placental 'Barrier' and Infections of the Fetus," *Birth Defects: Original Articles Series,* 1:74–76.

Enlow, Donald H. (1968): *The Human Face—An Account of the Postnatal Growth and Development of the Craniofacial Skeleton,* Hoeber Medical Division, Harper & Row, Publishers, Incorporated, New York.

Erdélyi, Robert (1957): "The Influence of Toxoplasmosis on the Incidence of Congenital Facial Malformations," *PRS,* 20: 306–310.

Erhardt, C. L., and F. G. Nelson (1964): "Reported Congenital Malformations in New York City, 1958 and 1959," *American Journal of Public Health,* 54:1489–1506.

Estlander, J. A. (1872): "Eine Methode aus der Einen Lippe Substanzverluste der Anderen zu Ersetzen," *Archiv für Klinische Chirurgie,* 14:622–631. Also in *PRS,* 42:361–364.

Ewers, S. R. (1968): "A Study of Prenatal Growth of the Human Bony Palate from 3 to 9 Months," *American Journal of Orthodontics,* 54:3–28.

Excerpta Medica Foundation (1963): *Third International Congress of Plastic Surgery,* International Congress Series, No. 58.

Fairbanks, Grant (1966): *Experimental Phonetics: Selected Articles,* University of Illinois Press, Urbana.

——— and D. C. Spriestersbach (1950): "A Study of Minor Organic Deviations in 'Functional' Disorders of Articulation: 1. Rate of Movement of Oral Structures," *Journal of Speech and Hearing Disorders,* 15:60–69.

Falk, Mervyn L., and George A. Kopp (1968): "Tongue Position and Hypernasality in Cleft Palate Speech," *CPJ,* 5:229–237.

Falter, Jane Werth, and Ralph L. Shelton, Jr. (1964): "Bulb Fitting and Placement in Prosthetic Treatment of Cleft Palate," *CPJ,* 1:441–447.

Fára, Miroslav, and Miluše Brousilová (1969): "Experiences with Early Closure of Velum and Later Closure of Hard Palate," *PRS,* 44:134–141.

——— and J. Šmahel (1967): "Postoperative Follow-Up of Restitution Procedures in the Orbicularis Oris Muscle after Operation for Complete Bilateral Cleft of the Lip," *PRS,* 40:13–21.

Fishbein, Morris, ed. (1961): *First International Conference on Congenital Malformations,* J. B. Lippincott Company, Philadelphia.

———, ed. (1963): *An Illustrated Medical and Health Encyclopedia,* H. S. Stuttman Company, Publishers, New York.

Fitzgibbon, John J. (1923): "The Correction of Congenital Cleft Palates by Appliances," *Dental Items of Interest,* 45:711–718.

Fletcher, Harvey (1929): *Speech and Hearing,* D. Van Nostrand Company, Inc., New York.

——— (1953): *Speech and Hearing in Communication,* D. Van Nostrand Company, Inc., New York.

Fletcher, Samuel G. (1966): "Cleft Palate: A Broader View," *Journal of Speech and Hearing Disorders,* 31:3–13.

Fogh-Andersen, Poul (1942): *Inheritance of Harelip and Cleft Palate,* Nyt Nordisk Forlag, Arnold Busck, Copenhagen, Denmark.

——— (1946): "Harelip and Cleft Palate: 1,000 Patients Submitted to Operation," *Acta Chirurgica Scandinavica,* 94:213–242.

——— (1961): "Incidence of Cleft Lip and Palate: Constant or Increasing?" *Acta Chirurgica Scandinavica,* 122:106–111.

——— (1965): "Rare Clefts of the Face," *Acta Chirurgica Scandinavica,* 129:275–281.

——— (1966): "Thalidomide and Congenital Cleft Deformities," *Acta Chirurgica Scandinavica,* 131:197–200.

Foster, Carol R., Jane J. Giddan, and Joel Stark (1969): *Assessment of Children's Language Comprehension,* research ed.,

Consulting Psychologists Press, Palo Alto, Calif.

Foster, T. D. (1957): "Malocclusions in 322 Patients with Cleft Lip and Palate Who Have Not Had Presurgical Dental Orthopaedic Treatment," *Report of the Forty-Third Congress, European Orthodontic Society,* 445–454.

Francis, W. W. (1963): "Repair of Cleft Palate by Philibert Roux in 1819," *Journal of the History of Medicine and Allied Sciences,* 18:209–219.

Frank, Barnett (1955): "A Rationale for Closer Cooperation between the Orthodontist and the Speech and Hearing Therapist," *American Journal of Orthodontics,* 41:571–582.

Fraser, F. Clarke (1955): "Thoughts on the Etiology of Clefts of the Palate and Lip," *Acta Genetica,* 5:358–369.

——— (1959): "Causes of Congenital Malformations in Human Beings," *Journal of Chronic Diseases,* 10:97–110.

——— (1960): "Some Experimental and Clinical Studies on the Causes of Congenital Clefts of the Palate and of the Lip," *Archives of Pediatrics,* 77:151–156.

——— (1967): "Cleft Lip and Cleft Palate," *Science,* 158(3808):1603–1606.

——— (1968): "Cleft Lip and Cleft Palate," *CPJ,* 5:187–194.

——— and Dorothy Warburton (1964): "No Association of Emotional Stress or Vitamin Supplement during Pregnancy to Cleft Lip or Palate in Man," *PRS,* 33:395–399.

Fraser, G. R., and J. S. Calnan (1961): "Cleft Lip and Palate: Seasonal Incidence, Birth Weight, Birth Rank, Sex, Associated Malformations, and Parental Age," *Archives of Disease in Childhood,* 36:420–423.

French, N. R., C. W. Carter, Jr., and Walter Koenig, Jr. (1930): "The Words and Sounds of Telephone Conversations," *Bell Telephone System Technical Publications,* Monograph B-491.

Fritzell, Björn (1963): "An Electromyographic Study of the Movements of the Soft Palate in Speech," *Folia Phoniatrica,* 15:307–311.

——— (1969): "The Velopharyngeal Muscles in Speech," *Acta Oto-Laryngologica,* Supplementum 250.

Fujiki, Yoshishige, and Takuro Wada (1967): "Synchronization of Cinefluorography and Speech Observations," *CPJ,* 4:291–299.

Fujino, Hiroshi, Katumi Tanaka, and Yoshiharu Sanui (1963): "Genetic Study of Cleft-Lips and Cleft-Palates Based upon 2,828 Japanese Cases," *Kyushu Journal of Medical Science,* 14:317–331.

Fukuhara, Tatsuo (1965): "New Method and Approach to the Genetics of Cleft Lip and Cleft Palate," *Journal of Dental Research,* 44:259–268.

Fulton, John T. (1957): "Closure of the Human Palate in Embryo," *American Journal of Obstetrics and Gynecology,* 74:179–182.

Garner, L. D. (1964): "An Orthodontic Approach to the Veau Type IV Cleft Lip and Palate Problem in the Preschool Child," *CPJ,* 1:82–87.

Garrison, Fielding H. (1917): *An Introduction to the History of Medicine,* W. B. Saunders Company, Philadelphia.

Gentry, John T., Elizabeth Parkhurst, and George V. Bulin (1959): "An Epidemiological Study of Congenital Malformations in New York State," *American Journal of Public Health,* 49:497–513.

Georgiade, N(icholas) (1964): "Early Utilization of Prosthetic Appliances in Cleft Palate Patients," *PRS,* 34:617–624.

———, ed. (1968–): *Cranio-Facial-Cleft Palate Bibliography,* National Library of Medicine and American Cleft Palate Association, Durham, N.C.

———, Richard A. Mladick, and Frank L. Thorne (1968): "Positioning of the Premaxilla in Bilateral Cleft Lips by Oral Pinning and Traction," *PRS,* 41:240–243.

———, ———, ———, and Raymond Massengill (1969): "Preliminary Evaluation of the Island Flap in Cleft Palate Repair," *CPJ,* 6:488–494.

———, Kenneth L. Pickrell, and Galen W. Quinn (1964): "Varying Concepts in Bone

Grafting of Alveolar Palatal Defects," *CPJ*, 1:43–51.

Gibbons, P., and H. Bloomer (1958): "A Supportive-Type Prosthetic Speech Aid," *Journal of Prosthetic Dentistry*, 8:362–369.

Gibson, Thomas (1955): "The Prostheses of Ambroise Paré," *British Journal of Plastic Surgery*, 8:3–8.

Gier, Ronald E., and Thomas B. Fast (1967): "Median Maxillary Anterior Alveolar Cleft," *Oral Surgery, Oral Medicine, and Oral Pathology*, 24:496–502.

Gilmore, Stuart I., and Susan M. Hofman (1966): "Clefts in Wisconsin: Incidence and Related Factors," *CPJ*, 3:186–199.

Glanz, Sanford (1959): "Correction of Secondary Cleft Lip Deformities with Closure of Naso-Oral Fistulas," *PRS*, 24:74–82.

Glover, Donald M. (1961): "A Long Range Evaluation of Cleft Palate Repair," *PRS*, 27:19–30.

Goetzinger, C. P., J. E. Embrey, R. Brooks, and G. O. Proud (1960): "Auditory Assessment of Cleft Palate Adults," *Acta Oto-Laryngologica*, 52:551–557.

Goldman, Ronald, and Macalyne Fristoe (1969): *Goldman-Fristoe Test of Articulation*, American Guidance Service, Circle Pines, Minn.

Goldwyn, Robert M. (1968a): "Johann Friedrich Dieffenbach (1794–1847)," *PRS*, 42:19–28.

——— (1968b): "Jonathan Mason Warren and His Contributions to Plastic Surgery," *PRS*, 41:1–7.

——— (1969): "Bernhard von Langenbeck: His Life and Legacy," *PRS*, 44:248–254.

Goljan, Kenneth R. (1968): "Induction of Cleft Palate by Means of Internal Radiation," *Journal of Dental Research*, 47:500.

Gonzalez, Juan B., and Arnold E. Aronson (1970): "Palatal Lift Prosthesis for Treatment of Anatomic and Neurologic Palatopharyngeal Insufficiency," *CPJ*, 7:91–104.

Goodstein, Leonard D. (1961): "Intellectual Impairment in Children with Cleft Palates," *Journal of Speech and Hearing Research*, 4:287–294.

Gordon, Benjamin Lee (1959): *Medieval and Renaissance Medicine*, Philosophical Library, Philadelphia.

Gorlin, Robert J. (1968): "Syndromes Associated with Facial Clefting," *Journal of Dental Research*, 47:935.

Graber, T. M. (1968): "Normal Occlusion," *Dental Clinics of North America*, July 1968, 273–290.

Graham, Malcolm D. (1964): "A Longitudinal Study of Ear Disease and Hearing Loss in Patients with Cleft Lips and Palates," *Annals of Otology, Rhinology, and Laryngology*, 73:34–47.

———, James W. Schweiger, and William H. Olin (1962): "Hearing Loss and Ear Disease in Cleft Palate Patients with Obturators," *PRS*, 30:348–358.

Green, Rodney I. (1959): "The Radiological Appearances of the Soft Palate with Reference to the Treatment of Cleft Palate," *Journal of the Faculty of Radiologists*, 10:27–39.

Greene, John C. (1963): "Epidemiology of Congenital Clefts of the Lip and Palate," *Public Health Reports*, 78:589–602.

——— (1968): "Epidemiologic Research—1964–1967," *Journal of the American Dental Association*, 76:1350–1356.

———, Jack R. Vermillion, and Sylvia Hay (1965): "Utilization of Birth Certificates in Epidemiologic Studies of Cleft Lip and Palate," *CPJ*, 2:141–156.

———, ———, ———, Stephen F. Gibbens, and Susan Kerschbaum (1964): "Epidemiologic Study of Cleft Lip and Cleft Palate in Four States," *Journal of the American Dental Association*, 68:387–404.

Gregg, N. M. (1942): "Congenital Cataract Following German Measles in the Mother," *Transactions of the Ophthalmological Society of Australia*, 3:35–46.

——— (1945): "Rubella during Pregnancy of Mother with Its Sequelae of Congenital

Defects in Child," *Medical Journal of Australia,* 1:313–315.

Gregory, Hugo H., ed. (1968): *Learning Theory and Stuttering Therapy,* Northwestern University Press, Evanston, Ill.

Griffith, B. Herold, Clarence W. Monroe, B. Jay Hill, William F. Waldrop, and Harvey White (1968): "Motion of the Lateral Pharyngeal Walls during Velo-Pharyngeal Closure," *PRS,* 41:338–342.

Gruber, Haskell, James S. Harvin, and Dewayne Hull (1966): "The Role of the Orthodontist on the Cleft Palate Team in a Military Hospital," *PRS,* 38:560–566.

Gutzmann, Hermann Albert Carl (1893): *Vorlesungen über die Störungen der Sprache und Ihre Heilung, Gehalten in den Lehrcursen über Sprachstörungen für Aertze und Lehrer,* H. Kornfeld, Berlin.

Gylling, Uno, and Atso I. Soivio (1962): "Frequency, Morphology, and Operative Mortality in Cleft Lip and Palate in Finland," *Acta Chirurgica Scandinavica,* 123:1–5.

——— and ——— (1965): "Submucous Cleft Palate: Surgical Treatment and Results," *Acta Chirurgica Scandinavica,* 129:282–287.

Hackbush, Florentine (1951): "Psychological Studies of Cleft Palate Patients," *American Association for Cleft Palate Rehabilitation Newsletter,* 1(4):7.

Hage, J. (1966): "Millard's Island Flap in Secondary Lengthening of Cleft Soft Palates," *British Journal of Plastic Surgery,* 19:317–321.

Hagerty, Robert, Donald A. Hess, and Willis K. Mylin (1968): "Velar Motility, Velopharyngeal Closure, and Speech Proficiency in Cartilage Pharyngoplasty: The Effect of Age at Surgery," *CPJ,* 5:317–326.

———, Milton J. Hill, Harold S. Pettit, and John J. Kane (1958): "Soft Palate Movement in Normals," *Journal of Speech and Hearing Research,* 1:325–330.

——— and F. S. Hoffmeister (1954): "Velopharyngeal Closure: An Index of Speech," *PRS,* 13:290–298.

Halfond, Murray M., and John J. Ballenger (1956): "An Audiologic and Otorhinologic Study of Cleft-Lip and Cleft-Palate Cases," *Archives of Otolaryngology,* 64:58–62.

Hall, M. E. (1938): "Auditory Factors in Functional Articulatory Speech Defects," *Journal of Experimental Education,* 7:110–132.

Hamacher, Edward N. (1967): "Roll-Y Pharyngoplasty and Palate-Lengthening Procedure," *CPJ,* 4:300–307.

Hamby, Wallace B. (1967): *Ambroise Paré, Surgeon of the Renaissance,* Warren H. Green, Inc., St. Louis.

Hamilton, W. J., J. D. Boyd, and H. W. Mossman (1962): *Human Embryology,* 3rd ed., The Williams & Wilkins Company, Baltimore.

Handelman, Chester S., and Samuel Pruzansky (1968): "Occlusion and Dental Profile with Complete Bilateral Cleft Lip and Palate," *Angle Orthodontist,* 38:185–198.

Hanson, Marvin (1964): "A Study of Velopharyngeal Competence in Children with Repaired Cleft Palates," *CPJ,* 1:217–231.

Hardy, James C., and Herbert J. Arkebauer (1966): "Development of a Test for Velopharyngeal Competence during Speech," *CPJ,* 3:6–21.

Harkins, Cloyd S. (1946): "The Responsibility of the Prosthodontist in the Treatment of the Cleft Palate Patient," *American Journal of Orthodontics and Oral Surgery,* 32:684–687.

——— (1960): *Principles of Cleft Palate Prosthesis,* Columbia University Press, New York.

———, Asa Berlin, Robert L. Harding, Jacob Longacre, and Richard M. Snodgrasse (1960): "Report of the Nomenclature Committee: Proposed Morphological Classification of Congenital Cleft Lip and Cleft Palate," *Cleft Palate Bulletin,* 10:11–16.

———, ———, ———, ———, and ——— (1962): "A Classification of Cleft Lip and Cleft Palate," *PRS,* 29:31–39.

——— and Herbert Koepp-Baker (1948): "Twenty-Five Years of Cleft Palate Prosthesis," *Journal of Speech and Hearing Disorders,* 13:23–30.

Harrington, Robert (1944): "A Study of the Mechanism of Velopharyngeal Closure," *Journal of Speech Disorders,* 9:325–345.

Harris, John W. S., and Ian P. Ross (1956): "Cortisone Therapy in Early Pregnancy: Relation to Cleft Palate" *Lancet,* 270 (6931):1045–1047.

Hay, Sylvia (1967): "Incidence of Clefts and Parental Age," *CPJ,* 4:205–213.

Hess, Donald A., Robert F. Hagerty, and Willis K. Mylin (1968): "Velar Motility, Velopharyngeal Closure, and Speech Proficiency in Cartilage Pharyngoplasty: An Eight Year Study," *CPJ,* 5:153–162.

——— and Eugene T. McDonald (1960): "Consonantal Nasal Pressure in Cleft Palate Speakers," *Journal of Speech and Hearing Research,* 3:201–211.

Hill, Milton J. (1956): "An Investigation of the Attitudes and Information Possessed by Parents of Children with Clefts of the Lip and Palate," *Cleft Palate Bulletin,* 6(1):3–4.

——— and R. G. Hagerty (1960): "Efficacy of Pharyngoplasty for Speech Improvement in Postoperative Cleft Palates," *Cleft Palate Bulletin,* 10:66–67.

——— and ——— (1962): "Speech Following Pharyngoplasty in Postoperative Cleft Palate Subjects," *Journal of Speech and Hearing Research,* 5:179–184.

His, Wilhelm (1880): *Anatomie Menschlicher Embryonen,* Verlag von F. C. W. Voget, Leipzig.

Hixon, Ernest H. (1951): "A Study of the Incidence of Cleft Lip and Cleft Palate in Ontario," *Canadian Journal of Public Health,* 42:508–511.

Hixon, T. J., J. H. Saxman, and H. Diane McQueen (1967): "A Respirometric Technique for Evaluating Velopharyngeal Competence during Speech," *Folia Phoniatrica,* 19:203–219.

Hochberg, Irving, and Jack Kabcenell (1967): "Oral Stereognosis in Normal and Cleft Palate Individuals," *CPJ,* 4:47–57.

Hoffman, Saul, David R. Wesser, Fanny Calostypis, and Bernard E. Simon (1968): "The Rotation-Advancement Technique (Millard) as a Secondary Procedure in Cleft Lip Deformities," *CPJ,* 5:37–43.

Holdsworth, W. G. (1963): *Cleft Lip and Palate,* 3rd ed., Grune & Stratton, Inc., New York.

Holland, Audrey L. (1967): "Some Applications of Behavioral Principles to Clinical Speech Problems," *Journal of Speech and Hearing Disorders,* 32:11–18.

Hollmann, Karl (1969): "Theoretical Study of the Inheritance of Cleft Lips, Jaws, and Palates," *PRS,* 44:167–170.

Holmes, Edgar M., and George F. Reed (1955): "Hearing and Deafness in Cleft-Palate Patients," *Archives of Otolaryngology,* 62:620–624.

Hoopes, John E., and Jacob I. Fabrikant (1968): "Objective Evaluation of Cleft Palate Speech," *PRS,* 42:214–224.

Hoppe, Wolfgang (1965): *Lippen-, Kiefer-, Gaumenspalten,* Ferdinand Enke Verlag, Stuttgart.

Horton, Charles E., Hugh H. Crawford, Jerome E. Adamson, Samuel Buxton, Reuben Cooper, and Jack Kanter (1964): "The Prevention of Maxillary Collapse in Congenital Lip and Palate Cases," *CPJ,* 1:25–30.

Hotz, Margaret M. (1969): "Pre- and Early Postoperative Growth-Guidance in Cleft Lip and Palate Cases by Maxillary Orthopedics (an Alternative Procedure to Primary Bone-Grafting)," *CPJ,* 6:368–372.

Howard, R. D. (1969): "An Improved Appliance for the Pre-Surgical Orthodontic Preparation of the Cleft Case for Secondary Bone-Grafting," *British Journal of Plastic Surgery,* 22:90–93.

Huddart, A. G. (1968): "Studies in the Form and Dimensions of the Pre-Deciduous Maxillary Arch in Unilateral Cleft Lip and Palate," *Dental Practitioner,* 18:449.

Humphrey, Tryphena (1969): "The Relation between Human Fetal Mouth Opening Reflexes and Closure of the Palate," *American Journal of Anatomy,* 125:317–344.

Hynes, Wilfred (1950): "Pharyngoplasty by Muscle Transplantation," *British Journal of Plastic Surgery,* 3:128–135.

——— (1967): "Observations on Pharyngoplasty," *British Journal of Plastic Surgery,* 20:244–256.

Ingalls, T. H., and F. R. Philbrook (1958): "Monstrosities Induced by Hypoxia," *New England Journal of Medicine,* 259:558–564.

International Medical Congress (1964): *Second International Conference on Congenital Malformations,* International Medical Congress, Ltd., New York.

Irwin, John V., ed. (1965): "Proceedings of the Conference: Communicative Problems in Cleft Palate," *ASHA Reports,* Number 1.

Isshiki, Nobuhiko, Iwao Honjow, and Masanori Morimoto (1968): "Effects of Velopharyngeal Incompetence upon Speech," *CPJ,* 5:297–310.

——— and Masanori Morimoto (1968): "Anterior Cleft Palate Closure by Turnover Flaps," *PRS,* 42:249–251.

Ivy, Robert H. (1950): "Recent Trends in Cleft Palate Treatment," *PRS,* 5:537–538.

——— (1957):"Congenital Anomalies," *PRS,* 20:400–411.

——— (1962a): Editorial note following "A Classification of Cleft Lip and Cleft Palate," *PRS,* 29:79.

——— (1962b): "The Influence of Race on the Incidence of Certain Congenital Anomalies, Notably Cleft Lip–Cleft Palate," *PRS,* 30:581–585.

——— (1967): "The Philtrum of the Upper Lip," *PRS,* 40:94–95.

——— (1968): "Congenital Deformities Recorded on Birth Certificates in Pennsylvania, 1961–1965, with Special Reference to Racial Influence on Incidence," *PRS,* 41:50–53.

Jacobson, Bailey, and Sheldon W. Rosenstein (1965): "Early Maxillary Orthopedics: A Combination Appliance," *CPJ,* 2:369–376.

Johanson, Bengt, and Åke Ohlsson (1961): "Bone Grafting and Dental Orthopaedics in Primary and Secondary Cases of Cleft Lip and Palate," *Acta Chirurgica Scandinavica,* 122:112–124.

Johns Hopkins Medical Institutions (1968–): *Communication Disorders,* Information Center for Hearing, Speech, and Disorders of Human Communication, Baltimore.

Johnson, Thomas H., Allan E. Green, and Edwin N. Rise (1967): "Nasopharyngography: Its Technic and Uses," *Radiology,* 88:1166–1169.

Johnson, Wendell, Spencer F. Brown, James F. Curtis, Clarence W. Edney, and Jacqueline Keaster (1967): *Speech Handicapped School Children,* 3rd ed., Harper & Row, Publishers, Incorporated, New York.

———, Frederic L. Darley, and D. C. Spriestersbach (1963): *Diagnostic Methods in Speech Pathology,* Harper & Row, Publishers, Incorporated, New York.

Jordan, Harvey Ernest, and James Ernest Kindred (1942): *Textbook of Embryology,* D. Appleton-Century Company, Inc., New York.

Jordan, Ronald E., Bertram S. Kraus, and C. Marshall Neptune (1966): "Dental Abnormalities Associated with Cleft Lip and/or Palate," *CPJ,* 3:22–55.

Kantner, Claude E. (1947): "The Rationale of Blowing Exercises for Patients with Repaired Cleft Palates," *Journal of Speech Disorders,* 12:281–286.

Kaplan, Ernest N., Richard P. Jobe, and Robert A. Chase (1969): "Flexibility in Surgical Planning for Velopharyngeal Incompetence," *CPJ,* 6:166–174.

Keating, John H., ed. (1890): *Cyclopaedia of the Diseases of Children, Medical and Surgical,* J. B. Lippincott Company, Philadelphia.

Keith, Sir Arthur (1940): "Concerning the Origin and Nature of Certain Malformations of the Face, Head, and Foot," *British Journal of Surgery,* 28:173–192.

Kelsey, Charles A., Fred D. Minifie, and Thomas J. Hixon (1969): "Applications of Ultrasound in Speech Research," *Journal of Speech and Hearing Research,* 12:564–575.

———, R. J. Woodhouse, and F. D. Minifie (n.d.): *Coarticulation in the Pharynx,* Department of Radiology, Department of Communicative Disorders, University of Wisconsin, Madison.

Kemper, John W. (1946): "The Responsibility of the Surgeon in Treating Palatal and Related Defects," *American Journal of Orthodontics and Oral Surgery,* 32:667–670.

Kennedy, W. P. (1967): "Epidemiological Aspects of the Problem of Congenital Malformations," *Birth Defects: Original Article Series,* 3:1–18.

Kernahan, Desmond A., and Richard B. Stark (1958): "A New Classification for Cleft Lip and Cleft Palate," *PRS,* 22:435–441.

Kessler, Howard E. (1951): "A Study of Cleft Palate and Hare Lip Cases in the Cleveland Public School System," *Oral Surgery, Oral Medicine, and Oral Pathology,* 4:1381–1385.

——— (1954): "The Relationship of Dentistry to Speech," *Journal of the American Dental Association,* 48:44–49.

Keys, Donnette (1960): "The Nebraska Cleft Palate Team," *Journal of the Nebraska Dental Association,* 36(4):6–9.

Kiehn, Clifford, John D. DesPrez, Arthur Tucker, and Margueritte Malone (1965): "Activation of the Incompetent Soft Palate by Means of Muscle Transplants: A Preliminary Report on Sixteen Cases," *CPJ,* 2:133–140.

Kilner, T. Pomfret (1958): "The Management of the Patient with Cleft Lip and/or Palate," *American Journal of Surgery,* 95:204–210.

Kingsley, Norman W. (1880): *A Treatise on Oral Deformities* (*as a Branch of Mechanical Surgery*), D. Appleton and Company, New York.

Kirk, Samuel A., James J. McCarthy, and Winifred D. Kirk (1968): *Illinois Test of Psycholinguistic Abilities,* rev. ed., University of Illinois Press, Urbana.

Kirkpatrick, John A. (1964): "Roentgen Evaluation of Velopharyngeal Closure," *CPJ,* 1:388–390.

——— and Richard W. Olmsted (1959): "Cinefluorographic Study of Pharyngeal Function Related to Speech," *Radiology,* 73:557–559.

Kiskadden, William S., A. M. Schechtman, and Clayton Brock (1949): "Theories of the Etiology of Congenital Deformities," *International Abstracts of Surgery,* 88:1–14.

Kitamura, Hironori (1966): "Epithelial Remnants and Pearls in the Secondary Palate in the Human Abortus: A Contribution to the Study of the Mechanism of Cleft Palate Formation," *CPJ,* 3:240–257.

Knox, George, and Fenton Braithwaite (1963): "Cleft Lips and Palates in Northumberland and Durham," *Archives of Disease in Childhood,* 38:66–70.

Kobes, Herbert R., and Samuel Pruzansky (1960): "The Cleft Palate Team—A Historical Review," *American Journal of Public Health,* 50:200–205.

Kobes, Von L., and G. Kittel (1966): "Eine Möglichkeit der Medico-Mechanischen, Aktiven Behandlung der Rhinolalia Aperta Functionalis," *Folia Phoniatrica,* 18:19–25.

Koepp-Baker, Herbert (1946): "The Responsibility of the Speech Correctionist in the Treatment of the Cleft Palate Patient Who Has Received Surgical or Prosthetic Treatment," *American Journal of Orthodontics and Oral Surgery,* 32:714–717.

Krantz, Henrietta C., and Florence M. Henderson (1947): "Relationship between Maternal Ancestry and Incidence of Cleft Palate," *Journal of Speech Disorders,* 12:267–278.

Kraus, Bertram S. (1960): "Prenatal Growth and Morphology of the Human Bony Palate," *Journal of Dental Research,* 39:1177–1199.

——— and Jay D. Decker (1960): "The Prenatal Inter-Relationships of the Maxilla and Premaxilla in the Facial Development of Man," *Acta Anatomica,* 40:278–294.

———, Hironori Kitamura, and Ralph A. Latham (1966): *Atlas of Developmental Anatomy of the Face,* Hoeber Medical Division, Harper & Row, Publishers, Incorporated, New York.

Krogman, Wilton M. (1954): "The Problem of the Cleft Palate Face," *PRS,* 14:370–375.

Lang, Brien R. (1967): "Modification of the Palatal Lift Speech Aid," *Journal of Prosthetic Dentistry,* 17:620–626.

Langman, Jan (1963): *Medical Embryology: Human Development—Normal and Abnormal,* The Williams & Wilkins Company, Baltimore.

Latham, R. A. (1966): "The Pathogenesis of Cleft Palate Associated with the Pierre Robin Syndrome. An Analysis of a Seventeen-Week Human Foetus," *British Journal of Plastic Surgery,* 19:205–214.

——— and W. R. Burston (1964): "The Effect of Unilateral Cleft of the Lip and Palate on Maxillary Growth Pattern," *British Journal of Plastic Surgery,* 17:10–17.

Lauterstein, Aubrey, and Mark Mendelsohn (1964): "An Analysis of the Caries Experience of 285 Cleft Palate Children," *CPJ,* 1:314–319.

Lee, Laura (1969): *Northwestern Syntax Screening Test,* Northwestern University Press, Evanston, Ill.

Leibowitz, Joshua O. (1958): "Amatus Lusitanus and the Obturator in Cleft Palates," *Journal of the History of Medicine and Allied Sciences,* 13:492–503.

Lejeune, J., M. Gautier, and R. Turpin (1959): "Etude des Chromosomes Somatiques de Neuf Enfants Mongoliens," *Comptes Rendus Hebdomadaires des Séances de l'Académie des Sciences,* 248:1721–1722.

LeMesurier, A. B. (1955): "The Quadrilateral Mirault Flap Operation for Hare-Lip," *PRS,* 16:422–433.

——— (1962): *Hare-Lips and Their Treatment,* The Williams & Wilkins Company, Baltimore.

Lencione, Ruth M., ed. (1968): *Cleft Palate Habilitation,* Syracuse University Press, Syracuse, N.Y.

Letterman, Gordon, Maxine Schurter, and Bahman Teimourian (1964): "Vilray Papin Blair's Early Concept of the Cleft Palate Problem," *CPJ,* 1:125–129.

Levin, Nathaniel M., ed. (1962): *Voice and Speech Disorders: Medical Aspects,* Charles C Thomas, Publisher, Springfield, Ill.

Lewin, Michael L. (1962): "The Management of Cleft Lip and Palate Cases in the Soviet Union," *PRS,* 29:22–30.

——— (1964): "Management of Cleft Lip and Palate in the United States and Canada," *PRS,* 33:383–393.

Lewis, Ruth (1961): "A Survey of the Intelligence of Cleft Palate Children in Ontario," *Cleft Palate Bulletin,* 11:83–85.

Lewis, Stephen R., John B. Lynch, and Truman G. Blocker, Jr. (1968): "Fascial Slings for Tongue Stabilization in the Pierre Robin Syndrome," *PRS,* 42:237–241.

Lifton, Jacob C. (1956): "Methods of Feeding Infants with Cleft Palates," *Journal of the American Dental Association,* 53:22–31.

Lillywhite, Herold (1956): "Teamwork in the Oregon Cleft Palate Program," *Journal of Speech and Hearing Disorders,* 21:18–24.

Lindsay, D. W., A. B. LeMesurier, and A. W. Farmer (1962): "A Study of the Speech Results of a Large Series of Cleft Palate Patients," *PRS,* 29:273–288.

Linthicum, Fred H., Harold Body, and Jacqueline Keaster (1959): "Incidence of Middle Ear Disease in Children with Cleft Palate," *Cleft Palate Bulletin,* 9:23–25.

Lintz, Lois Brian, and Dorothy Sherman (1961): "Phonetic Elements and Perception of Nasality," *Journal of Speech and Hearing Research,* 4:381–396.

Lis, Edward F., Samuel Pruzansky, Herbert Koepp-Baker, and Herbert R. Kobes (1956): "Cleft Lip and Cleft Palate: Perspectives in Management," *Pediatric Clinics of North America,* November 1956, 995–1028.

Liston, Robert (1846): *Elements of Surgery,* 4th Am. ed., Ed. Barrington and Geo. D. Haswell, Philadelphia.

Litzow, Thaddeus, and Frederic L. Darley (1966): "Evaluation of Velopharyngeal Competence after Primary Repair of the Palate," *Mayo Clinic Proceedings,* 41:524–535.

Loeb, William J. (1964): "Speech, Hearing, and the Cleft Palate," *Archives of Otolaryngology,* 79:4–14.

Longacre, J. J., ed. (1968): *Craniofacial Anomalies: Pathogenesis and Repair,* J. B. Lippincott Company, Philadelphia.

Loretz, Wayne, W. W. Westmoreland, and Lloyd F. Richards (1961): "A Study of Cleft Lip and Cleft Palate Births in California, 1955," *American Journal of Public Health,* 51:873–877.

Luban, Joseph (1955): "Speech and the Cleft Palate Patient," *American Journal of Orthodontics,* 41:121–136.

Lubit, Erwin, and Robert S. Larsen (1969): "The Lubit Palatal Exerciser: A Preliminary Report," *CPJ,* 6:120–133.

Lubker, James F. (1968): "An Electromyographic-Cinefluorographic Investigation of Velar Function during Normal Speech Production," *CPJ,* 5:1–18.

——— and Kenneth L. Moll (1965): "Simultaneous Oral-Nasal Air Flow Measurements and Cinefluorographic Observations during Speech Production," *CPJ,* 2:257–272.

——— and Hughlett L. Morris (1968): "Predicting Cinefluorographic Measures of Velopharyngeal Opening from Lateral Still X-Ray Films," *Journal of Speech and Hearing Research,* 11:747–753.

Lufkin, Arthur Ward (1938): *A History of Dentistry,* Lea & Febiger, Philadelphia.

Luse, Eleanor, J. Heisse, and J. Foley (1964): "The Vocal Approach in the Correction of Cleft Palate Speech," *Folia Phoniatrica,* 16:123–129.

Lutz, Kenneth R., and Fred B. Moor (1955): "A Study of Factors in the Occurrence of Cleft Palate," *Journal of Speech and Hearing Disorders,* 20:271–276.

Lynch, Henry T., compiler (1969): *International Directory of Genetic Services,* 2nd ed., The National Foundation, New York.

McCabe, Peter A. (1966): "A Coding Procedure for Classification of Cleft Lip and Cleft Palate," *CPJ,* 3:383–391.

McCroskey, R. L., Jr. (n.d.): *Some Effects of Anesthetizing the Articulators under Conditions of Normal and Delayed Side-Tone,* OSU Research Foundation and U.S. Naval School of Aviation Medicine, Bureau of Medicine and Surgery, Project NM001 104 500, Report No. 65, Pensacola, Fla.

McDonald, Eugene T. (1964): *Articulation Testing and Treatment, A Sensory-Motor Approach,* Stanwix House, Pittsburgh.

——— and Herbert Koepp-Baker (1951): "Cleft Palate Speech: An Integration of Research and Clinical Observations," *Journal of Speech and Hearing Disorders,* 16:9–20.

McEvitt, William G. (1952): "Cleft Lip and Palate and Parental Age," *PRS,* 10:77–82.

——— (1968): "Micrognathia and Its Management," *PRS,* 41:450–455.

———, Kenneth W. Sproule, J. Hilliard Hicks, and Eugene P. Hawthorne (1969): "Closure of Anterior Cleft Palate by Spontaneous Tissue Growth," *PRS,* 44:125–133.

McIntosh, Rustin, Katharine K. Merritt, Mary R. Richards, Mary H. Samuels, and Marjorie T. Bellows (1954): "The Incidence of Congenital Malformations: A Study of 5,964 Pregnancies," *Pediatrics,* 14:505–522.

MacMahon, Brian, and Thomas McKeown (1953): "The Incidence of Harelip and Cleft Palate Related to Birth Rank and Maternal Age," *American Journal of Human Genetics,* 5:176–183.

MacNalty, Sir Arthur Salusbury, ed. (1961): *The British Medical Dictionary,* The Caxton Publishing Company, Ltd., London.

McNeil, C. Kerr (1954): *Oral and Facial Deformity,* Pitman Publishing Corporation, New York.

McWilliams, Betty Jane (1954): "Some Factors in the Intelligibility of Cleft-Palate Speech," *Journal of Speech and Hearing Disorders,* 19:524–527.

——— (1956): "Some Observations of Environmental Factors in Speech Development of Children with Cleft Palate," *Cleft Palate Bulletin,* 6(1):4–5.

——— (1958): "Articulation Problems of a Group of Cleft Palate Adults," *Journal of Speech and Hearing Research,* 1:68–74.

——— and Doris P. Bradley (1965): "Ratings of Velopharyngeal Closure during Blowing and Speech," *CPJ,* 2:46–55.

——— and Bertram Girdany (1964): "The Use of Televex in Cleft Palate Research," *CPJ,* 1:398–401.

———, Ross H. Musgrave, and Phyllis A. Crozier (1968): "The Influence of Head Position upon Velopharyngeal Closure," *CPJ,* 5:117–124.

Machida, Junji (1967): "Air Flow Rate and Articulatory Movement during Speech," *CPJ,* 4:240–248.

Mader, John B. (1954): "The Relative Frequency of Occurrence of English Consonant Sounds in Words in the Speech of Children in Grades One, Two, and Three," *Speech Monographs,* 21:294–300.

Maisels, David O. (1966): "Early Orthopaedic Treatment of Clefts of the Primary and Secondary Palates: A Surgeon's View," *CPJ,* 3:76–86.

——— (1967): "The Timing of the Various Operations Required for Complete Alveolar Clefts and Their Influence on Facial Growth," *British Journal of Plastic Surgery,* 20:230–243.

Makuen, G. Hudson (1901): "Cleft Palate and Its Relation to Speech," *Transactions of the Twenty-Third Annual Meeting of the American Laryngological Association,* 116–122.

Malson, T. S. (1957): "Nonobstructing Speech Aid during Growth and Orthodontic Treatment," *Journal of Prosthetic Dentistry,* 7:403–415.

——— (1969): "Prosthesis for the Newborn," *Journal of Prosthetic Dentistry,* 21:384–387.

Maltz, Maxwell (1946): *Evolution of Plastic Surgery,* Froben Press, New York.

Marcks, Kerwin M., Allan E. Trevaskis, and Milton Tuerk (1955): "100 Palatoplasties," *PRS,* 16:352–361.

Marks, Carol Rea (1968): "Tongue Thrusting and Interdentalization of Speech Sounds among Cleft Palate and Noncleft Palate Subjects," *CPJ,* 5:48–56.

Martone, Alexander L., and John W. Black (1962): "An Approach to Prosthodontics through Speech Science," *Journal of Prosthetic Dentistry,* 12:629–636.

Mason, Francis (1877): *On Harelip and Cleft Palate,* J. & A. Churchill, London.

Mason, R. M., and S. A. Hoster (1968): "Clinical, Radiographic, and Speech Findings in Speakers with Primary Palate Clefts and Congenital Palatopharyngeal Incompetence," paper presented at 44th Annual Convention, American Speech and Hearing Association.

Massengill, R(aymond), Jr., and M. Bryson (1967): "A Study of Velopharyngeal Function as Related to Perceived Nasality of Vowels, Utilizing a Cine-Fluorographic Television Monitor," *Folia Phoniatrica,* 19:45–52.

———, Kenneth Pickrell, and Judith Fetterrolf (1968): "Relationship between Articulation Errors and Other Factors in Children with Cleft Palates," *PRS,* 41:564–567.

———, Galen W. Quinn, Kenneth L. Pickrell, and Carole Levinson (1968): "Therapeutic Exercise and Velopharyngeal Gap," *CPJ,* 5:44–47.

Masters, F. W., H. G. Bingham, and D. W. Robinson (1960): "The Prevention and Treatment of Hearing Loss in the Cleft Palate Child," *PRS,* 25:503–509.

Mather, K., and U. Philip (1940): "The Inheritance of Harelip and Cleft Palate in Man," *Annals of Eugenics,* 10:403–416.

Matthews, David, and W. Grossman (1964): "Restoration of the Collapsed Maxillary Arch by Rapid Expansion and Bone Grafting," *CPJ,* 1:430–440.

Matthews, Jack, and Margaret C. Byrne (1953): "An Experimental Study of Tongue Flexibility in Children with Cleft Palates," *Journal of Speech and Hearing Disorders,* 18:43–47.

Mazaheri, Mohammad (1958): "Statistical Analysis of Patients with Congenital Cleft Lip and/or Cleft Palate at the Lancaster Cleft Palate Clinic," *PRS,* 21:193–203.

——— (1962): "Indications and Contraindications for Prosthetic Speech Appliances in Cleft Palate," *PRS,* 30:663–669.

———, Robert L. Harding, and Surender Nanda (1967): "The Effect of Surgery on Maxillary Growth and Cleft Width," *PRS,* 40:22–30.

——— and R. T. Millard (1965): "Changes in Nasal Resonance Related to Differences in Location and Dimension of Speech Bulbs," *CPJ,* 2:167–175.

———, ———, and Duane M. Erickson (1964): "Cineradiographic Comparison of Normal to Noncleft Subjects with Velopharyngeal Inadequacy," *CPJ,* 1:199–209.

———, Surender Nanda, and Viken Sassouni (1967): "Comparison of Midfacial Development of Children with Clefts with Their Siblings," *CPJ,* 4:334–341.

——— and Pradeep P. Sahni (1969): "Techniques of Cephalometry, Photography, and Oral Impressions for Infants," *Journal of Prosthetic Dentistry,* 21:315–323.

Means, Beverly Jane, and John Irwin (1954): "An Analysis of Certain Measures of Intelligence and Hearing in a Sample of the Wisconsin Cleft Palate Population," *Cleft Palate Bulletin,* 4(2):4.

Mecham, Merlin (1959): *Verbal Language Development Test,* American Guidance Service, Circle Pines, Minn.

———, J. Lorin Jex, and J. Dean Jones (1967): *Utah Test of Language Development,* Communication Research Associates, Salt Lake City.

Meinhold, Von G. (1964): "Zur Objektivierung der Postoperativen Sprachfunktion bei Patienten mit Gaumenspalten," *Folia Phoniatrica,* 16:81–96.

Merkeley, Howard J. (1959): "Cleft Palate Prosthesis," *Journal of Prosthetic Dentistry,* 9:506–513.

Meskin, Lawrence H., Robert J. Gorlin, and Robert J. Isaacson (1964): "Abnormal Morphology of the Soft Palate: I. The Prevalence of Cleft Uvula," *CPJ,* 1:342–346.

———, Samuel Pruzansky, and Warren H. Gullen (1968): "An Epidemiologic Investigation of Factors Related to the Extent of Facial Clefts: 1. Sex of Patient," *CPJ,* 5:23–29.

Metrakos, Julius D., Katherine Metrakos, and Hamilton Baxter (1958): "Clefts of the Lip and Palate in Twins," *PRS,* 22:109–122.

Mettler, Cecilia C. (1947): *History of Medicine,* The Blakiston Company, Philadelphia.

Metzger, James T. (1957): "Consideration of Factors in Determining the Age for Closure of Congenital Palatal Clefts," *Cleft Palate Bulletin,* 7(1):7–8.

Milham, Samuel, Jr. (1963): "Underreporting of Incidence of Cleft Lip and Palate," *American Journal of Diseases of Children,* 106:185–188.

Milisen, Robert, and Associates (1954): "The Disorder of Articulation: A Systematic Clinical and Experimental Approach," *Journal of Speech and Hearing Disorders,* Monograph Supplement 4.

Millard, D. Ralph (1962): "Wide and/or Short Cleft Palate," *PRS,* 29:40–57.

——— (1963a): "The Island Flap in Cleft Palate Surgery," *Surgery, Gynecology, and Obstetrics,* 116:297–300.

——— (1963b): "The Triad of Columella Deformities," *PRS,* 31:370–384.

——— (1964a): "Composite Lip Flaps and Grafts in Secondary Cleft Deformities," *British Journal of Plastic Surgery,* 17:22–29.

——— (1964b): "Rotation-Advancement Principle in Cleft Lip Closure," *CPJ,* 1:246–252.

——— (1966): "A New Use of the Island Flap in Wide Palate Clefts," *PRS,* 38:330–335.

——— (1968): "Extensions of the Rotation-Advancement Principle for Wide Unilateral Cleft Lips," *PRS,* 42:535–544.

———, George Balber, and Betty W. Philips (1967): "A Data Collection System for Cleft Lip and Palate: 1. Surgical Evaluation," *CPJ,* 4:277–290.

——— and Kenneth A. McNeill (1965): "The Incidence of Cleft Lip and Palate in Jamaica," *CPJ,* 2:384–388.

——— and Sydney Williams (1968): "Median Lip Clefts of the Upper Lip," *PRS,* 42:4–14.

Millard, Robert T., ed. (1964): *An Integrated Program Concerned with Habilitation-Rehabilitation of Oral-Facial-Communicative Disorders,* Lancaster Cleft Palate Clinic, Lancaster, Pa.

Miller, E. R. (1959): "Cinefluorography in Practice," *Radiology,* 73:560–565.

Minifie, Fred. D., Thomas J. Hixon, Charles A. Kelsey, and Robert J. Woodhouse (1969): *Lateral Pharyngeal Wall Movement during Speech Production,* Department of Communicative Disorders, Department of Rehabilitative Medicine, Department of Radiology, University of Wisconsin, Madison.

Moffat, Helen M. (1951): "Counseling Parents of Cleft Palate Children," *American Association for Cleft Palate Rehabilitation Newsletter,* 1(4):7–8.

Moll, Kenneth L. (1962): "Velopharyngeal Closure on Vowels," *Journal of Speech and Hearing Research,* 5:30–37.

——— (1964a): "Cineradiography in Research and Clinical Studies of the Velopharyngeal Mechanism," *CPJ,* 1:391–397.

——— (1964b): " 'Objective' Measures of Nasality," *CPJ,* 1:371–373.

——— (1965): "A Cinefluorographic Study of Velopharyngeal Function in Normals during Various Activities," *CPJ,* 2:112–122.

——— and Thomas H. Shriner (1967): "Preliminary Investigation of a New Concept of Velar Activity during Speech," *CPJ,* 4:58–69.

Moller, Karlind T., Clark D. Starr, and Richard R. Martin (1969): "The Application of Operant Conditioning Procedures to the Facial Grimace Problem," *CPJ,* 6:193–201.

Monie, I. W., and A. Cacciatore (1962): "The Development of the Philtrum," *PRS,* 30:313–321.

Monroe, Clarence W. (1966): "Midline Cleft of the Lower Lip, Mandible, and Tongue, with Flexion Contracture of the Neck: Case Report and Review of the Literature," *PRS,* 38:312–319.

———, B. Herold Griffith, Sheldon W. Rosenstein, and Bailey N. Jacobson (1968): "The Correction and Preservation of Arch Form in Complete Clefts of the Palate and Alveolar Ridge," *PRS,* 41:108–112.

Morimitsu, K. Jack (1958): "A Review of Prosthetic Therapy of the Cleft Palate Patient," *Cleft Palate Bulletin,* 8(2):7–10.

Morley, Muriel E. (1967): *Cleft Palate and Speech,* 6th ed., The Williams & Wilkins Company, Baltimore.

Morris, Henry (1953): *Human Anatomy,* 11th ed., The Blakiston Division of McGraw-Hill Book Company, New York.

Morris, Hughlett L. (1962): "Communication Skills of Children with Cleft Lips and Palates," *Journal of Speech and Hearing Research,* 5:79–90.

———, ed. (1965): *Cleft Lip and Palate: Criteria for Physical Management,* 1963 Conference, University of Iowa, Iowa City.

——— (1966): "The Oral Manometer as a Diagnostic Tool in Clinical Speech Pathology," *Journal of Speech and Hearing Disorders,* 31:362–369.

——— and Jeanne K. Smith (1962): "A Multiple Approach for Evaluating Velopharyngeal Competency," *Journal of Speech and Hearing Disorders,* 27:218–226.

——— and D. C. Spriestersbach (1967): "The Pharyngeal Flap as a Speech Mechanism," *PRS,* 39:66–70.

———, ———, and Frederic L. Darley (1961): "An Articulation Test for Assessing Competency of Velopharyngeal Closure," *Journal of Speech and Hearing Research,* 4:48–55.

Moss, James P. (1968): "Rapid Expansion of the Maxillary Arch," *Journal of Practical Orthodontics,* 11:165–171.

Moss, Melvin L. (1956): "Malformations of the Skull Base Associated with Cleft Palate Deformity," *PRS,* 17:226–234.

———, Bertram E. Bromberg, In Chul Song, and Gilbert Eisenman (1968): "The Passive Role of Nasal Septal Cartilage in Mid-Facial Growth," *PRS,* 41:536–541.

Muir, I. F. K. (1966): "Repair of the Cleft Alveolus," *British Journal of Plastic Surgery,* 19:30–36.

Mukherji, Murari Mohan (1969): "Cheek Flap for Short Palates," *CPJ,* 6:415–420.

Munson, S. E., and Anna M. May (1955): "Are Cleft Palate Persons of Sub-Normal Intelligence?" *Journal of Educational Research,* 48:617–621.

Murphy, Douglas P. (1947): *Congenital Malformations,* 2nd ed., J. B. Lippincott Company, Philadelphia.

Murray, R. W. (1904): "Geographical Distribution of Harelip and Cleft Palate," *Lancet,* Vol. 1 for 1904 (4212):1423.

Musgrave, Ross H. (1963): "Observations on the Repair of the Unilateral Cleft Lip," *Cleft Palate Bulletin,* 13:4–7.

Mylin, Willis K., Robert F. Hagerty, and Donald A. Hess (1968): "The Pin-Retained Prosthesis in Cleft Palate Orthopedics," *CPJ,* 5:219–228.

Mysak, Edward D. (1966): *Speech Pathology and Feedback Theory,* Charles C Thomas, Publisher, Springfield, Ill.

National Institutes of Health (1969): *The National Institute of Dental Research Directory of U.S. Facilities Providing Cleft Lip and Cleft Palate Services,* U.S. Department of Health, Education, and Welfare, Washington, D.C.

Neel, James V. (1958): "A Study of Major Congenital Defects in Japanese Infants," *American Journal of Human Genetics,* 10:398–445.

Neumann, B. (1967): "Measurement of Changes Produced by Presurgical Treatment of Unilateral Clefts," *Report of the Forty-Third Congress, European Orthodontic Society,* 315–323.

Neuner, Otto (1969): "Special Problems in Full Rehabilitation of the Nasal Base and Upper Lip in Single and Double Clefts," *CPJ,* 6:384–398.

Nylén, Bengt O. (1961): "Cleft Palate and Speech," *Acta Radiologica,* Supplementum 203.

Obregon, Gonzalo, and Jeanne K. Smith (1959): "The Posterior Pharyngeal Flap Palatoplasty: II. Analysis of 29 Patients," *Archives of Otolaryngology,* 69:174–175.

O'Hara, A. Edward (1963): "Roentgen Evaluation of Patients with Cleft Palate," *Radiologic Clinics of North America,* 1:1–11.

Oldfield, Michael C. (1949): "Modern Trends in Hare Lip and Cleft Palate Surgery with a Review of 500 Cases," *British Journal of Surgery,* 37:178–194.

——— (1959): "Some Observations on the Cause and Treatment of Hare-Lip and Cleft Palate, Based on the Treatment of 1,041 Patients," *British Journal of Surgery,* 46:311–321.

——— and G. T. Tate (1964): "Cleft Lip and Palate: Some Ideas on Prevention and

Treatment, Based on 1,166 Cases," *British Journal of Plastic Surgery,* 17:1–9.

Olin, William H. (1960): *Cleft Lip and Palate Rehabilitation,* Charles C Thomas, Publisher, Springfield, Ill.

Olinger, Nathaniel A. (1942): "Surgical Prosthesis," *American Journal of Orthodontics and Oral Surgery,* 28:222–238.

Orban, Balint J., ed. (1957): *Oral Histology and Embryology,* 4th ed., The C. V. Mosby Company, St. Louis.

Orticochea, Miguel (1968): "Construction of a Dynamic Muscle Sphincter in Cleft Palates," *PRS,* 41:323–327.

Ortiz-Monasterio, F., Alfonso Serrano R., Gustavo Barrera P., Hermann Rodriguez-Hoffman, and Enrique Vinageras (1966): "A Study of Untreated Adult Cleft Palate Patients," *PRS,* 38:36–41.

Osborne, G. S., and S. Pruzansky (1968): "The Effect of Cervical Anomalies on Nasopharyngeal Depth," paper presented at 44th Annual Convention, American Speech and Hearing Association.

Owsley, John Q., Lucie I. Lawson, Earl R. Miller, and Harry M. Blackfield (1966): "Experience with the High Attached Pharyngeal Flap," *PRS,* 38:232–242.

Ozerovic, B., and M. Markovic (1967): "Our Experiences in Early and Late Presurgical Orthopaedic Treatment of Congenital Clefts of Lip and Palate," *Report of the Forty-Third Congress, European Orthodontic Society,* 325–336.

Padgett, Earl Calvin (1930): "The Repair of Cleft Palate after Unsuccessful Operations," *Archives of Surgery,* 20:453–472.

Palmer, John M., and Martin R. Adams (1962): "The Oral Image of Children with Cleft Lips and Palates," *Cleft Palate Bulletin,* 12:72–76.

Pannbacker, Mary (1968): "Congenital Malformations and Cleft Lip and Palate," *CPJ,* 5:333–339.

——— (1969): "Hearing Loss and Cleft Palate," *CPJ,* 6:50–56.

Paradise, Jack L., and Charles D. Bluestone (1968): "On the Universality of Otitis Media in Infants with Cleft Palate," paper presented at 26th Annual Meeting, American Cleft Palate Association.

Passavant, Philippus Gustavus (1869): "Ueber die Verschliessung des Schlundes beim Sprechen," *Archiv für Pathologische Anatomie und Physiologie und für Klinische Medicin,* 46:1–31, figures.

Patten, Bradley M. (1953, 1968): *Human Embryology,* 2nd ed., The Blakiston Division of McGraw-Hill Book Company, New York; 3rd ed., McGraw-Hill Book Company, New York.

Peat, John H. (1968): "A Cephalometric Study of Tongue Position," *American Journal of Orthodontics,* 54:339–351.

Peer, Lyndon A., Walter H. Bryan, Lyon P. Strean, John C. Walker, W. G. Bernhard, and George C. Peck (1958): "Induction of Cleft Palate in Mice by Cortisone and Its Reduction by Vitamins," *Journal of the International College of Surgeons,* 30:249–254.

———, Lyon P. Strean, John C. Walker, Jr., William G. Bernhard, and George C. Peck (1958): "Study of 400 Pregnancies with Birth of Cleft Lip-Palate Infants," *PRS,* 22:442–449.

Peet, Eric W., and T. J. S. Patterson (1963): *The Essentials of Plastic Surgery,* F. A. Davis Company, Philadelphia.

Pennisi, Vincent R., William R. Shadish, and Horace Klabunde (1969): "Orbicularis Oris Muscle in the Cleft Lip Repair," *CPJ,* 6:141–153.

Petersen, William F. (1934): "The Distribution of Congenital Malformations in the United States," *American Journal of Obstetrics and Gynecology,* 28:70–77.

Petit, P., and J. Psaume (1967): "Expansion Pré-Opératoire et Greffon Osseux dans le Traitement du Bec-de-Lièvre," *Report of the Forty-Third Congress, European Orthodontic Society,* 341–348.

Phair, Gretchen Mueller (1947): "The Wisconsin Cleft Palate Program," *Journal of Speech Disorders,* 12:410–414.

Philips, Betty Jane W., and Kenneth R. Bzoch (1969): "Reliability of Judgments of Articulation of Cleft Palate Speakers," *CPJ,* 6:24–34.

——— and Robert J. Harrison (1969a): "Articulation Patterns of Preschool Cleft Palate Children," *CPJ,* 6:245–253.

——— and ——— (1969b): "Language Skills of Preschool Cleft Palate Children," *CPJ,* 6:108–119.

Pickerill, H. P. (1950–1951): "The Other Side of the Lantern: A Series of Operations by Lord Lister," *British Journal of Plastic Surgery,* 3:216–221.

Pickrell, Kenneth, Galen Quinn, and Raymond Massengill (1968): "Primary Bone Grafting of the Maxilla in Clefts of the Lip and Palate: A Four Year Study," *PRS,* 41:438–443.

Pierce, George Warren, K. F. Terwilliger, Vincent Pennisi, and E. Horace Klabunde (1955): "Early Orthodontic Treatment in Cleft Palate Children," *PRS,* 16:3–15.

Pitanguy, Ivo, and Talita Franco (1967): "Nonoperated Facial Fissures in Adults," *PRS,* 39:569–577.

Pitzner, Joan C., and Hughlett L. Morris (1966): "Articulation Skills and Adequacy of Breath Pressure Ratios of Children with Cleft Palate," *Journal of Speech and Hearing Disorders,* 31:26–40.

Platt, James H. (1947): "The History and Principles of Obturator Design," *Journal of Speech Disorders,* 12:111–123.

Platt, L. Jay, and J. Douglas Noll (1969): "Nonphonetic Influences on Velar Position: Effects of Vocal Frequency and Vocal Effort," paper presented at 1969 International Congress on Cleft Palate.

Plummer, George (1952): "Anomalies Occurring in Children Exposed *in Utero* to the Atomic Bomb at Hiroshima," *Pediatrics,* 10:687–693.

Powell, William J., and Hilger Perry Jenkins (1968): "Transverse Facial Clefts: Report of Three Cases," *PRS,* 42:454–459.

Prins, David, and H. Harlan Bloomer (1965): "A Word Intelligibility Approach to the Study of Speech Change in Oral Cleft Patients," *CPJ,* 2:357–368.

——— and ——— (1968): "Consonant Intelligibility: A Procedure for Evaluating Speech in Oral Cleft Subjects," *Journal of Speech and Hearing Research,* 11:128–137.

Pruzansky, Samuel (1953): "Description, Classification, and Analysis of Unoperated Clefts of the Lip and Palate," *American Journal of Orthodontics,* 39:590–611.

———, ed. (1961): *Congenital Anomalies of the Face and Associated Structures,* Charles C Thomas, Publisher, Springfield, Ill.

——— (1964): "Pre-Surgical Orthopedics and Bone Grafting for Infants with Cleft Lip and Palate: A Dissent," *CPJ,* 1:164–187.

——— and Howard Aduss (1964): "Arch Form and the Deciduous Occlusion in Complete Unilateral Clefts," *CPJ,* 1:411–418.

——— and ——— (1967): "The Prevalence of Arch Collapse and Malocclusion in Complete Unilateral Cleft Lip and Palate," *Report of the Forty-Third Congress, European Orthodontic Society,* 365–382.

Public Health Service (1966): *Research Explores Cleft Palate,* Public Health Service Publication No. 1487, Health Information Series No. 135, Washington, D.C.

Quigley, Lawrence F., Jr., F. R. Shiere, Richard C. Webster, and Carolus M. Cobb (1964): "Measuring Palatopharyngeal Competence with the Nasal Anemometer," *CPJ,* 1:304–313.

Quinn, Galen W., Kenneth L. Pickrell, and Raymond Massengill, Jr. (1967): "Rapid Expansion Procedures—Cleft Lip-Palate," paper presented at 25th Annual Meeting, American Cleft Palate Association.

Randall, P(eter) (1957): "The Management of Cleft-Lip and Cleft-Palate Patients,"

American Journal of Medical Science, 233:204–219.

——— (1959): "A Triangular Flap Operation for the Primary Repair of Unilateral Clefts of the Lip," *PRS,* 23:331–347.

———, Wilton M. Krogman, and Soona Jahina (1965): "Pierre Robin and the Syndrome That Bears His Name," *CPJ,* 2:237–246.

———, A. Edward O'Hara, and Frank P. Bakes (1958): "A Simplified X-Ray Technique for the Study of Soft Palate Function in Patients with Poor Speech," *PRS,* 21:345–356.

Rayne, John (1966): "An Improved Technique for Buccal Inlays in Cleft Lip and Palate Cases," *British Journal of Plastic Surgery,* 19:124–127.

Rees, Thomas D., Chester A. Swinyard, and John Marquis Converse (1962): "The Prolabium in the Bilateral Cleft Lip: An Electromyographic and Biopsy Study," *PRS,* 30:651–662.

Reidy, J. P. (1964): "Pharyngoplasty in Speech," *British Journal of Plastic Surgery,* 17:389–399.

Rhone, J. W. (1894): "Duplex Obturator," *International Dental Journal,* 15:545–549.

Richardson, William P., and A. C. Higgins (1964): "A Survey of Handicapping Conditions and Handicapped Children in Alamance County, North Carolina," *American Journal of Public Health,* 54:1817–1830.

Ricketts, R. M. (1954): "The Cranial Base and Soft Structures in Cleft Palate Speech and Breathing," *PRS,* 14:47–61.

——— (1968): "Esthetics, Environment, and the Law of Lip Relation," *American Journal of Orthodontics,* 54:272–289.

Ridley, Doris R. (1968): "Class III Occlusions in Patients with Clefts of Lip and Palate," *Dental Practitioner,* 19:25–36.

Riesman, David (1935): *The Story of Medicine in the Middle Ages,* Paul B. Hoeber, Inc., New York.

Riley, Glyndon D. (1966): *The Riley Articulation and Language Test,* Western Psychological Services, Beverly Hills, Calif.

Ritter, E. Gene (1962): "A Cinefluorographic and Spectrographic Study of Perceived Nasality," unpublished doctor's dissertation, University of Missouri-Columbia.

Robertson, N. R. E., and R. Hilton (1968): "A Method of Demonstrating Changes Produced by Presurgical Oral Orthopaedics," *Dental Practitioner,* 18:449–450.

——— and A. Jolleys (1968): "Effects of Early Bone Grafting in Complete Clefts of Lip and Palate: Preliminary Report," *PRS,* 42:414–421.

Roe, Vivian, and Robert Milisen (1942): "The Effect of Maturation upon Defective Articulation in Elementary Grades," *Journal of Speech Disorders,* 7:37–50.

Rogers, Blair O. (1967): "Palatal Surgery Prior to von Graefe's Pioneering Staphylorrhaphy (1816): An Historical Review of the Early Causes of Surgical Indifference to Repairing the Cleft Palate," *PRS,* 39:1–19.

Rosen, Morton S., and Kenneth R. Bzoch (1958): "The Prosthetic Speech Appliance in Rehabilitation of Patients with Cleft Palate," *Journal of the American Dental Association,* 57:203–210.

Rosenstein, Sheldon W., and Bailey N. Jacobson (1967): "Early Maxillary Orthopedics: A Sequence of Events," *CPJ,* 4:197–204.

Rosenzweig, Sanford (1966): "Psychological Stress in Cleft Palate Etiology," *Journal of Dental Research,* 45:1585–1593.

Ross, R. B., and Malcolm C. Johnston (1967): "The Effect of Early Orthodontic Treatment on Facial Growth in Cleft Lip and Palate," *CPJ,* 4:157–164.

——— and W. K. Lindsay (1965): "The Cervical Vertebrae as a Factor in the Etiology of Cleft Palate," *CPJ,* 2:273–281.

Rouse, Verna V. (1956): "A Study of the Articulation of a Group of Children with Cleft Lips and Palates," *Cleft Palate Bulletin,* 6(3):6–9.

Rubin, Leonard, Richard Walden, Bertram Bromberg, and Gene Pressel (1961): "Summary of Pharyngeal Flap: Statistical Evaluation," *Cleft Palate Bulletin,* 11:4–5.

Ruess, Aubrey L. (1965): "A Comparative Study of Cleft Palate Children and Their Siblings," *Journal of Clinical Psychology,* 21:354–360.

Rush, James (1827): *Philosophy of the Human Voice,* J. B. Lippincott and Company, Philadelphia.

Sakurai, Edwin H., David F. Mitchell, and Louis A. Holmes (1966): "Bilateral Oblique Facial Clefts and Amniotic Bands: A Report of Two Cases," *CPJ,* 3:181–185.

Sanders, J. (1934): "Inheritance of Harelip and Cleft Palate," *Genetica,* 15:433–510.

Santiago, Arturo (1969): "Classification of Cleft Lip and Palate for Machine Record Coding," *CPJ,* 6:434–439.

Sataloff, Joseph, and Margaret Fraser (1952): "Hearing Loss in Children with Cleft Palates," *Archives of Otolaryngology,* 55: 61–64.

Savara, B. S., and I. J. Singh (1968): "Norms of Size and Annual Increments of Seven Anatomical Measures of Maxillae in Boys from Three to Sixteen Years of Age," *Angle Orthodontist,* 38:104–120.

Sayegh, C. (1964): "The Etiology of Congenital Malformations, Part 2," *Birth Defects: Abstracts of Selected Articles,* 1(7): No. 370.

Sayler, Helen K. (1949): "The Effect of Maturation upon Defective Articulation in Grades Seven through Twelve," *Journal of Speech and Hearing Disorders,* 14:202–207.

Schaeffer, J. Parsons, ed. (1942): *Morris' Human Anatomy,* 10th ed., The Blakiston Company, Philadelphia.

Schalit, Albert (1946): "Obturator of Choice for Congenital Cleft Palate," *American Journal of Orthodontics and Oral Surgery,* 32:688–713.

Schrudde, J. (1965): "Primary Osteoplasty for Clefts of the Lip, Palate, and Jaw," *British Journal of Plastic Surgery,* 18:183–187.

Schuchardt, Karl, ed. (1966): *Treatment of Patients with Clefts of Lip, Alveolus, and Palate,* Georg Thieme Verlag, Stuttgart.

Schultz, Richard C. (1964): "A Survey of European and Scandinavian Bone Grafting Procedures for Cleft Palate Deformities," *CPJ,* 1:188–190.

Schwartz, Martin F. (1968): "The Acoustics of Normal and Nasal Vowel Production," *CPJ,* 5:125–140.

Schwartz, Ralph (1954): "Familial Incidence of Cleft Palate," *Journal of Speech and Hearing Disorders,* 19:228–238.

Schweckendiek, Wolfram, and Claus Danzer (1970): "Psychological Studies in Patients with Clefts," *CPJ,* 7:533–539.

Scott, James (1968): "Aspects of Comparative Dental Anatomy," *Dental Magazine and Oral Topics,* 85:59–62.

Sesgin, M. Ziya, and Richard B. Stark (1961): "The Incidence of Congenital Defects," *PRS,* 27:261–267.

Shames, George H., Herbert Rubin, and Joan K. Shames (1968): "Correlates to Language Development in Cleft Palate Children," paper presented at 26th Annual Meeting, American Cleft Palate Association.

Shapiro, Raymond N., William Eddy, John Fitzgibbon, and Gerald O'Brien (1958): "The Incidence of Congenital Anomalies Discovered in the Neonatal Period," *American Journal of Surgery,* 96:396–400.

Shelton, Ralph L., Jr., and J. F. Bosma (1962): "Maintenance of the Pharyngeal Airway," *Journal of Applied Physiology,* 17:209–214.

———, Alta R. Brooks, and Karl A. Youngstrom (1964): "Articulation and Patterns of Palatopharyngeal Closure," *Journal of Speech and Hearing Disorders,* 29:390–408.

———, ———, and ——— (1965): "Clinical Assessment of Palatopharyngeal Closure," *Journal of Speech and Hearing Disorders,* 30:37–43.

———, Arthur F. Lindquist, Linda Chisum, William B. Arndt, Karl A. Youngstrom, and Sheldon L. Stick (1968): "Effect of

Prosthetic Speech Bulb Reduction on Articulation," *CPJ,* 5:195–204.

——— and Ralph S. Lloyd (1963): "Prosthetic Facilitation of Palatopharyngeal Closure," *Journal of Speech and Hearing Disorders,* 28:58–66.

Sherman, Dorothy (1954): "The Merits of Backward Playing of Connected Speech in the Scaling of Voice Quality Disorders," *Journal of Speech and Hearing Disorders,* 24:312–321.

———, Duane C. Spriestersbach, and J. Douglas Noll (1959): "Glottal Stops in the Speech of Children with Cleft Palates," *Journal of Speech and Hearing Disorders,* 24:37–42.

Shiere, F. R., and J. H. Fisher (1964): "Neonatal Orthopedic Correction for Cleft Lip and Palate Patients: A Preliminary Report," *CPJ,* 1:17–24.

Shriner, Thomas H., and Dorothy Sherman (1967): "An Equation for Assessing Language Development," *Journal of Speech and Hearing Research,* 10:41–48.

Sidney, Ruth Ann, and Jack Matthews (1956): "An Evaluation of the Social Adjustment of a Group of Cleft Palate Children," *Cleft Palate Bulletin,* 6(4):10.

Silberg, Stanley L. (1968): "The Incidence of Clefts of the Lip and Palate in Missouri, 1953–1964," personal communication, May 8, 1968.

Skolnik, Emanuel M. (1958): "Otologic Evaluation in Cleft Palate Patients," *Laryngoscope,* 68:1908–1949.

Skoog, Tord (1965a): "The Pharyngeal Flap Operation in Cleft Palate," *British Journal of Plastic Surgery,* 18:265–282.

——— (1965b): "The Use of Periosteal Flaps in the Repair of Clefts of the Primary Palate," *CPJ,* 2:332–339.

——— and Robert H. Ivy, eds. (1957): *Transactions of the International Society of Plastic Surgeons,* The Williams & Wilkins Company, Baltimore.

Slaughter, W. B., and S. Pruzansky (1954): "The Rationale for Velar Closure as a Primary Procedure in the Repair of Cleft Palate Defects," *PRS,* 13:341–357.

———, ———, and Harold L. Harris (1956): "Cleft Lip and Cleft Palate: Surgical Considerations," *Pediatric Clinics of North America,* November 1956, 1029–1047.

Sloan, Robert F., Stanley W. Brummett, Joseph L. Westover, Robert M. Ricketts, and Franklin L. Ashley (1964): "Recent Cinefluorographic Advances in Palatopharyngeal Roentgenography," *American Journal of Roentgenology, Radium Therapy, and Nuclear Medicine,* 92:977–985.

Sloane, Howard N., Jr., and Barbara D. MacAulay, eds. (1968): *Operant Procedures in Remedial Speech and Language Training,* Houghton Mifflin Company, Boston.

Slutsky, Harry (1969): "Maternal Reaction and Adjustment to Birth and Care of Cleft Palate Child," *CPJ,* 6:425–429.

Smith, James W. (1961): "Clinical Experiences with the Vermilion Bordered Lip Flap," *PRS,* 27:527–543.

Smith, Jeanne K. (1969): "Contraindications for Speech Therapy for Cleft Palate Speakers," *CPJ,* 6:202–204.

Smith, Robert M., and Betty Jane McWilliams (1968): "Psycholinguistic Abilities of Children with Clefts," *CPJ,* 5:238–249.

Spina, Victor (1966): "The Advantages of Two Stages in Repair of Bilateral Cleft Lip," *CPJ,* 3:56–60.

Spira, Melvin, Sonia Findlay, S. Baron Hardy, and Frank J. Gerow (1969): "Early Maxillary Orthopedics in Cleft Palate Patients: A Clinical Report," *CPJ,* 6:461–470.

Spriestersbach, D(uane) C., Frederic L. Darley, and Hughlett L. Morris (1958): "Language Skills in Children with Cleft Palates," *Journal of Speech and Hearing Research,* 3:279–285.

———, ———, and Verna Rouse (1956): "Articulation of a Group of Children with Cleft Lips and Palates," *Journal of Speech and Hearing Disorders,* 21:436–445.

———, Dean M. Lierle, Kenneth L. Moll,

and William F. Prather (1962): "Hearing Loss in Children with Cleft Palates," *PRS,* 30:336–347.

———, Kenneth L. Moll, and Hughlett L. Morris (1961): "Subject Classification and Articulation of Speakers with Cleft Palates," *Journal of Speech and Hearing Research,* 4:362–372.

——— and Gene R. Powers (1959a): "Articulation Skills, Velopharyngeal Closure, and Oral Breath Pressure of Children with Cleft Palates," *Journal of Speech and Hearing Research,* 2:318–325.

——— and ——— (1959b): "Nasality in Isolated Vowels and Connected Speech of Cleft Palate Speakers," *Journal of Speech and Hearing Research,* 2:40–45.

——— and Dorothy Sherman, eds. (1968): *Cleft Palate and Communication*, Academic Press, Inc., New York.

Stark, Richard B. (1954): "The Pathogenesis of Harelip and Cleft Palate," *PRS,* 13:20–39.

——— (1962): *Plastic Surgery*, Harper & Row, Publishers, Incorporated, New York.

———, ed. (1968): *Cleft Palate: A Multidiscipline Approach,* Hoeber Medical Division, Harper & Row, Publishers, Incorporated, New York.

———, Margie de Forest, Edna Harris, and Heinz Vollenweider (1962): "Investigation of Possible Causative Factors Producing Human Maldevelopment," *PRS,* 30:543–553.

———, Clayton R. DeHaan, Stanley P. Frileck, and Paul D. Burgess, Jr. (1969): "Primary Pharyngeal Flap," *CPJ,* 6:381–383.

——— and Norbert A. Ehrmann (1958): "The Development of the Center of the Face with Particular Reference to Surgical Correction of Bilateral Cleft Lip," *PRS,* 21:177–192.

——— and D. A. Kernahan (1959): "A Classification for Cleft Lip and Cleft Palate Based upon Newer Concepts of Embryology," *Cleft Palate Bulletin,* 9:45–46.

Stedman's Medical Dictionary (1966): 21st ed., The Williams & Wilkins Company, Baltimore.

Steffensen, W. H. (1952): "Palate Lengthening Operations," *PRS,* 10:380–387.

Stevenson, Alan C., Harold A. Johnston, M. I. Patricia Stewart, and Douglas R. Golding (1966): *Congenital Malformations: A Report of a Study of Series of Consecutive Births in 24 Centres,* World Health Organization, Supplement to Volume 34, *Bulletin of the World Health Organization,* Geneva.

Stiegler, Eleanor J., and Mildred F. Berry (1958): "A New Look at the Etiology of Cleft Palate," *PRS,* 21:52–73.

Stool, Sylvan E., and Peter Randall (1967): "Unexpected Ear Disease in Infants with Cleft Palate," *CPJ,* 4:99–103.

Stoppany, G. A. (1909): "Cleft Palates and Obturators," *Dental Review,* 23:1035–1039.

Strean, Lyon P., and Lyndon A. Peer (1956): "Stress as an Etiologic Factor in the Development of Cleft Palate," *PRS,* 18:1–8.

Streeter, George L. (1942): "Developmental Horizons in Human Embryos: Description of Age Group XI, 13 to 20 Somites, and Age Group XII, 21 to 29 Somites," *Contributions to Embryology,* 30:213–245.

Stryker, Stephanie, Betty Philips, and Robert J. Harrison (1968): "Speech and Language Measures on Pre-School Cleft Palate Children," paper presented at 26th Annual Meeting, American Cleft Palate Association.

Šubrt, Ivan, Jaroslav Červenka, and Miloš Křeček (1966): "Cytogenetic Study of Cleft Lip and Palate," *CPJ,* 3:362–367.

Subtelny, J. Daniel (1955): "Width of the Nasopharynx and Related Anatomic Structures in Normal and Unoperated Cleft Palate Children," *American Journal of Orthodontics,* 41:889–909.

——— (1957): "A Cephalometric Study of the Growth of the Soft Palate," *PRS,* 19:49–62.

——— (1962): "A Review of Cleft Palate Growth Studies Reported in the Past 10 Years," *PRS,* 30:56–67.

——— (1966): "Orthodontic Treatment of Cleft Lip and Palate, Birth to Adulthood," *Angle Orthodontist,* 36:273–292.

——— and Herbert Koepp-Baker (1956): "The Significance of Adenoid Tissue in Velopharyngeal Function," *PRS,* 17:235–250.

———, Robert M. McCormack, Joanne D. Subtelny, Joseph H. Worth, Lester M. Cramer, James C. Runyon, and Robert M. Rosenblum (1968): "Synchronous Recording of Speech with Associated Physiological and Pressure-Flow Dynamics: Instrumentation and Procedure," *CPJ,* 5:93–116.

Subtelny, Joanne D. (1964): "Physio-Acoustic Considerations in the Radiographic Study of Speech," *CPJ,* 1:402–410.

———, George H. Kho, Robert M. McCormack, and J. Daniel Subtelny (1969): "Multidimensional Analysis of Bilabial Stop and Nasal Consonants—Cineradiographic and Pressure-Flow Analysis," *CPJ,* 6:263–289.

———, Herbert Koepp-Baker, and J. Daniel Subtelny (1961): "Palatal Function and Cleft Palate Speech," *Journal of Speech and Hearing Disorders,* 26:213–224.

———, Mamoru Sakuda, and J. Daniel Subtelny (1966): "Prosthetic Treatment for Palatopharyngeal Incompetence: Research and Clinical Implications," *CPJ,* 3:130–158.

——— and J. Daniel Subtelny (1959): "Intelligibility and Associated Physiological Factors of Cleft Palate Speakers," *Journal of Speech and Hearing Research,* 2:353–360.

Sullivan, David E. (1961): "Bilateral Pharyngoplasty as an Aid to Velopharyngeal Closure," *PRS,* 27:31–37.

Sweitzer, Richard S., Jay Melrose, and Hughlett L. Morris (1968): "The Air-Bone Gap as a Criterion for Identification of Hearing Losses," *CPJ,* 5:141–152.

Takagi, Yasuaki, June L. McCalla, and James F. Bosma (1966): "Prone Feeding of Infants with the Pierre Robin Syndrome," *CPJ,* 3:232–239.

———, Robert E. McGlone, and Robert T. Millard (1965): "A Survey of the Speech Disorders of Individuals with Clefts," *CPJ,* 2:28–31.

Taub, Stanley (1966): "The Taub Oral Panendoscope: A New Technique," *CPJ,* 3:328–346.

Taylor, J. A. (1922): *History of Dentistry,* Lea & Febiger, Philadelphia.

Templin, Mildred, and Frederic L. Darley (1969): *The Templin-Darley Test of Articulation,* 2nd ed., University of Iowa, Iowa City.

Tennison, C. M. (1952): "The Repair of the Unilateral Cleft Lip by the Stencil Method," *PRS,* 9:115–120.

Thaler, Seth, and Howard W. Smith (1968): "Submucous Cleft Palate," *Archives of Otolaryngology,* 88:184–189.

Thilander, Birgit, and Sten Stenström (1967): "Treatment of Primary Cleft Lip and Palate Cases in the Light of the Results of Experimental Animal Study," *Report of the Forty-Third Congress, European Orthodontic Society,* 349–364.

Thomas, James Blake (1968): *Introduction to Human Embryology,* Lea & Febiger, Philadelphia.

Trasler, Daphne G., B. E. Walker, and F. C. Fraser (1956): "Congenital Malformations Produced by Amniotic-Sac Puncture," *Science,* 124(3219):439.

Trauner, Richard, and Martin Trauner (1967a): "Results of Cleft Lip Operations," *PRS,* 40:209–219.

——— and ——— (1967b): "Results of Cleft Palate Operations," *PRS,* 39:168–174.

Travis, Lee Edward, ed. (1957): *Handbook of Speech Pathology,* Appleton-Century-Crofts, Inc., New York.

Tretsven, Venus E. (1963): "Incidence of Cleft Lip and Palate in Montana Indians," *Journal of Speech and Hearing Disorders,* 28:52–57.

——— (1965): "Impressions Concerning Clefts in Montana Indians of the Past," *CPJ,* 2:229–236.

Truax, Rhoda (1944): *Joseph Lister,* Bobbs-Merrill Company, New York.

Trusler, Harold M., Thomas B. Bauer, and John M. Tondra (1955): "The Cleft Lip-Cleft Palate Problem," *PRS,* 16:174–188.

Tulenko, John F. (1968): "Cleft Lip Nasal Deformity in the Absence of Cleft Lip: A Case Report," *PRS,* 41:35–37.

Tünte, Wilhelm (1969): "Is There a Secular Increase in the Incidence of Cleft Lip and Cleft Palate?" *CPJ,* 6:430–433.

Vallance-Owen, J., Fenton Braithwaite, J. S. P. Wilson, J. R. G. Edwards, and D. G. Maurice (1967): "Cleft Lip and Palate Deformities and Insulin Antagonism," *Lancet,* Vol. 2 for 1967: 912–914.

Van Demark, Duane R. (1964): "Misarticulations and Listener Judgments of the Speech of Individuals with Cleft Palates," *CPJ,* 1:232–245.

——— (1966): "A Factor Analysis of the Speech of Children with Cleft Palate," *CPJ,* 3:159–170.

——— (1969): "Consistency of Articulation of Subjects with Cleft Palate," *CPJ,* 6:254–262.

——— and Ann Ahlstrand Van Demark (1967): "Misarticulations of Cleft Palate Children Achieving Velopharyngeal Closure and Children with Functional Speech Problems," *CPJ,* 4:31–37.

Van der Woude, Anne (1954): "Fistula Labii Inferioris Congenita and Its Association with Cleft Lip and Palate," *American Journal of Human Genetics,* 6:244–256.

Van Gelder, L. (1965): *Het Zachte Gehemelte bij de Spraak,* De Erven F. Bohn, Haarlem, Netherlands.

Van Hattum, Rolland J. (1958): "Articulation and Nasality in Cleft Palate Speakers," *Journal of Speech and Hearing Research,* 1:383–387.

Van Praagh, William (1888): "Defective Articulation the Result of Cleft Palate," *Transactions of the Odontological Society of Great Britain,* 20:330–338.

Van Riper, Charles (1947, 1963): *Speech Correction: Principles and Methods,* 2nd ed., 4th ed., Prentice-Hall, Inc., Englewood Cliffs, N.J.

——— and John V. Irwin (1958): *Voice and Articulation,* Prentice-Hall, Inc., Englewood Cliffs, N.J.

Vaughan, Harold Stearns (1940): *Congenital Cleft Lip, Cleft Palate, and Associated Nasal Deformities,* Lea & Febiger, Philadelphia.

Veau, Victor (1931): *Division Palatine,* Masson et Cie., Paris.

——— and Mme. Borel-Maisonny (1943): "Radioscopie et Staphylorraphie," *Mémoires de l'Académie de Chirurgie,* 69:36–42.

——— and Georges Politzer (1936): "Embryologie du Bec-de-Lièvre: Le Palais Primaire," *Annales d'Anatomie Pathologique,* 13:275–326.

———, with Jacques Récamier (1938): *Bec-de-Lièvre,* Masson et Cie., Paris.

Vilar-Sancho, B. (1962): "A Proposed New International Classification of Congenital Cleft Lip and Cleft Palate," *PRS,* 30:263–266.

Vincent, C. J. (1960): "The Pedodontist in Cleft Palate Rehabilitation," *Cleft Palate Bulletin,* 10:68–69.

Vini Coff, Alan R. (1960): "Clinical Evaluation of Cleft Palate Patients and Their Speech," *PRS,* 25:496–502.

Viparelli, V., and G. Mastrangelo (1964): "Malformations after Electroshock?" *Birth Defects: Abstracts of Selected Articles,* 1(7): No. 353.

Voelker, Charles H. (1934): "Phonetic Distribution in Formal American Pronunciation," *Journal of the Acoustical Society of America,* 5:242–246.

Walden, Richard H., Robert K. Dean, Michael Morrissey, Leonard Rubin, Bertram E. Bromberg, and Sidney LaPook (1968): "Autogenous Vomer Grafts for Premaxillary Stabilization," *PRS,* 41:444–449.

Walker, Bruce E. (1959): "Effects on Palate Development of Mechanical Interference with the Fetal Environment," *Science,* 130(3381):981.

Wallace, A. B., ed. (1960): *Transactions of the International Society of Plastic Surgeons,* E. & S. Livingstone, Ltd., Edinburgh and London.

——— (1966): "Canadian-Franco-Scottish Co-Operation: A Cleft-Palate Story," *British Journal of Plastic Surgery,* 19:1–14.

Wallace, Anthony F. (1966): "Esser's Skin Flap for Closing Large Palatal Fistulae," *British Journal of Plastic Surgery,* 19:322–326.

Wallace, Helen M., and Susan T. Fisher (1966): "Use of Congenital Malformation Data Reported on Live Birth Certificates," *Public Health Reports,* 81:631–638.

Wang, Mark K. H. (1962): "A Follow-Up Study of Unilateral Cleft Lips Repaired by the Modified LeMesurier's and Tennison's Technique," *PRS,* 30:329–335.

Warbrick, J. G. (1960): "The Early Development of the Nasal Cavity and Upper Lip in the Human Embryo," *Journal of Anatomy,* 94:351–362.

Warkany, Josef (1958): "Production of Congenital Malformations by Dietary Measures," *Journal of the American Medical Association,* 168:2020–2023.

——— (1959): "Congenital Malformations in the Past," *Journal of Chronic Diseases,* 10:84–96.

——— and H. Kalter (1957): "Experimental Cleft Palate: Interpretations and Misinterpretations," *Cleft Palate Bulletin,* 7(3):9.

——— and ——— (1962): "Maternal Impressions and Congenital Malformations," *PRS,* 30:628–637.

Warren, D(onald) W. (1965): "A Physiologic Approach to Cleft Palate Prosthesis," *Journal of Prosthetic Dentistry,* 15:770–778.

——— and James L. Devereux (1966): "An Analog Study of Cleft Palate Speech," *CPJ,* 3:103–114.

———, Luis F. Duany, and Newton D. Fischer (1969): "Nasal Pathway Resistance in Normal and Cleft Lip and Palate Subjects," *CPJ,* 6:134–140.

——— and Arthur B. DuBois (1964): "A Pressure Flow Technique for Measuring Velopharyngeal Orifice Area during Continuous Speech," *CPJ,* 1:52–71.

——— and F. A. Hofmann (1961): "A Cineradiographic Study of Velopharyngeal Closure," *PRS,* 28:656–669.

——— and Stephen B. Mackler (1968): "Duration of Oral Port Constriction in Normal and Cleft Palate Speech," *Journal of Speech and Hearing Research,* 11:391–401.

——— and William E. Ryon (1967): "Oral Port Constriction, Nasal Resistance, and Respiratory Aspects of Cleft Palate Speech: An Analog Study," *CPJ,* 4:38–46.

———, Matthew T. Wood, and Doris P. Bradley (1969): "Respiratory Volumes in Normal and Cleft Palate Speech," *CPJ,* 6:449–460.

Watson, Charles G. (1964): "Personality Adjustment in Boys with Cleft Lips and Palates," *CPJ,* 1:130–138.

Weatherley-White, R. C. A., William C. Dersch, and Ruth M. Anderson (1964): "Objective Measurement of Nasality in Cleft Palate Patients: A Preliminary Report," *CPJ,* 1:120–124.

———, Richard B. Stark, and Clayton R. DeHaan (1966): "Acoustic Analysis of Speech Validation Studies," *CPJ,* 3:291–300.

Webster, Richard, Richard J. Coffey, Robert E. Kelleher, and Lawrence F. Quigley, Jr. (1961): "The Value of Pharyngeal Flap Surgery," *Cleft Palate Bulletin,* 11:5–6.

Weinberger, Bernhard Wolf (1948): *An Introduction to the History of Dentistry,* The C. V. Mosby Company, St. Louis.

Weiss, Curtis Elmer (1968): "An Investigation of the Effects of Disrupted Lingual Taction on Acoustic and Physiological Parameters of Articulation," unpublished doctor's dissertation, University of Missouri-Columbia.

Wells, Charlotte G. (1945): "A Speech Training Center for Cleft Palate Children," *Quarterly Journal of Speech,* 31:68–73.

West, Robert, and Merle Ansberry (1968):

The Rehabilitation of Speech, 4th ed., Harper & Row, Publishers, Incorporated, New York.

Westlake, Harold, and David Rutherford (1966): *Cleft Palate,* Prentice-Hall, Inc., Englewood Cliffs, N.J.

Whillis, J. (1930): "A Note on the Muscles of the Palate and the Superior Constrictor," *Journal of Anatomy,* 65:92–95.

Wilhelmsen, Hans R., and Ross H. Musgrave (1966): "Complications of Cleft Lip Surgery," *CPJ,* 3:223–231.

Williams, Arthur C., Bernard N. Rothman, and Ira H. Seidman (1968): "Management of a Feeding Problem in an Infant with Cleft Palate," *Journal of the American Dental Association,* 77:81–83.

Williams, H. Bruce (1968): "A Method of Assessing Cleft Lip Repairs: Comparison of LeMesurier and Millard Techniques," *PRS,* 41:103–107.

——— and F. M. Woolhouse (1962): "Comparison of Speech Improvement in Cases of Cleft Palate after Two Methods of Pharyngoplasty," *PRS,* 30:36–42.

Williams, P. L., C. P. Wendell-Smith, and Sylvia Treadgold (1966): *Basic Human Embryology,* J. B. Lippincott Company, Philadelphia.

Wilson, James G. (1959): "Experimental Studies on Congenital Malformations," *Journal of Chronic Diseases,* 10:111–130.

Wolstenholme, G. E. W., and Celia M. O'Connor, eds. (1960): *Ciba Foundation Symposium on Congenital Malformation,* Little, Brown and Company, Boston.

——— and Ruth Porter, eds. (1967): *Mongolism,* Ciba Foundation Study Group No. 25, Little, Brown and Company, Boston.

Wood, Pauline J., and B. S. Kraus (1962): "Prenatal Development of the Human Palate: Some Histological Observations," *Archives of Oral Biology,* 7:137–150.

Woolf, C. M., R. M. Woolf, and T. R. Broadbent (1963): "A Genetic Study of Cleft Lip and Palate in Utah," *American Journal of Human Genetics,* 15:209–215.

———, ———, and ——— (1965): "Lateral Incisor Anomalies: Microforms of Cleft Lip and Palate?" *PRS,* 35:543–547.

Wylie, Howard Lee, and Betty Jane McWilliams (1965): "Guidance Material for Parents of Children with Clefts," *CPJ,* 2:123–132.

Yules, Richard B., and Robert A. Chase (1969): "Pharyngeal Flap Surgery: A Review of the Literature," *CPJ,* 6:303–308.

———, William H. Northway, and Robert A. Chase (1968): "Quantitative Ciné Radiographic Evaluation of Velopharyngeal Incompetence," *PRS,* 42:58–64.

———, Jacque Welch, Julie Urbani, and Ross Elliott (1968): "Untraining Hypernasality," paper presented at 26th Annual Meeting, American Cleft Palate Association.

Zemlin, Willard R. (1968): *Speech and Hearing Science: Anatomy and Physiology,* ©Prentice-Hall, Inc., Englewood Cliffs, N.J.

Zimmerman, Leo M., and Ilza Veith (1967): *Great Ideas in the History of Surgery,* 2nd rev. ed., Dover Publications, Inc., New York.

Index

- Acquired clefts, 7–8, 12
- Adenoids, 128, 208
- Age:
  - for orthodontics, 163
  - for presurgical maxillary orthopedics, 152–153
  - for surgery: to the palate, 140, 142, 156
    - to the prepalate, 140, 142, 148, 150
- Airflow measurements, 69, 209–210
- Airstream:
  - assessment of direction of, 211–212
  - normal control of, 64
  - remedial procedures for control of, 243–247
- Alveolar clefts (*see* Prepalatal clefts)
- Anesthesia, 11, 15, 18
- Appliances, dental, 6, 21, 164–167
- Articulation:
  - control of velopharyngeal valve in, 64–65
  - correlation with resonance, 135–137, 264–266
  - remedial procedures, 247–264
    - consonant sounds, 247–262
    - vowel sounds, 262–264
  - typical errors, 131–135, 140
- Artificial palate, 16–17, 167–171
- Assessment:
  - forms, 184–199, 201–207, 212, 214, 217–219
  - general principles, 177–181
  - information needed, 183–199
    - auditory acuity, 193–194
    - family history, 191–192
    - general impressions, 199
    - identification, 184–185
    - intelligence, 191–193
    - language, 194–196
    - malformations at birth, 185–186
    - orthodontic management, 188–189
    - physical management, 190–191
    - previous speech training, 197–198
    - prosthodontic management, 188
    - radiologic studies, 196–197
    - surgical management, 187
  - of skills in oral communication, 200–221
    - additional steps, 219–221
    - status of structures, 201–207
      - dental and alveolar, 202
      - labial, 201–202
      - laryngeal, 206
      - lingual, 203
      - palatal, 204
      - pharyngeal, 205–206
      - respiratory, 206–207
  - summary, 219
  - use of structures for speech, 211–218
    - articulatory activities, 213–216
    - intelligibility, 216–218
    - velopharyngeal valving, 211–213
    - visual aspects, 218
- Associated anomalies, 118–120
- Audiologist, 2, 7, 179, 193–194

- Birth order, 81–82
- Bone grafting, 155–156

- Causal factors:
  - agreement on, 92–94
  - drugs, 86–88
  - early beliefs, 71–74
  - environment, 71–72, 77, 81–92
  - geography, 83
  - inheritance, 72, 77–81
  - maternal impressions, 72–74
  - nutrition, 85–86
  - pressure changes, 90
  - problems in determining, 74–77
  - questions remaining, 94–97
  - race, 83–84
  - radiation, 88
  - season of birth, 82–83
  - stress, 90–92
  - superstitions, 73–74
  - viral infections, 89–90
- Cinefluorography, 61, 208–209
- Classifications of clefts:
  - American Cleft Palate Association, 106–112, 114
  - Davis and Ritchie, 104–105
  - Kernahan and Stark, 106
  - other systems, 104
  - prior to 1958, 104–106
  - Veau, 104–105
- Cleft lip (*see* Prepalatal clefts)
- Cleft palate (*see* Palatal clefts)
- Communication among team members, 3, 145–146, 174–175, 182
- Consonant sounds:
  - deviations in cleft palate speakers, 131–135
  - normal production and use, 60–61
  - remedial procedures for errors on, 247–262

- Dental anomalies, 125–126
- Dentistry:
  - historical figures, 16–17
  - orthodontics, 163–167
  - prosthodontics, 167–171
- Dentition:
  - in bone grafting, 155
  - prenatal development of, 54–55
- Diagnosis (*see* Assessment)
- Dieffenbach, Johann, 13–14, 20, 157
- Dorrance, George Morris, 16, 158
- Down's syndrome, 80

- Effects of clefts:
  - on community, 116
  - on family, 117–118
  - on individual, 118–142
    - accompanying malformations, 118–120
    - appearance, 124–125
    - dental problems, 125–126
    - growth, 120–121
    - health, 120–121

Effects of clefts:
on individual: hearing, 126–129
intelligence, 121–123
language, 139–140
social adjustment, 123–124
speech, 129–139
Electromyography, 69, 208–209
Embryology, 39–60
Environmental factors, prenatal, 71–77, 81–92
Etiology (*see* Causal factors)
Eustachian tube, 128
Evaluation (*see* Assessment)

Facial clefts, 112, 114
Fauchard, Pierre, 12, 16
Fitzgibbon, John J., 17, 24–25, 171
Flap:
Abbe, 16, 151–152
bone, 157
cheek, 159
island, 159
mucoperiosteal, 157
nasolabial, 159
periosteal, 159
pharyngeal, 159–161
vomer, 158–159
Wardill, 158
Fogh-Andersen, Poul, 4, 28–29, 35, 37, 77–80
Forms for assessment:
information from specialists, 185–198
purposes, 181–183
for speech assessment, 200–219
Franco, Pierre, 3, 9, 18
Fusion of palate:
failure of, 98–99, 101
in normal prenatal development, 50–53, 55, 57

Genetic factors (*see* Causal factors)
Growth:
adaptation to, 269–270
effects of clefts on, 120–121
postnatal, 49–50
prenatal, 40–47

Habilitation (*see* Management)
Hard palate:
prenatal development of, 55–58
surgery to, 156–159
Harelip, 3–4
(*See also* Prepalatal clefts)
Health, 120, 140
Hearing:
assessment of, 179, 193–194
problems associated with clefts, 126–129, 141
Heredity, as causal factor in clefts, 72–73, 77–81
History of management of clefts, 7–26

Implants, pharyngeal, 161–162
Incidence of congenital clefts:
problems in determining, 29–33
by race, 33–34
range of, 29–30
reported between 1960 and 1968, 28
by sex, 37
by type, 35, 37
Incisive foramen, 4–5, 50, 57
Infection, as barrier to surgery, 11
Inheritance (*see* Heredity)
Instrumentation:
in assessment, 180–181, 208–211
nasality meter, 209
oral manometer, 210
oral panendoscope, 209
oscilloscope, 209
sound spectrograph, 209
ultrasound, 69, 205, 209
Intelligence:
assessment of, 191–193
of children with congenital clefts, 121–123
Intelligibility:
assessment of, 216–218
remedial procedures, 264–266, 270–273
typical problems in children with clefts, 137–138

Kingsley, Norman W., 22

Labial clefts (*see* Prepalatal clefts)
Language:
assessment of, 194–196
of children with congenital clefts, 139–140
defined, 130
in new situations, 179
remedial procedures, 271–273
Lip pits (*see* Van der Woude's syndrome)
Listener judgments, 180–181, 211, 216
Lister, Joseph, 13, 15, 20

Management:
dental, 152–155, 163–171
general sequence of, 146–147
before 1900, 7–22
speech, 171–174, 222–274
surgical, 147–163
Maxillary orthopedics, 152–155
Measurement of velopharyngeal closure, 68–69
Mesodermal penetration:
failure of, 99–100
in normal prenatal development, 53
Mongolism (*see* Down's syndrome)
Musculature of velopharyngeal closure, 61–63

Nasality:
in normal speech, 64
perceived, 69
Nasopharynx, depth of, 61
Nose:
"cleft lip," 112–113
nares constriction, 124, 218

Obturator:
 for acquired clefts, 12
 care of, 171, 173–174, 233
 construction of, 16–18, 21–22, 169–171
 effects on hearing, 127
 for feeding, 168
 Fitzgibbon, 171
Occult cleft, 36, 38
Operant conditioning, 226–227, 229, 232–233, 238, 271
Orofacial area:
 abnormal development, 98–101
 normal development, 40–47, 50–59
Orofacial-digital (OFD) syndrome, 120
Orthodontics:
 defined, 6
 phases, 163
 procedures, 163–167
 purposes, 163, 165
Orthodontist:
 contribution to team, 163–167
 information from, 189
Otologist, information from, 193–194

Palatal clefts:
 causal factors, 77–94
 defined, 4–6
 illustrated, 111–112
 incidence of, 34–37
 management before 1900, 9–16
 modern surgical procedures, 156–159
 obturation for, 169–171
Palatal insufficiency, 112, 114
Palatopharyngeal closure (*see* Velopharyngeal valve)
Palatoplasty (*see* Management, surgical)
Paré, Ambroise, 3, 9, 10, 12, 18
Parents:
 age of, 82
 questions from, 70
 suggestions to, 70–71, 146, 223, 273
Passavant, Philippus Gustavus, 13, 21–22, 63, 65–66
Passavant's pad (bar, cushion), 21, 61–62, 66, 208
Pathogenesis, 74, 98–101
Personality, 123–124, 141, 179
Pharyngoplasty:
 Hynes, 161
 implants, 161–162
 pharyngeal flap, 159–161
Pharynx, 58, 205
Philtrum, 53–54
Phonation, 60, 206
Pierre Robin syndrome, 112–113, 162
Plastic surgery:
 defined, 6
 goals of, 130
 before 1900, 8–16
 procedures, 147–162
Premaxilla, 9, 55, 108, 110, 150–152, 155
Prenatal development (*see* Embryology)
Prepalatal clefts:
 alveolar, 4
  classification of, 108
  illustrated, 108
 causal factors, 77–92
 classification of, 107–109
 defined, 3–4
 illustrated, 107–110
 incidence of, 35, 37
 labial, 4
  classification of, 107–108
  illustrated, 107
  incidence of, 35, 37
  variant terms for, 3–4
 obturation of, 168–169
 surgical repair of, 8–9, 147–156
Pressure for articulation, 64
Primary palate, 106
Prolabium, 108, 110, 150
Prostheses:
 construction of, 170–171
 decision to use, 169
 defined, 6
 management of, 171
 parts of, 169
 prior to 1900, 12, 16–17
 purposes, 167–168
Prosthodontic management, 6, 167–171
Prosthodontist:
 contribution to team, 167–171
 information from, 188
Psychologist, information from, 192–193
Psychosocial factors, 123–124

Race, effect on incidence of clefts, 33–34, 83–84
Radiography, 68–69, 196–197
Rare clefts, 112–113
Remedial procedures for speech disorders:
 adaptation to change, 269–270
 articulatory activities, 247–264
 automatization of speech, 270–273
 awareness of structures, 229–233
 control of structures, 233–239
 correlation of articulation and resonation, 264–266
 direction of airstream, 243–247
 goals, 225–226
 motivation, 228–229
 planning, 223–225
 prior to 1940, 20–25
 self-monitoring, 266–269
 velopharyngeal closure, 239–243
 (*See also* Management)
Resonance:
 correlation with articulation, 135–137, 264–266
 in speech, 130
 typical problems, 135–137
Respiration, assessment of, 206–207
Roux, Philibert, 13–14, 19–20

Secondary palate, 106
Sensory channels in remediation, 266–269

Sex differences in cleft types, 36–38
Social adjustment, 123–124, 141
Soft palate, thickness of, 61
Speech:
  aid, 6, 170–171
  bulb, 6, 170–171
  effects of clefts on, 129–139
  remedial procedures, 20–21, 23–25, 222–274
Speech pathologist:
  as clinician, 222–274
  contribution to team, 171–174
  as diagnostician, 173, 200–221
  information from, 197–198
Stark, Richard B., 4, 100, 106
Submucosal cleft, 36–37, 112–113
Superstitions, 73–74
Surgeons:
  contribution to team, 147–163
  information from, 185–188
  after 1900, 16, 19–20, 147–163
  before 1900, 10–16
  oral, 6
  plastic, 6
Surgical procedures:
  Beverly Douglas, 162
  for closure of palatal cleft, 156–163
    Dieffenbach-Warren, 157
    Dieffenbach-Warren-von Langenbeck, 157
    Dorrance, 158
    Esser, 159
    Ganzer-Veau-Ruppe, 158
    Gillies-Fry, 158
    Millard, 159
    pharyngeal flap, 159
    Rosenthal, 159
    V-Y advancement, 158
    Veau, 158
    Veau-Wardill-Kilner, 157–158
    von Langenbeck, 157
    W-V flap, 158
    Wardill-Kilner, 158
  for closure of prepalatal cleft, 148–152
    Abbe, 151–152
    cosmetic surgery, 151
    Hagedorn, 149
    LeMesurier, 149
    linear closure, 150–151
    Millard, 149, 151
    Mirault, 149
    rotation-advancement, 149
    Tennison, 149, 151
    Z-plasty, 150
  fascial sling, 162
  goals, 130, 147–149, 151, 157

Team:
  in assessment, 176
  contributions of team members, 147–174
  history of, 144
Team:
  members of, 145–146
  opinions on team management, 144–145
  problems, 145
Teratogenic agents, 47, 75, 84
Teratology, 7, 76
Terminology:
  general, 3–7
  referring to palatopharyngeal aperture, 67
  used by dentists, 163–171
  used by embryologists, 41–45
  used by surgeons, 6, 147–163
Therapy (*see* Remedial procedures for speech disorders)
Tongue:
  assessment of motility and control of, 203
  participation in velopharyngeal closure, 208–209
  position in cleft patients, 208, 247
  prenatal development, 55, 58
Twinning, 80–81
Types of clefts:
  classification, 114
  illustrated, 107–112
  incidence by, 35, 37
  palatal, 108–110
  prepalatal, 107–108
  rare, 110–114

Ultrasound, 69, 205, 209
Uvula:
  bifid, 36
  musculature of, 63

Van der Woude's syndrome, 113, 118–119
Veau, Victor, 3, 5, 25, 67, 99–100, 104–105, 150, 157–158
Velopharyngeal incompetence, assessment of, 207–213
Velopharyngeal valve, sphincter: assessment of efficiency of, 207–213
    functions in speech, 63–68
    measurements of function of, 68–69
    musculature of, 61–63
    normal function of, 65–68
    remedial procedures for inefficiency of, 239–243
Velum:
  articulate, 17
  movable, 17
Voice:
  assessment, 206
  effects of clefts on, 138–139
von Graefe, Karl Ferdinand, 13–14, 19–20
von Langenbeck, Bernhard, 13–14, 157
Vowel sounds:
  normal production and use of, 60–61
  remedial procedures, 262–264

Whillis, J., ring of, 63